PRAISE FOR

GET OFF YOUR SUGAR

"Sugar consumption is at an all-time high. This toxic, addictive substance contributes to cancer, heart disease, diabetes, obesity, and autoimmune diseases. Breaking the sugar habit is one of the biggest health challenges we face. That's why I recommend reading *Get Off Your Sugar*! But don't stop at reading. Grab a copy to gift to your loved ones as well. Dr. Gioffre has done a stellar job of putting together a succinct, science-backed plan in his new book that will put you back in the driver's seat of your health. If you are a sugarholic, this book is a must-own."

—DR. PETER OSBORNE, bestselling author of *No Grain, No Pain*

"Dr. Daryl's Get Off Your Sugar approach has not only changed my life, it has deepened my understanding of beauty from the inside out. If I've learned one thing in all of my experience, it's that what you put in your body is much more important than what you put on your face. This book will give you the power to transform your skin, energy, and health."

—BOBBI BROWN, beauty guru, founder of *Beauty Evolution*,
and author of *Beauty from the Inside Out*

"This is an urgently needed book everyone should read now. Our health and immune function truly depend on us getting off of sugar and improving alkalinity as Dr. Daryl Gioffre shares. This elemental necessity is essential for our willpower and to empower us to make good choices in our daily lives every day."

—ANNA CABECA, DO, Ob/Gyn, bestselling author
of *The Hormone Fix* and *Keto-Green 16*

"Consuming sugar is like pouring gasoline on a fire in our bodies! It triggers an explosive level of inflammation in the body that increases pain, suppresses your immune system, lowers energy levels, and impairs your brain. Perhaps even worse, it causes an addiction as strong as any drug in the world. In this book, Dr. Gioffre shows you how to break free from your sugar addiction, use your own body fat for fuel, and build internal resistance so you can live at your best."

—DR. DAVID JOCKERS, DNM, DC, MS, founder of DrJockers.com
and author of *The Keto Metabolic Breakthrough*

"I've seen the difference food can make in the lives of people all around the globe. Every bite you take fuels illness or contributes to health. If you want to get off the fast track to chronic disease and take a step into a brighter future, then *Get Off Your Sugar* is for you."

—OCEAN ROBBINS, bestselling author of *31-Day Food Revolution* and CEO, Food Revolution Network

"I applaud Dr. Gioffre for his work. I've spent a lot of time studying the effects of sugar and exposing it for the health robber that it is. Its link to heart disease, attack on peripheral nerves, paralysis of the immune system, and competition with vitamin C have caused untold damage that can only be reversed by limiting your sugar intake. Dr. Gioffre not only identifies the problem but gives you a plan to overcome your sugar addiction. I especially love the chapter on re-mineralizing the body and highlighting my favorite mineral, magnesium, as the most important mineral to replace."

—CAROLYN DEAN, MD, ND, author of *The Magnesium Miracle*, *Sugar Without the Icing*, and eighteen other health books, which are available for free download at www.drcarolyndeanlive.com

"Dr. Gioffre provides cutting-edge information to tackle the most dangerous health crisis of our time: obesity. Using the strategies in this book, especially as they pertain to stress eating, you can conquer obesity and live the life you always dreamed."

—JACK WOLFSON, DO, FACC, author of *The Paleo Cardiologist*

"After being addicted to junk food for years, which then led me to rock bottom with my health, I can attest that sugar fuels cancer and other illnesses. However, healing is possible with nutrient-rich foods. In Dr. Gioffre's new book *Get Off Your Sugar*, you will learn how to kick sugar cravings and be on your way to becoming the healthiest version of yourself. *Get Off Your Sugar* is full of recipes and strategies to make it easy to kiss sugar good-bye for good!"

—LIANA WERNER-GRAY, nutritionist and author of *The Earth Diet*, *Cancer-Free with Food*, and *Anxiety-Free with Food*

"Dr. Daryl is one of the most passionate pioneers of health who is always on the pursuit of helping others get off sugar. His quest for true answers to healing our bodies is remarkable. Dr. Daryl's knowledge is packaged up in this book in an eloquent way that is an easy to understand yet fun to read! After reading *Get Off Your Sugar*, you will be inspired to take charge of your life and never touch the white stuff again!"

—MARIA EMMERICH, international bestselling author

"In *Get Off Your Sugar*, Dr. Daryl lays out an easy-to-follow plan to do just that: end sugar and carb addition. Food is medicine! This is simply a must-read for anyone wanting to improve their metabolic health. You will learn to overcome the cravings and get your mojo back!"

—DORIAN GREENOW, "Mister Mojo," aka Dorian, founder of Keto-Mojo

GET
OFF
YOUR
SUGAR

ALSO BY DR. DARYL GIOFFRE:

Get Off Your Acid

GET OFF YOUR SUGAR

Burn the Fat, Crush Your Cravings,
and Go From STRESS EATING
to STRENGTH EATING

Dr. Daryl Gioffre

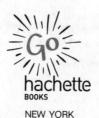

hachette
BOOKS

NEW YORK

Hachette Go, an imprint of Hachette Books
Hachette Book Group
1290 Avenue of the Americas
New York, NY 10104
HachetteGo.com
Facebook.com/HachetteGo
Instagram.com/HachetteGo

First Edition: January 2021

Hachette Books is a division of Hachette Book Group, Inc.

The Hachette Go and Hachette Books name and logos are trademarks of Hachette Book Group, Inc.

The publisher is not responsible for websites (or their content) that are not owned by the publisher.

Print book interior design by Linda Mark.

Library of Congress Cataloging-in-Publication Data
Names: Gioffre, Daryl, author.
Title: Get Off Your Sugar: Burn the Fat, Crush Your Cravings, and Go From Stress Eating to Strength Eating / Dr. Daryl Gioffre.
Description: First edition. | New York : Hachette Go, 2021. | Includes bibliographical references and index.
Identifiers: LCCN 2020025283 | ISBN 9780738286228 (trade paperback) | ISBN 9780738286211 (ebook)
Subjects: LCSH: Sugar-free diet. | Detoxification (Health) | Nutrition.
Classification: LCC RM237.85 .G54 2021 | DDC 613.2/8332—dc23
LC record available at https://lccn.loc.gov/2020025283

ISBNs: 978-0-7382-8622-8 (paperback), 978-0-7382-8621-1 (ebook)

Printed in the United States of America

LSC-C

Printing 1, 2020

This book is dedicated to my wife, Chelsea,
and my two children, Brayden and Alea.

Chelsea, my rock, my warrior, my love.
None of it would be possible without you.

Brayden and Alea, you are my whole heart and whole world.
The goal of everything I do is to help create a better world for you.

Contents

PHASE 3: **FEED—90 DAYS**

Foreword

by Kelly Ripa

LOOK: I MAY NOT BE A DOCTOR, BUT I CAN DEFINITELY ATTEST TO HOW DR. DARYL has helped change my life.

For years I had a candy drawer at home that I kept fully stocked and would dip into whenever I felt the faintest urge for sugar. I knew that sugar isn't good for you, but I figured that everybody needed to have *some* kind of vice, right? What was so bad about rewarding myself with something sweet?

What I didn't fully appreciate is just how addictive sugar truly is.

When I first met Dr. Daryl (my daughter Lola's pediatrician recommended him after Lola came home sick from camp), he taught me how important it was to get acidic foods out of my daughter's diet, and out of my diet too. I did his alkaline cleanse and saw great results—some recurring aches and pains that I had chalked up to getting older completely went away. I was so inspired, I got rid of the candy drawer. If only my cravings had disappeared with it! Sadly, they didn't. When life got super busy with work, or the kids, or both, the urge to eat jelly beans would come on so strong it took everything I had not to send my husband out to the deli to pick some up.

When I talked to Dr. Daryl about my cravings, he explained that sugar is **eight times** more addictive than cocaine. That helped me feel better about having them, but I still didn't know how I would prevent the cravings from happening in the first place.

That's why I was thrilled when Dr. Daryl told me he'd developed a program to help people quit sugar. Keeping cravings at bay while feeling full, happy, and not in any way deprived? Sign me up!

I've followed Dr. Daryl's Get Off Your Sugar program for a little over a year. It's doable, it's delicious, and I've seen the proof that it works too: Last year, when I turned fifty, Dr. Daryl tested my biological age, and it showed I had the physical health of a thirty-five-year-old. Clearly, we're doing something right!

I love how Dr. Daryl focuses on what you need to *add* to your diet instead of what to take away, but I think what really makes his approach so powerful is that he helps you get off—and stay off—the stress-eating roller coaster. I know it's so hard not to rely on your favorite sweet treats when life gets tough, and it can be difficult to manage everything life throws at you, but hear me out: thanks to Dr. Daryl, you're holding in your hands a proven strategy and plan that will help you through the tough times. When you strength eat every day, you're better equipped to handle challenges that arise, whether that's a global pandemic or something closer to home. You also don't need to rely on your willpower to fight through your cravings—you can save your strength for other things! (And you don't have to give up all the things you love; as Dr. Daryl says, "it's not about deprivation, it's about moderation.")

Whether you are ready to completely overhaul your diet or you already eat pretty healthy but could use some guidance to get off the sweet stuff, the Get Off Your Sugar program will help your energy skyrocket, your sleep quality improve, and your weight find its natural balance. A few short weeks from now, your friends will start asking what you've been doing because they'll notice an undeniable glow! Better yet, you'll know that you're taking great care of your health (and if you're a parent, modeling for your kids how they can do it too). It's a delicious paradox: when you get off your sugar, life gets truly sweet.

Introduction

The Problem That Just Won't Go Away

HOW MANY TIMES HAVE YOU DECIDED TO CLEAN UP YOUR DIET AS A NEW YEAR'S resolution? It's a pretty popular commitment to make—in December 2018, 54 percent of Americans listed "eat healthier" as their top resolution.

Two of those Americans were Jennifer Lopez and her boyfriend, New York Yankees slugger Alex Rodriguez, who in January 2019 announced that they would be giving up all sugar and carbs for ten days and challenged their fans to join them in their no-sugar challenge.

There was a lot of excitement when they first made their announcement. J.Lo and A-Rod even appeared on the *Today Show*, where they invited hosts Hoda Kotb and Carson Daly (and anyone else watching at home) to join them. It seemed like a great way to start the new year—how hard could ten days of clean eating be?

Turns out, it was more than hard—it was punishing. Only a couple of days in, J.Lo and A-Rod were struggling. They shared in their social media posts about their progress that they were tired, hungry, and basically just trying to hang on for all ten days. They weren't alone: Carson Daly got only one day in to the challenge before falling off the wagon. Hoda made better progress, but by Day 5, she confessed that she was "always starving."

J.Lo and A-Rod did make it all ten days, but they had to rely on substitutes, such as sugar-free jelly, to keep them going. As soon as the challenge was over, A-Rod posted a picture on his Instagram of not one, not two, but three large pepperoni pizzas, a box of French fries, a huge plate of chicken wings, and two big plates of pastries with the caption "How did you break the 10-day challenge?" These two paragons of fitness and healthy living may have raised awareness, but they didn't create lasting change.

We all know sugar is bad for us. We know it contributes to tooth decay and belly fat. You may know that the American Heart Association counsels folks to keep their sugar consumption low because of its tie to heart health. But still, we all eat it all day, every day, whether that's in the forms we typically think of when we think of sugar—such as ice cream, cookies, and candy—or in its more hidden forms—in flavored yogurts, enhanced waters, and condiments. Why can't we cut the cord on something we know is damaging us?

The reason that sugar is so hard to quit is because it is addicting. In fact, a peer-reviewed study published in the journal *PLoS One* showed that sugar is eight times as addictive as cocaine! The cold-turkey approach—while noble and attention-getting—is just too steep a mountain to climb. I guarantee you that 80 percent of people who try a J.Lo–type challenge wouldn't make it to ten days (and I'm being generous).

The real problem with sugar isn't that it's delicious, it's that it completely overrides your body's programming for health. It hijacks your hormones and your brain and makes you not just crave sugar but actually need it on a cellular level to keep going. And like any true addiction, it's nearly impossible to beat with willpower alone.

Sugar creates the problem—the exhaustion, the accelerated aging, the loss of libido, the achy joints—and then appears to offer the solution to the problem—the hit of energy and a fleeting sense of being invincible. It's an attempt to quiet a craving that makes the next round of cravings only worse.

When new clients come to see me at my Park Avenue Wellness Center in New York City or Newport Beach, they tell me they feel like they're ninety years old, even when they're only in their late thirties or early forties. In addition to their stiff joints and nonexistent sex drive, they're often struggling with perimenopause symptoms. Their hair lacks luster. Their skin is dry and noticeably wrinkled. They've put on weight that has accumulated around their middle and doesn't seem to budge no matter what they do. They are finding it harder and harder to will themselves through their busy days.

In nearly every case, when I ask them to write down what they've eaten in the last forty-eight hours (an exercise I'll walk you through in Chapter 1), we find that they are stress eating with loads of sugar—sugar in the morning to get going, sugar at lunch to stay motivated, sugar in the afternoon to pull themselves out of a slump, sugar at night to celebrate having gotten through the day. They don't even realize just how much sugar they're eating and how addicted they've gotten.

The thing is, being addicted to sugar is not your fault. Sugar is hidden in nearly every processed food. It creates its own self-perpetuating cycle of cravings. And it makes your body work harder just to keep going. Sugar is not just ingrained in our brain, it's baked into our culture. We turn to sugar when we're celebrating and when we're sad; when we need a pick-me-up in the afternoon and when we're relaxing in the evening with a pint of Ben & Jerry's. There's always some sugar-based treat that's the latest craze, whether it's fruit smoothies, cupcakes, or donuts. Heck, you can hardly buy a pair of kid's pajamas that doesn't have some kind of sweet treat on it. Sugar really is as American as apple pie. It's also a drug that no one realizes is a drug.

It's no wonder so many of us are struggling with it.

You know sugar's bad for you. You want to stop. You just don't know how. Just because being addicted to sugar isn't your fault doesn't mean there's nothing you can do about it. But it takes more than just wanting to stop. You've also got to know how to do it. And very, very few people have ever been taught how to outsmart sugar and give their body what it needs to grow out of its addiction. This book aims to change all that.

Creating lasting change in your sugar habits and health *is* possible. When I finally kicked my decades-long sugar addic-

tion, it actually wasn't hard, once I altered my strategy. When I finally began doing things differently, I started off slowly, with just a small change here and there. I ditched the deprivation mindset that left me addicted nearly my entire life. Instead, I added more healthy foods, and with time, the good stuff started crowding out the bad. Every step I took gave me more energy and reduced my cravings. And that's how I got off my sugar. Seriously, if I can do it, *I know* you can.

HOW I GOT OFF MY SUGAR

Growing up, my nickname was "Candyman." I always had a big bag of candy with me, which made me really popular on the bus to the soccer games. I drank fruit juices morning, noon, and night. When I ate my Honey Nut Cheerios in the morning, I added a spoonful of sugar *to every bite I ate*! When I got to college, I replaced my round-the-clock fruit juices with Coca-Cola and kept right on eating the sugary cereals and sweet treats. Even as an adult, I had little jars of M&M's tucked away throughout my house—even on my bedside table. Chelsea—then my fiancée, now my wife—clued me in that I would even reach over into the jar and shove a handful of candy into my mouth while I was still sleeping.

I knew I had a serious problem with sugar. I very much wanted to stop eating it. (It was around this time that I earned a new nickname, "Sugar Blues," when my brother snapped a picture of me reading the book *Sugar Blues* in one hand with a box of Lucky Charms in the other.) But I just couldn't do it. I didn't realize the truth—that my "sugar habit" was really a "sugar addiction." I had willpower in spades; after all, that's how I could run around the soccer field, even in the midst of a huge sugar crash. But willpower wasn't enough for me, and it isn't enough for the vast majority of people either.

One thing I had going for me when I was a young adult was that I continued to play competitive soccer, so the sugar didn't result in weight gain (although it did contribute to my frequent injuries and my low energy levels). It wasn't until I became a chiropractor and stopped exercising so much that the weight crept on. Ten pounds turned to 20, turned to 30, until I was carrying 42 extra pounds. I was the shoemaker with no shoes, a walking contradiction who one minute was telling a patient to stop the sugar because it's inflaming their joints and then walking back to my office to eat a candy bar.

I did my best to ignore how different my body had become, until one day I was leaning over to adjust a patient and my pants ripped up the back seam. I'm not talking a little tear, it was a full on explosion that I still don't understand how I managed to hide from my patient. Luckily, I had another pair of slacks in my office, but that painful moment showed me what I had been willfully ignoring—that sugar was taking a huge toll on my body. My pride was hurt, but my eyes were opened.

Very soon after that day, I attended an event that espoused the alkaline diet and drinking green juice. I vowed to give it a try. I almost spit out my first green juice.

My taste buds were so acclimated to the sickly sweetness of soda and candy that it tasted like swamp water to me. But I kept drinking it anyway, and something amazing happened. In a few days, I started to think green juice tasted good. About that time was when I noticed that my pants had gotten looser.

I kept making small but powerful adjustments to my diet, my exercise plan, and my life, and in three weeks, my life-long addiction and sugar cravings were completely gone! In three and a half months, I was down 42 pounds. And I never felt deprived or sorry for myself. All I felt was more energy than I had ever had.

Since then, I've given myself a new nickname: "health investigator." In addition to my doctorate in chiropractic and functional nutrition, I became a live blood microscopist because I wanted to know how the lifestyle choices people make affected their health and energy, down to the cellular level. I became a certified raw food chef. To this day, I regularly pore over the research, talk to my colleagues, and attend conferences so I can keep adding to my knowledge base.

When I was addicted to sugar, I didn't hold back in my quest for satisfying my sweet tooth. Now I use that same devotion and tenacity to research health and implement what my studies reveal.

FINDING LIFE AFTER SUGAR

Once I figured out how to ditch my sugar cravings, I took all that information and brought it to my chiropractic and nutrition patients—and I've worked with nearly

120,000 of them over my twenty years of practice. When I started sharing with them my approach to weaning off sugar, they started losing weight and holding their adjustments longer. I've seen proof that my "add, don't take away" way of changing dietary habits is doable. And better yet, it's sustainable. It might take a little longer than going cold turkey, but that's okay because my Get Off Your Sugar approach actually lasts.

I codified my investigations and my experience into a powerful yet easy-to-follow program.

Because I've been able to work with so many patients in real time, and have lived the program myself, I've learned that no plan will work if it doesn't anticipate the fact that because sugar is an addiction, when you're coming off it you're very likely to experience cravings that can feel irresistible and can block your progress. That's why the Get Off Your Sugar program arms you with strategies for snacking as well as gives you a list of snacks that will satisfy you without derailing you. Even better, it starts by getting more minerals into your body, which helps you not develop the cravings in the first place. There's a reason why we start out with minerals—like nearly every American, you are likely mineral-deficient, and this is why you have the cravings you have and honestly why most people fail. They removed the poison, but they never provided the antidote.

My intention with my program is to basically hold you by the elbow and guide you around obstacles and toward health in the most doable and direct manner possible.

WHY THE GET OFF YOUR SUGAR PROGRAM WORKS

The Get Off Your Sugar program isn't your typical diet. Most diets are deprivation-based—they tell you all the things you need to remove. I take an "add" approach; I show you all the things to add to your diet so that you naturally crowd out the many sources of sugar. Even more important, the things you'll add will help your body heal itself from the inside out and will naturally reduce your cravings so that it gets easier and easier to stick with the program. When you add in the good stuff, your body works better, and everything in your life feels a little easier. Motivation and willpower will get you started, but it's consistency and habit that will keep you going.

I promise that I have put a ton of thought, experimentation, and experience into what step comes first and will tell you only as much as you need to know to take a new action without overwhelming you.

Because it takes 21 days to create a new habit, the heart of the Get Off Your Sugar program is, you guessed it, 21 days. To keep you engaged and progressing smoothly, I've broken these 21 days into 7 steps. That means you'll spend three days on each step, so you have to focus on only one new thing at any given time. I designed it this way to help you acclimate slowly to a new way of eating. Like eating an elephant, the way to build a new habit is one bite at a time. I've learned through working with my patients that this step-by-step approach works. Also, there's a stacking effect because each step builds in the step that comes before and lays a foundation for the one that comes after.

For each step, I'll explain why that particular strategy is important, I'll tell you exactly what you'll be adding over the next three days, and I'll show you how to do it with a daily action plan so that by the time you get to Day 21, you'll have more energy, less weight, better digestion, and no cravings.

But I won't leave you hanging there. Because it takes ninety days to turn a habit into a lifestyle, I'll also walk you through the first three months of your life after sugar, helping you navigate around the things that every one of us faces and that can cause you to get off track—things like going on vacation, facing a crunch time at work, or even a stressful global panademic. I'll also help you understand how to calibrate your eating plan so that you don't have to forgo all sugar forevermore, but you will know when and how often to indulge so that you won't slide back into old patterns. Better yet, my program will help you turn on your fat-burning engine so that you won't *need* sugar to get through your day; you'll be able to access the energy that's stored in your fat cells but that never gets accessed when you're eating and burning sugar.

The beautiful news is that once you get habituated to the steps I share in these pages, the Get Off Your Sugar program basically runs itself. And that leaves you with so much more time and mental and physical energy to go about enjoying your health and your life.

WHAT'S POSSIBLE WHEN YOU KICK THE SUGAR HABIT

When you break your sugar addiction, you do two important things:

1. You cut out a major contributor to acidity, inflammation, brain fog, aging, and chronic disease.
2. You add the things your body needs to heal itself.

Once you begin to strength eat, big things start happening: Your energy increases. You lose weight. Your digestion improves. You sleep better. Your body just plain *feels* better. You'll notice the changes on a physical level (and so will your health-care provider, because the results of your blood tests improve too). But there are also things that will happen on a deeper level that you can only imagine now—things like having the clarity and the energy to make a much-needed career change, perhaps, or to improve your most important relationships. It goes way beyond mere physical health.

Health is more than just the absence of disease; it's about physical, mental, and emotional well-being. It's the difference between not being sad and being happy. Are you ready to go beyond being not sick, and experience true health?

one

Why Sugar Is So Easy to Love and So Hard to Give Up

I'M PROBABLY NOT TELLING YOU ANYTHING YOU DON'T ALREADY KNOW WHEN I SAY that America is in the midst of a cataclysmic health crisis.

More than 100 million American adults—nearly one in three—has diabetes or prediabetes, according to the Centers for Disease Control.[1] Nearly half of all American adults have heart disease, per the American Heart Association.[2] And our kids aren't faring much better: nearly one-third of American children are either overweight or obese and thus on track to develop diabetes and heart disease at ever earlier ages.[3]

I'm not including this information here because I want to scare you, because fear isn't a great motivator for long-term change. Rather, I want you to understand *why* we are where we are. Because once you understand the root cause, you can address it. And so far, we have been trying to manage symptoms once they appear—lose the weight, fight the fatigue, or lower the cholesterol. And that is the equivalent of snipping the wires to the smoke alarm that's going off, instead of putting out the fire.

Like any fire, the one that's destroying our health has many factors that keep it going—stress is the oxygen that feeds it, and environmental toxins are the lighter fluid that make it flame higher. But the fuel that ignites the fire in the first place is sugar.

HIJACKED BY SUGAR

According to the World Atlas, Americans eat more sugar than people in any other country in the world, with the average American eating just over 130 pounds of sugar in a year.[4] A 2015 study published in the journal *Lancet Diabetes & Endocrinology* found that 74 percent of American food products contain regular or low-calorie sweeteners.[5] This goes a long way toward explaining why the average American consumes about 20 teaspoons of added sugar a day—more than three times more than the 6 teaspoons a day my colleague Dr. Robert Lustig, a neuroendocrinologist and an expert on sugar's effects on the body, says is the most your liver can metabolize in a day. Anything above that small amount gets stored as fat.[6]

RECOMMENDED DAILY SUGAR INTAKE FROM THREE DIFFERENT SOURCES

* **US Dietary Guidelines**, 2015–2020: Less than 10 percent of daily caloric intake, which translates to 12.5 teaspoons a day for a person eating 2,000 calories per day[7]

* **World Health Organization**, 2015: Less than 5 percent of daily caloric intake, which translates to about 6 teaspoons a day[8]

* **American Heart Association**: 6 teaspoons a day for women, 9 teaspoons a day for men[9]

Those 130 pounds a year translate to more than 38 teaspoons of sugar every day, which no matter which source of official health guidance you look to—the US Dietary Guidelines, the World Health Organization, or the American Heart Association—exceeds the daily recommended sugar intake by at least 250 percent and as much as 533 percent.

Why are we eating so much sugar when we know how bad it is for us and when so many of us are already facing ill health effects from it? Is it because we lack willpower? Are we too crunched for time to eat any other way? I know these are common excuses, but they aren't the root cause. The reason we're eating so many more pounds of sugar each year than could ever be considered a good idea is simple: *we are addicted*.

A DAY IN THE LIFE OF AMERICAN SUGAR CONSUMPTION

A lot of my patients tell me, "Oh, I don't eat much sugar," thinking that it comes only in the form of cakes, cookies, and candy bars. Very few people realize just how much sugar is lurking in the foods we eat every single day. Take a look at this typical daily food intake; you'll see for yourself how easy it is for your sugar intake to be through the roof without your even realizing it.

FOOD	GRAMS OF SUGAR
Breakfast	
Orange juice (1 cup)	26 g
Honey Nut Cheerios with milk (1 cup of each)	40 g
Mid-morning snack	
Low-fat yogurt	23 g
Lunch	
Apple juice (1 cup)	24 g
Turkey sandwich from Subway (6-inch on 9-grain bread with lettuce, tomatoes, onions)	3 g
Banana (medium)	12 g
Midafternoon snack	
Protein bar	30 g
Dinner	
Pizza	5 g
Salad (with store-bought dressing)	6 g
Soda	36 g
Dessert	
Ice cream (one cup)	28 g

Grand total for one day: 233 grams
. . . which equals 54.6 teaspoons

ADDICTION ISN'T A WEAKNESS; IT'S A NATURAL PHYSIOLOGICAL RESPONSE

Your body can burn either sugar (in the form of glycogen) or fat for fuel. But because we overconsume sugar all day, every day, and we rarely go more than a couple of hours without eating, your body has become dependent on using sugar as fuel and has lost its ability to burn fat. And because sugar is like kindling on a fire, a couple of hours after eating, your body will tell you that you need to re-fuel, *stat*. In search of more glucose, you'll reach for the high-carb, high-sugar foods.

In those moments when your sugar levels are crashing, your brain will sense what's happening and panic because it knows it needs more glucose to keep running. So, it pushes you into a state of fight-or-flight and cues the adrenal glands to release the stress hormone, cortisol. Cortisol signals you to eat more sugar so that the brain can keep doing its thing. Stress leads you to reach for sugar, and then sugar keeps you locked in the stress response.

Another issue that makes sugar so addictive is that insulin lights up the brain receptors for dopamine, a neurotransmitter associated with pleasure. Want to know what else stimulates your dopamine receptors? Addictive drugs, such as cocaine and opioids. Really, according to your brain, sugar is no different than drugs. In fact, it's time we start calling a spade a spade: sugar *is* a drug, and right now, it's America's drug of choice. As JJ Virgin, author of *JJ Virgin's Sugar Impact Diet*, pointed out when I interviewed her for my Get Off Your Sugar online summit, said, "Sugar is addictive, expensive, and it plays a major role in disease. The more sugar you have, the more you need to get the same high (or even just to function). Without it, you feel awful, and your brain is in a fog."

I'm telling you this because I want you to understand that your sugar addiction is not your fault. It's a hard-wired physiological response. As if that weren't bad enough, sugar has a strong emotional pull over us too.

Sugar is our first taste in life, whether that's via breast milk or formula. We associate it from the very start with both survival and comfort. When we are kids, parents use sugar to pacify us, or to motivate us to put our shoes on. And ever since our very first birthday cake, we learn that any milestone is best celebrated with a sugary treat.

It's 100 percent true that to truly change your relationship to sugar, you will have to find a different means of adding sweetness to your life—to start celebrating with special outings instead of candies and cakes, to let the people you love know you care by giving them something other than a plate of cookies, to nurture yourself through the down moments by reading an inspiring book instead of reaching for the pint of ice cream.

The food industry knows both our physiological and our emotional attachment to sugar all too well and goes to great lengths to exploit them. They have spent millions and millions of dollars to hire consultants, such as Howard Moskowitz, a mathematician and experimental psychologist, to toy with the ratio of sugar, salt, and fat in hundreds of different food products to find what Moskowitz calls the "bliss point," which means the food is sweet enough to crave but not so sweet that you want to stop eating it. *New York Times* investigative reporter Michael Moss, who interviewed Moskowitz for his 2013 book *Salt Sugar Fat*, told NPR:

> It's not that they engineer bliss points for sweetness in things like soda, ice cream, cookies—things we know and

expect to be sweet. The food companies have marched around the grocery store adding sweetness, engineering bliss points to products that didn't used to be sweet. So now bread has added sugar and a bliss point for sweetness. Yogurt can be as sweet as ice cream for some brands. And pasta sauce—my gosh, there are some brands with the equivalent of sugar from a couple of Oreo cookies in one half-cup serving.

And what this does, nutritionists say, is create this expectation in us that everything should be sweet. And this is especially difficult for kids who are hard-wired to the sweet taste. So when you drag their little butts over to the produce aisle and try to get them to eat some of that stuff we all should be eating more of—Brussels sprouts and broccoli, which have some of the other basic tastes like sour and bitter—you get a rebellion on your hands.[10]

WHY WILLPOWER WON'T WORK (FOR LONG)

Over the last decade or two, we've come to realize that drug addicts and alcoholics aren't addicted because they lack willpower; it's because they have a disease that has taken control of their brain. We are now coming to understand that sugar addiction acts the same way. Which means it's darn near impossible to just decide you're going to stop eating sugar and never touch the stuff again. Especially because research has shown that the executive function portion of your brain—which is responsible for things like self-regulation—works less well when you're hungry, tired, and stressed. And that's exactly when the quick-pick-me-up of a pint of ice cream or big bowl of pasta is the most irresistible.

You may know one or two people who one day decided to change their diet and that was seemingly all it took, but those folks are outliers. That's one of the reasons why contestants on *The Biggest Loser* were nearly all found to have regained some, if not all, of their weight back six years after appearing on the show—even when will-power does work in the short term (and, in the case of these reality TV show contestants, a heaping helping of public accountability and professional support from physical trainers, nutritionists, and doctors), it rarely works in the long term.[11] The fact is that the vast majority of people simply *cannot* quit sugar cold turkey; and those who can feel awful while they're doing it.

To truly go from stress eating to strength eating, you have to give your body what it needs to break free from the addiction to sugar—minerals to help quell the cravings; healthy fats to encourage the switch to fat-burning so the drive to replenish glucose is lessened; the right proteins to provide long-lasting energy; and lifestyle changes that give you alternative tools to keep yourself feeling fulfilled, rewarded, and relaxed. It's not like flipping a switch; it's a slow build where you add more of the good things so that the unhealthy things you've been eating naturally start to fall away.

SIX BIG TRUTHS ABOUT SUGAR THAT ARE KEEPING YOU FAT, EXHAUSTED, AND MENTALLY DRAINED

Eating sugar makes you fat. The US medical establishment and mainstream media have been blaming fat for making us fat and sick since the 1950s, when Ancel Keys published his first of many studies that examined the diet of countries where rates of cardiovascular disease were low and posited that it was because the people in these countries ate low amounts of saturated fat. Keys's findings have since been refuted, but in his era he was hailed as a prophet.

This demonizing of saturated fat led to the adoption of many food products that have now been shown to be devastating to heart and total health, including margarine (which was nearly all hydrogenated fat) and foods that have been manipulated to be "low fat." When you remove the fat, your food tastes like cardboard, so guess what you have to put into foods to make them palatable? Sugar and salt. The war on fat is a primary reason that 74 percent of food products available today have sugar in them.[12]

Even now, with the ketogenic trend, people are still afraid that eating fat makes you fat. But eating fat helps train your body to burn fat for fuel—and when that happens, you can access all those calories that have been stored in your fat cells and you lose weight. Eating sugar, on the other hand, contributes to overeating and storing any extra calories as fat, all the while never feeling satisfied or full and constantly battling cravings for ever higher amounts of sugar.

Eating sugar makes you addicted. As I've mentioned, when you eat sugar, your body metabolizes glucose into the bloodstream, which then triggers the pancreas to secrete insulin, otherwise known as your fat-storing hormone. Over time, your insulin receptors get burned out and stop receiving insulin's messages to lower blood glucose levels, and the only way your body knows to respond in that instance is to pump out more and more insulin, which only exacerbates the problem. High levels of insulin also increase levels of leptin, a hormone secreted by your fat cells that tells your brain when it's time to eat. The result is that your brain is constantly getting the signal that you need more food. As if that's not bad enough, glucose lights up the pleasure centers in your brain, and over time, it dulls those pleasure centers so that it takes more and more glucose to elicit the same pleasurable response. It all adds up to the fact that eating sugar makes you want to keep taking bite after bite, and to do it day after day after day. Add to the mix the carefully calibrated blend of flavors used by the food industry to make their products compulsively eatable, with sugar hidden everywhere, and you can't stop eating sugar, even when you try.

When you eat a lot of sugar, you burn sugar only for fuel, not fat. Your body has the ability to burn two kinds of fuel: sugar and fat. If you are metabolically flexible, you can burn both as a primary energy source. But when you consistently eat a lot of sugary, high-carb foods, you get stuck in a cycle where you never reach the point where you need to burn fat, and over time, your ability to do so weakens. Your body carries around 160,000 calories it can access at any time—5 percent of those calories are stored in the form of sugar, while 95 percent are stored in your fat. Why the big difference in numbers? The sugar-burning system was designed to be used only in flight-or-fight situations (a.k.a. emergencies, to get you out of danger), because sugar burns quickly, like lighting a tissue on fire. Like that tissue, sugar is also a dirty fuel—it leaves a lot of damaging free radicals in its wake, like dark, dirty smoke that then floats throughout your body, causing damage to otherwise healthy cells.

Burning fat, on the other hand, is like burning a big, dry log—it's a low and slow burn that doesn't produce a lot of smoke or ash. We're designed to be able to shift between burning fat and burning sugar—fat for when we are settled into normal daily life and sugar for those rare times when we need quick energy to run away from or face a threat. With our chronic stress levels, and our carb- and sugar-rich diets, most of us of have been in sugar-burning mode for so long that our bodies have forgotten how to burn fat. This makes it harder to lose weight and change our eating habits, because if we eat sugar, we burn sugar, and if we burn sugar, we're going to crave sugar to keep the fire stoked, because our bodies will burn through those 5 percent of calories in a pretty short time.

Put another way, running on sugar is a little like being a car with an engine that makes a lot of noise, never seems to shift into a higher gear, and leaves a cloud of dirty exhaust in its wake, whereas burning fat is more like being an efficient electric car that can recharge itself as it goes and leaves no emissions in its wake. You have to ask yourself, do you want to run like a Model T or a Tesla?

All sugars are not created equal. To be clear, all sugars, whether they are naturally occurring, such as those found in fruit, or added during processing, such as those found in packaged foods, trigger the same hormonal cascade that keeps you hungry, fat, and foggy. But a 2015 review of numerous studies, published in the *Mayo Clinic Proceedings*, concluded that one type of sugar—fructose—is harder on the body than others.[13] The digestive tract can't absorb fructose as well as it can glucose, sucrose, and other forms of sugar, meaning more of it gets sent to your liver, where it then contributes to a whole host of chronic diseases, including insulin resistance, fatty liver disease, triglyceride production, and type 2 diabetes. It's like thinking you're going to take a nice, manageable little swim in an ocean of sugar, and instead you get swept away in a tsunami.

The study also found that added sugars are more harmful than naturally occurring sugars. For example, fructose is often found in fruit, but when you eat a piece of fruit, you also get a healthy dose of fiber to slow the absorption of the sugar, as well as an array of phytonutrients and minerals that can counteract some of its harmful effects in the body. When you drink just fruit juice, however, that fiber is stripped away and you can consume in one small glass of orange juice, the amount of fructose found in four oranges. It's glorified sugar water. To make matters worse, the food industry has latched on to high-fructose corn syrup as a primary ingredient in sodas and processed foods, and it is 55 percent fructose. When it comes to sugar, nobody does it better than nature.

There are multiple sources of sugar in our diet. Three other categories are raising our blood sugar levels and keeping us stuck in burning sugar while also decimating our gut health (which I talk more about in Chapter 2). I call them weapons of mass destruction because their first letters spell out WMDs: wheat, meat, and dairy, and of course the *s* at the end stands for sugar—which all of these foods end up being metabolized into. These three mainstays of the American diet are typically grown using tons of chemical pesticides and fertilizers (in the case of wheat, as well as the grains that are used to feed the cows, pigs, and chickens we then consume) in addition to antibiotics and hormones (in the case of meat and dairy). Dairy is high in lactose, a sugar that 65 percent of the population has trouble digesting; if you overeat meat, the excess protein gets converted into glucose in your liver via the process known as gluconeogenesis; and wheat is high in

Six Big Truths continue on page 10

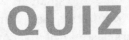

QUIZ

HOW SUGAR-ADDICTED ARE YOU?

Instead of asking about your sugar consumption, this quiz asks you to assess the physical and mental symptoms of sugar addiction you may be experiencing. It is designed to help you clearly hear what your body is trying to tell you.

For each question, give yourself a score of 0 through 10, with 0 meaning "absolutely not, never ever" and 10 being "absolutely yes, all the time, and a lot." Because you can't change a habit you don't know you have, it's important to be honest when answering the following questions, as they can help you see how bad things really are. At the end of the quiz, add up the numbers you gave for answers and check your results against the ranges listed at the bottom of this quiz.

1. Do you feel tired, even after a good night's sleep?

    My score: ____

2. Does your energy plummet in the afternoon?

    My score: ____

3. Do you rely on snacks and/or caffeine to stay energized and focused throughout the day?

    My score: ____

4. Have you gained weight in the last six months, or are you having trouble losing weight?

    My score: ____

5. Do you crave sweets or carb-rich foods, such as bread or pasta?

    My score: ____

6. Do you find that you have to eat more and more ice cream, chocolate, or other high-sugar food to satisfy your sweet tooth?

    My score: ____

7. Do you experience headaches, brain fog, or unexplained moodiness?

    My score: ____

8. Do you regularly experience skin breakouts, or is your hair dry and brittle?

    My score: ____

9. Do you regularly feel guilty, bloated, exhausted, or sick to your stomach after eating?

    My score: ____

10. Do you seem to catch every virus that crosses your path?

    My score: ____

0–25 points: Doing Great

According to this quick symptom assessment, you likely aren't addicted to sugar. The Get Off Your Sugar program can absolutely still help you optimize your health; you just won't have the big hurdle of sugar cravings to get in your way.

26–50 points: Facing a Crossroads

If you answered the questions honestly, it seems you're doing pretty well at keeping your sugar consumption in check. Don't let this knowledge act like a permission slip to eat more of the sweet stuff, however, because the more you eat it, the more it disrupts your gut health, immunity, and hormonal balance, and the harder it will be to avoid the trap of stress eating. Completing the Get Off Your Sugar program will help you crush any cravings you may experience and improve your overall health in the short and the long term.

51–75 points: Flirting with Disaster

Things could be worse, but they could also be so much better. This may be the first time you're realizing that your constant illnesses, breakouts, fatigue, moodiness, or cravings are related to sugar. If you don't take steps to wean yourself off it, things are only going to get worse, and likely more quickly than you would ever imagine. Be thankful that you're catching it now, before you're a full-on sugarholic, and that you've found a program that will help you override your cravings so that you can experience a post–sugar addiction life and all the energy and vitality that comes with it.

Quiz continues

76–100 points: Full-on Stress Eater Sugarholic

Here's the bad news: you are addicted to sugar and your health is paying the price. But there is good news: you're holding in your hands all the information you need to finally get off this merry-go-round and break free from your cravings, lose the weight, restore your immunity, slow down the aging clock, and feel more energized than perhaps you ever have before. If this news is coming as a shock to you, know you're not alone—so many Americans are suffering at the hands of sugar without realizing it, because sugar is in so many foods we eat. Be kind to yourself—you were brave to take this quiz. Know that that level of openness will serve you well as you follow the Get Off Your Sugar program, and keep going . . . you're about to start feeling a whole heck of a lot better.

carbs, which means it's high in glucose. Each of these foods keeps you trapped in a cycle where you eat sugar, burn sugar, and crave sugar. To make matters worse, these foods are metabolized into acid—wheat to sulfuric acid; meat to sulfuric, phosphoric, and nitric acids; and dairy to lactic acid. Your body needs minerals to neutralize these acids, causing further mineral deficiency and more cravings for sugar. As a result, we typically eat so much of these foods that they crowd out most of the mineral-rich vegetables in our diet. The WMDs are the number one reason you are still getting too much sugar in your diet, even if you don't eat typical sugar-filled sweets.

The body doesn't NEED sugar. You may have heard that the brain requires glucose for fuel, but actually ketones—the fatty acids produced when your body burns fat for fuel—are its preferred source of fuel.

Our bodies require sugar only to fuel the action we take as a response to stress, and we have five hormones that can mobilize glucose (including the stress hormones cortisol and epinephrine); they are capable of producing all we need. We don't need to get it from food.

THREE THINGS SUGAR DOES THAT OTHER FOODS DON'T

1. **Prematurely ages your cells.** If you put a fish in healthy water, it stays healthy. But if you put it in a toxic pond, over time its health is going to be affected. Your cells are the same way—they can be only as healthy as the environment they live in. Sugar creates lactic acid and contributes to an acidic internal environment that causes oxidative stress and inflammation. Unless you dramatically reduce your

sugar intake, the inside of your body is essentially a dirty fishbowl. In an acidic environment, cells break down prematurely. Externally, you can see evidence of this breakdown in your wrinkled skin, dry hair, and brittle nails. Internally, if this destruction isn't interrupted it can turn into chronic disease, such as Alzheimer's, heart disease, cancer, or diabetes, which all have inflammation at their root.

2. **Compromises your liver.** As you eat more sugar, your body releases more insulin, which then triggers fat storage. There are only so many places fat can be stored; the liver is one of them. Your liver is your major organ of detoxification, and when it gets riddled with fatty deposits, it has to work that much harder to regenerate itself, detoxify your blood, and pull excess glucose out of the bloodstream.

3. **Impairs brain function.** Glucose and insulin interfere with the healthy functioning of your brain, which is designed to run on fat, not sugar, as 60 percent of your brain is made up of fat. All that excess glucose can lead to insulin resistance in your brain, which is associated with Alzheimer's (also known as type 3 diabetes), brain fog, difficulty focusing, and ADD or ADHD in kids and adults. (More on this in Chapter 2.)

HOW TO BECOME A SUGAR DETECTIVE

Because sugar hides in so many forms, a first step toward truly reducing your sugar intake is to become a conscious shopper. And to do that, you must learn how to read a nutritional label and decode the information it provides so that you can see just how much sugar you are feeding yourself and your family.

Food manufacturers are required to list ingredients in the order of quantity, so whatever appears in the biggest amount is listed first, then every other ingredient is listed in decreasing order so that the last ingredient occurs in the least amount. There are *at least* sixty-two different names for sugar, and companies will use several different forms of it so that they never have to list "sugar" as one of the first ingredients. (Refer to the list on page 12 to see all sixty-two.)

Luckily, in 2016, the US Food and Drug Administration established a requirement for food manufacturers to add a line item to the nutrition label for "added sugars," which shows just how many grams of the various forms of sugar have been added to the product.

Sadly the implementation of this requirement has encountered many delays, and the labels won't be required on all food products until 2021. Hopefully, seeing that number in bold will help people choose products with lower amounts of added sugars and encourage manufacturers to add less in the first place.

GUIDELINES TO GAUGE THE AMOUNT OF SUGAR PER SERVING

Another way food manufacturers try to downplay the amount of sugar in their foods is to use an unrealistically small serving size. For example, if you look at a small bottle of a fruit smoothie and see that it lists only 20 grams of sugar, you may think, "Hey, this isn't bad." But you may not notice that the label also says there are 2.5 servings per bottle, which means there are actually 50 grams of sugar in a bottle that most people would consider to be a single serving. That means you'll exceed the daily recommended limit of 24 to 36 grams in one drink. It pays to learn how to read labels!

* **Low sugar content:** 5 grams per 100-gram serving amount, or 5 percent of ingredients

* **Medium sugar content:** 5 to 20 grams per 100-gram serving, or 20 percent sugar

* **High sugar content:** anything over 20 grams of sugar per 100-gram serving

Although having the added sugars listed separately on the nutritional label is a positive development—hopefully, it will influence both consumers and manufacturers to opt for fewer added sugars—it doesn't represent the total number of sugars in any given product, as there are also naturally occurring sugars, such as those found in fruits. For example, all yogurt contains lactose, which is a naturally occurring sugar found in milk. Flavored yogurts contain lactose as well as added sugars. To see how many grams of all types of sugar there are, you have to calculate the number of net carbs a product has (more about this on page 13).

SUGAR SPOTTER: LEARN THE 62 NAMES OF SUGAR

By familiarizing yourself with this list of sixty-two alternative names for sugar, you'll be making yourself a more educated consumer than the vast majority of the population, and you'll make it that much easier to avoid this addictive ingredient. (And here's a shortcut for you if you're not able to commit this entire list to memory—anything that ends in the suffix "-ose" is sugar.)

Agave nectar
Agave syrup
Barley malt
Barbados sugar
Beet sugar
Brown sugar
Buttered syrup
Cane juice
Cane sugar
Caramel
Coconut sugar
Corn syrup
Corn syrup solids
Confectioners' sugar
Carob syrup
Castor sugar
Date sugar
Dehydrated cane juice
Demerara sugar
Dextran
Dextrose

Diastatic malt
Diastase
Ethyl maltol
Evaporated cane juice
Flo malt
Free-flowing brown sugars
Fructose
Fruit juice
Fruit juice concentrate
Galactose
Glucose
Glucose solids
Golden sugar
Golden syrup
Granulated sugar
Grape sugar
High-fructose corn syrup
Honey
Icing sugar

Invert sugar	Powdered sugar
Lactose	Raw sugar
Malt	Refiner's syrup
Maltodextrin	Rice syrup
Maltose	Sorghum
Malt syrup	Sucanat
Mannitol	Sucrose
Maple syrup	Treacle
Molasses	Turbinado sugar
Muscovado sugar	Versatose
Panocha	Yellow sugar

WHAT IS A NET CARB?

Net carb refers to the total number of grams of carbohydrates a food contains minus the grams of fiber it contains. A carbohydrate is what's known as a macronutrient, or major category of nutrient—the other two macronutrients are protein and fat. A carbohydrate is a starch. Potatoes, grains (including bread and pasta), and beans are all starchy foods and high in carbohydrates. Sugar is also a form of carbohydrate; so is fiber. All carbs, with the exception of fiber, will get transformed into glucose by your body during the digestion process. Fiber doesn't because it isn't fully digested by the body and therefore doesn't impact blood sugar. So, to truly see how much sugar you are exposing yourself to, you need to subtract the total grams of fiber from the total grams of carbohydrates.

When you consume sugar with fiber, the fiber slows digestion, and as a result,

also minimizes the spike in blood sugar that consuming carbohydrates otherwise triggers. Fiber is often found in foods that naturally contain a lot of carbohydrates—such as fruits and root vegetables—and if you eat them in tandem, the carbs won't have as detrimental an effect on your blood sugar. Fiber also feeds your friendly gut bacteria and promotes elimination. In short, it's almost always a good idea to eat more fiber and less sugar, and keeping track of your net carbs is a simple way to gauge how well you're doing. Unfortunately, "net carbs" is a number that you have to calculate for yourself as it doesn't appear on a nutrition label.

Keep in mind that on the Get Off Your Sugar program, your ideal goal is to keep your net carbs under 50 grams per day.

As an example, a Hostess cupcake (which has practically no fiber and plenty of added sugars) has 29 grams of net carbs, a banana (which is fairly low fiber and has lots of natural sugars) has 23.8 grams net carbs, and an avocado (which is high in fiber and low in natural sugars) has 3.65 grams net carbs. It doesn't take a rocket scientist to see that you want to eat more foods like avocados, what I call "God's butter," and what my wife, Chelsea, has nicknamed "the new banana."

NET CARB GUIDELINES FOR WEIGHT LOSS AND MAINTENANCE

When it comes to weight loss, expert on keto-style eating and author of *The Primal Blueprint* Mark Sisson says you want to keep net carbs under 50 grams per day to initially nudge your body to start burning fat and lose up to 1 pound a day; between 50 and 100 grams per day is the sweet spot for slow and steady weight loss (approximately 1 or 2 pounds per week); and 100 to 150 grams per day for maintaining a healthy weight. Once you go higher than 150 grams of net carbs a day, you're creating inflammation and likely gaining weight.

SUGAR DETECTIVE RULES

✴ The four most important numbers on a nutrition label are total sugars, carbohydrates, fiber, and number of servings.

✴ 4 grams of sugar = 1 teaspoon.

✴ If you can't pronounce it, you can't digest it.

✴ Any product with a long list of ingredients (more than 4 or 5) is likely highly processed, not something you should be putting into your body.

SUGAR'S HIDING PLACES

Remember, the World Health Organization recommends keeping your sugar intake to 6 teaspoons or less a day. When you see how many teaspoons are actually *in* the foods and drinks so many of us have each day, you see just how easy it is to exceed that limit, and you can understand how the American average daily sugar consumption is 20 teaspoons!

BREAKFAST FOODS	
1 packet of instant oatmeal, maple syrup flavored	3 teaspoons
Yoplait strawberry yogurt	4.75 teaspoons
100 grams of Honey Nut Cheerios	6.67 teaspoons
100 grams of Special K	2.57 teaspoons
100 grams of granola	6 teaspoons
Medium-size banana	2.48 teaspoons
Bagel (4½ inches across)	1.2 teaspoons
SNACKS	
Grapes	3.14 teaspoons
Average protein bar	7.5 teaspoons
Bottled smoothies	Up to 24 teaspoons
BEVERAGES	
Coca-Cola (12-ounce can)	7.25 teaspoons
Red Bull	5.35 teaspoons

BEVERAGES	
Tonic water (12-ounce can)	6.4 teaspoons
Orange juice (1 cup)	5.25 teaspoons
Low-fat milk (1 cup)	2.5 teaspoons
Sports drink (20 ounces)	8 teaspoons
Sweet tea (12 ounces)	8.25 teaspoons
Vanilla almond milk (1 cup)	2.6 teaspoons
Large flavored coffee	Up to 25 teaspoons
Starbucks Pumpkin Spice Latte (tall)	5 teaspoons
CONDIMENTS	
Barbecue sauce (2 tablespoons)	3.5 teaspoons
Ketchup (2 tablespoons)	2 teaspoons
Prego tomato sauce (½ cup)	2 teaspoons
Newman's Own Honey Dijon Salad Dressing (2 tablespoons)	1.2 teaspoons

NEW NAME FOR BREAKFAST: DESSERT

Maybe you've occasionally had breakfast for dinner as a fun way of spicing up dinnertime with your kids, but most of us frequently do the reverse and have dessert for breakfast (something I got a chance to talk about when I went on *Live with Kelly and Ryan*!).

Here's what I mean: a Boston cream donut, a bagel with cream cheese, and coffee loaded with sugar and fake creamer are all the equivalent of eating cake or drinking a milk shake first thing in the morning. Once you've started the day on a sweet note, you're primed to keep craving sugar throughout the day.

I understand it can be hard to find a nonsweet breakfast option, especially when you're at a conference or work meeting. When a supersweet breakfast is your only choice, you have two strategies to make it better: your best option is to skip it! (You'll learn more about the power of intermittent fasting in Chapter 10.) But if you're not ready to start fasting yet, have half of that sweet breakfast instead of the whole thing, and pair it with a source of plant-based protein, such as hemp seeds or chia seeds and/or a source of healthy fats, such as half an avocado or a small handful of raw nuts. That'll slow down your digestion and keep your blood sugar more stable, so you stay satisfied longer.

,As you move through the Get Off Your Sugar program, you'll wean yourself off sugar and those first-thing-in-the-morning cravings will fade.

TRACK YOUR SUGAR

Now that you've gotten clear on your own symptoms of sugar addiction, let's determine how much sugar you are actually consuming—not how much you *think* you are. I can tell you that most people who come to my office tell me they don't eat many sweets, but when we sit down and do this exercise, they see that their perception is far different from the reality.

Recently, a mom came in with her son who was experiencing ADD, sleep issues, and constipation. I asked her about his diet and his sugar consumption, and she said, "Oh, we eat pretty healthy." But when she listed what her child had eaten in the last two days, everything she mentioned had massive amounts of sugar, including frozen waffles with maple syrup, Honey Nut Cheerios, flavored yogurts, and bagels. Until you learn how to be a sugar detective, it's common to underestimate just how much sugar you're eating, and to do it in a massive way.

I want you to turn to page 202 and use the chart there to write down everything that passed your lips in the last 48 hours. This exercise was the kick start to my journey to get off my sugar. *Please* don't skip this one and take it seriously.

This is different from keeping a food diary, where you write down everything you eat as you eat it. This exercise, where you look back at what you ate, will show you what your current diet actually is.

As you write down everything you ate and drank, I encourage you to be brutally honest and not leave anything out or fudge what or how much you actually ate. Don't forget little things, such as the creamer you put in your coffee and the condiments you had on your sandwich, as they are often significant sources of hidden sugars.

Once you've written everything down, look up the nutritional content of everything at nutritiondata.self.com, or enter it into an online food tracking tool, such as cronometer.com, which will calculate all kinds of data for you, including how many grams of sugar you consumed each day.

More likely than not, you are consuming a ton more sugar than you think you are. You will be *amazed* at where your sugar is hiding and coming from—I'm willing to bet that like most things, 20 percent of the foods and drinks you consume provide 80 percent of the sugar you're eating. Don't panic, though: very soon you will learn how to *swap* out the acidic, sugar-laden foods so many of us eat every day, for foods that have a similar taste and feel, minus the sugar tsunami (so you won't feel deprived!).

WHY HAVE OTHER DIETS FAILED YOU?

Perhaps you've tried other eating plans to help you get back to feeling good again. There is certainly no shortage of them! But even if they've given you some short-term results, you've likely found yourself right back where you started, just like those contestants from *The Biggest Loser*.

The key to maintaining a healthy weight over the long term is restoring your body's ability to burn fat. There are many popular diets designed to help you do just that, including the ketogenic (a.k.a. keto) and Paleo eating plans, which, like my Get Off Your Sugar program, are low carb. There is one crucial ingredient that even these widely adopted strategies miss, and that is mixing things up, or what's formally known as "diet variation." Just as your body will get used to doing the same workout over and over so that over time your efforts become less effective, it will also acclimate to any given eating strategy. So, even if you do manage to overcome your sugar addiction and find a way to eat that gets you into fat burning and helps you lose weight and reduce inflammation, if you never alter what you eat or when you eat it, you'll eventually start gaining weight again.

My good friend and chiropractic colleague Dr. Dan Pompa is an expert in cellular detoxification, nutritional ketosis, and fasting. He has done a ton of great work to explain and popularize the importance of diet variation, and it's something that I've baked into the Get Off Your Sugar program and that is missing from so many other popular eating plans. Diet variation isn't about eating less, it's about switching up what you eat and how often you eat it. It is designed to mimic how our ancient ancestors ate—some days, they'd had a successful hunt or harvest and so they feasted; others days, they were traveling or waiting on the growing season to return and so they fasted. As a result, our bodies have evolved to thrive when we eat different foods and different amounts of foods at different times.

The truth is, any time you change your diet, whether you are following keto, Paleo, or vegan, you will experience some positive results. The question is, do these diets last? Only if you **keep changing things up**. If you keep eating the same keto fats or the same seven vegetables, your body gets stuck. We need to continually eat different foods in different intervals (in cycles of feasting and fasting). Research has even shown that diet variation is more important than the diet itself![14]

You have to keep your body on its toes or else it will plateau (which is why I devote a full step in the Get Off Your Sugar program to build diet variation into your toolbox of new dietary habits, in Chapter 10).

HOW DOES THE GET OFF YOUR SUGAR PROGRAM COMPARE TO MOST POPULAR EATING PLANS?

Like the Get Off Your Sugar program, many of the most popular eating strategies today—including keto and Paleo—share a focus on eating foods that are high in fat, moderate in protein, and low in carbs. Here are the similarities and the differences between the four most popular eating plans today:

Ketogenic

Main points: Like the Get Off Your Sugar program, a ketogenic diet is a high-fat, moderate-protein, and low-carb diet specifically designed to turn you into a fat burner. Because the diet is low carb, it is also essentially low sugar.

Potential problems: I love an eating plan that helps you transition to burning fat.

But people eating a keto diet tend to overrely on dairy, which contains a lot of naturally occurring sugar and is also typically loaded with hormones and antibiotics (see page 88 for more on why I avoid dairy), and meat. As you'll learn in Chapter 8, when you eat more protein than your body needs to replenish and repair itself (and this amount is a lot lower than you might think), the excess is converted into glucose by the liver. That's right, it turns to *sugar*! Also because keto is highly focused on limiting the number of carbs you consume, and every vegetable—even dark, leafy green ones—contain carbs, many people eating keto will avoid vegetables as much as possible. Without the fiber, minerals, and phytonutrients that vegetables provide, a high-fat diet can lead to a condition called *metabolic endotoxemia*: without these important nutrients, bad bacteria can flourish in your gut, ultimately penetrating the gut wall and leaking into the bloodstream, bringing the endotoxins they contain with them. These endotoxins then trigger an immune response and drive up inflammation throughout the body.[15] Not exactly a side effect that you want when you're seeking to improve your health!

Also, a keto diet isn't generally a healthy long-term strategy (unless you are using it as a treatment plan for a major disease, such as brain cancer or epilepsy). And in my experience, people are either 100 percent keto, or they are back to their sugar-burning ways. *Note:* You do *not* want to be in ketosis 24/7; it's not healthy, and eventually, the body will go into starvation mode.

The Get Off Your Sugar program will teach you how to do keto the right way, with the right foods, in their right ratios, with diet variation and adding some feast and partial fast days, if you choose to go there.

Paleo

Main points: Eating only foods that our ancestors ate—meaning meat, fish, vegetables, and fruits with very few grains, no dairy (unless it is fermented), and no processed foods.

Potential problems: I think it's great that the Paleo eating plan avoids two of the biggest weapons of mass destruction—namely, wheat and dairy. The biggest issue I have with the Paleo diet is an overconsumption of animal protein, specifically meat, which gets turned into sugar by the liver. Also, most animals are fed a diet high in pro-inflammatory omega-6 fatty acids (primarily from soy and corn), which then get incorporated into their meat.

Vegetarian and Vegan

Main points: In most cases, vegetarians eat no meat from animals, fish, or seafood. (Some eat eggs, fish, and/or seafood, whereas some don't.) This is different from the vegan diet, which avoids *all* animal products, including eggs, dairy, and, for some vegans, even honey.

Potential problems: I love vegans and vegetarians—in fact, my wife is a vegan!—and I myself am a pescatarian (the only meat I occasionally eat is wild-caught omega-3 fish). But just because you don't eat meat, or perhaps any animal products at all, doesn't mean your diet is healthy. Many vegetarians and vegans overrely on refined carbs—breads, pasta, rice, and potatoes. And as you now know, eating too many carbs is the same thing as eating too much sugar. The vegetarians I see in my practice often have come to rely on eating the same foods over and over, so this eating plan also suffers from a lack of diet variability. However, if you do it the right way, as you'll learn by following the Get Off Your Sugar program, your health will flourish. (Because I recommend not eating dairy and making most, if not all, of your protein plant-based, the Get Off Your Sugar program is very vegetarian- and vegan-friendly.)

Mediterranean

Main points: Based on the traditional diets of cultures around the Mediterranean Sea, this approach to eating primarily olive oil, vegetables, fruits, nuts, seeds, legumes, potatoes, whole grains (including bread), herbs, spices, fish, and seafood; with moderate consumption of cheese, yogurt, poultry, and eggs. Red meat is eaten only sparingly, and processed foods, including processed meats, refined oils, and added sugars are avoided.

Potential problems: All those whole grains, beans, and legumes are carb heavy, and the dairy has a lot of naturally occurring sugar. Also many people don't have the enzymes necessary to digest beans (which typically leads to bloating and gas). (*Note:* I am okay with beans, as you will later see, as long as they are sprouted to remove the lectins and the antinutrients they contain.) This nutritional approach has only a moderate intake of fats, which won't help you transition into fat-burning mode.

GET OFF YOUR SUGAR

Main points: My program is a high-fat, moderate-protein (primarily from plant-based sources), and low-carb way of eating that focuses on also being high in minerals and fiber. High-fat, high-fiber diets have been shown to lower the inflammation associated with metabolic endotoxemia by feeding our healthy gut bacteria.[16] Crucially, it also builds variability in both actual foods eaten and timing of when those foods are eaten so that your body—or you—don't get bored and stop seeing results. As a result, you downregulate inflammation, reset your microbiome, and get rid of old damaged cells—all from improving the quality of the foods you eat and varying when you choose to eat them.

CHAPTER 1 ACTION PLAN

❉ Take the How Sugar-Addicted Are You? Quiz (page 8) and assess your results.

❉ Write down every bit of food and drink you've had in the last 48 hours in the chart on page 202, then use an online tool, such as nutritiondata.self .com or cronometer.com, to see how many teaspoons of sugar that adds up to (remember that 4 grams equals 1 teaspoon).

❉ Be sure to read the nutritional labels of your favorite products and see whether they are a low-sugar, medium-sugar, or high-sugar food.

I was addicted to sugar. In the morning I would wake up, and the first thing I would do was grab a piece of chocolate. I loved it all, cake, pie, especially apple, and my favorite, cookies. I would start out with just a little piece and end up eating everything. I thought I was in shape, but I was always tired. I had aches and pains—even the bottom of my feet were sore! I had a hard time concentrating. In addition to all of this, I suffered from acid reflux (I was on Prevacid for six years).

I was desperate. I searched the Internet and found Dr. Daryl. I did my first cleanse in 2015. I felt so much better, and I was surprised that the recipes were so delicious and easy to make! I now eat organic fruits and vegetables with lots of greens. No more processed foods and especially, no sugar. Dr. Daryl changed my life! He taught me how to make healthy choices. Now my skin is glowing, and I have an amazing amount of energy. I no longer take Prevacid. Eating healthy is my life now. Most importantly, I don't have the sugar cravings. I crave vegetables!   —Helene S.

two

How Sugar Drains
Your Whole-Body Health

Maybe you want to get off your sugar because you know that it's contributing to your weight gain. Maybe you don't like the way it makes you feel after the high has worn off. Maybe you're tired of the cravings and just want to get your life back.

These are all great reasons. But to really steel your resolve, I want to show you how sugar impacts the major organs and systems in your body and the resulting role it plays in every major disease. Having this knowledge will help fuel you through the seven steps I outline in Phase 2 of this book, so that you, too, can experience the level of health that's possible when you get off your sugar.

YOUR GUT ON SUGAR

Your gut comprises 80 percent of your immune system and 80 percent of your nervous system, and it is considered to be your second brain. Most important, particularly as pertains to sugar, your gut houses trillions of bacteria, both good and bad. Your gut bugs are what produce the neurotransmitters your body needs to function. A full 95 percent of your serotonin—a neurotransmitter responsible for regulating appetite, mood, sleep, and relaxation; 50 percent of your dopamine—the neurotransmitter associated with pleasure; and 30 other neurotransmitters, are manufactured by the microbes in your gut. They help determine whether a substance you ingested is friend or foe. You may think you're 100 percent human, but really, you have more bacteria than cells. If aliens abducted a human and analyzed what made us live and breathe, they'd say a human was nothing more than a bunch of bacteria housed in a funny suit of skin, muscle, and bones.

Tons of research now tells us that our gut bacteria determine varying aspects of health. I'm talkin' the health of your skin, your immune system, how many calories you burn, your weight, your chances of developing a disease, and more.

You have trillions of gut bacteria living inside your GI tract. Most bugs are beneficial, meaning they give health benefits, some are neutral, and some are considered harmful and may cause disease or unwanted symptoms.

When you are healthy and balanced, your bacteria thrive in the rich environment of the gut and you enjoy the multiple benefits the bacteria provide. But bacteria are switch-hitters that can be either beneficial or pathogenic. Stressors, such as sugar, antibiotics, stress, grains, decreased probiotics, and artificial sweeteners; medications, such as protein-pump inhibitors (PPIs, often prescribed for reflux); and chemicals, such as glyphosate, acidify and inflame the gut terrain, pushing more bacteria to the dark side. The only lasting way to get rid of the bad guys is to stop eating the foods that make our inner terrain unhealthy.

Let me ask you a question: If you have a pail filled with garbage and a bunch of rats, who brought who? Did the rats bring the garbage, or did the garbage bring the rats? That's right: the garbage brought the rats. You can poison the rats (in regard to bacteria that's gone bad, by giving antibiotics), but they will come back. And when they come back, you'll be even worse off, because your intervention made the terrain more toxic. It's only when you stop the poison and clean out the trash that the rats will go away. **You've got to maintain your terrain.**

Sugars (and artificial sweeteners) are the most toxic offenders of the gut because they destroy the terrain. Sugar breaks down to lactic acid, which, as you can probably guess from its name, is acidic. Think what acid does—it's corrosive; it can cut through metal. Over time, eating sugar creates leaky holes in your gut, which gives free entry for all kind of things to get into your bloodstream, such as toxins, fungus, mold, undigested proteins, yeast, and their mycotoxins.

It's estimated that 80 percent of people have some level of permeability in their gut lining, but in my experience, it's more like 100 percent, albeit in different degrees. It's pretty much impossible to escape leaky gut in our modern toxic age; however, we can do our best to minimize its potentially dangerous and devastating effects on our health.

In my practice, I look at my patients' blood under the microscope, and I can see some level of these invaders in their blood cells. These toxic particles throw off the pH balance of your blood. Your blood pH, the most important number in your body, needs to be tightly regulated within a narrow range of 7.35 to 7.45, ideally at 7.4; if it goes too far beyond that in either way, you will die. So, when something throws your blood pH off, your body will do whatever it takes to balance the pH, such as taking minerals from your bones, muscles, and mouth to buffer the toxic exposure.

Imagine what your pool looks like if its pH goes off—that's when you start breeding mosquitos and seeing blooms of weird green algae. The same thing happens inside your body when your pH balance is off. And just like the pool with a pH that has veered off course, your body becomes a cesspool that rusts and rots from the inside out.

||||||||||||||||||||||||||||||||||||||||||||||||||||||||||||||||||||||||||||||||||||||||||||

THE GUT IS A PATHWAY
TO THE BRAIN

A 2015 study published in *Neuroscience* found that mice who were fed a high-sugar diet for twelve days experienced changes in their gut bacteria that correlated to a significant loss of cognitive flexibility (the ability to adapt to changing circumstances). They also experienced diminished long-term and short-term memory.[1] Think about that next time you realize you forgot to send that email or can't find your keys—it may help give you the resolve to finally get off your sugar!

||||||||||||||||||||||

YOU'RE NOT CRAVING SUGAR, YOUR GUT BUGS ARE

Eating a lot of sugary foods breeds unhealthy bacteria, toxins, parasites, fungus, mold, and yeast. These are living organisms that have to eat, and they *love* sugar. In fact, they *need* it to survive. That's why I say that if you're craving sugar, it's not really even technically *you* who is doing the craving; it's your gut bugs.

A whopping 97 percent of women and 68 percent of men report experiencing cravings for certain foods. Given that our gut microbes coevolved with us and constantly depend on the incoming food that we eat to provide for their own sustenance, it's really no surprise that they are able to preferentially shape our eating preferences to improve their own chances of survival.[2]

One incredibly common strain of unfriendly microbes is yeast; specifically, *Candida albicans*, also known as candida. Everyone has candida in their body; it lives in your intestines and at low levels is harmless. But an overgrowth can wreak havoc on your body, including your blood, and affect every area of your health. Many people have a candida overgrowth and don't even know it! I don't just mean a vaginal yeast infection—both men and women can have an overgrowth, and it can take over lots of different parts of your body. In fact, if you have a vaginal yeast infection, that likely means the yeast is systemic and overgrown throughout your whole body. And yeast makes every health issue you have worse; it's the equivalent of the gasoline that causes a fire to rage out of control.

Candida needs sugar for a variety of reasons. It uses it to shore up its cell walls, which is made up of 80 percent carbohydrates. It also uses sugar to transform into a more dangerous, fungal form that is capable of penetrating more deeply into your gut lining.[3] Also, candida is protected by something called a biofilm, which is kind of like an invisibility cloak that makes these organisms invisible to your immune system. And about a third of the material used to make the biofilm is glucose.[4]

To make things worse, yeast also has to poop, and its waste products (called mycotoxins) are acidic, which only add fuel to the fire. When candida is overgrown, you get bloating, acid reflux, constipation, diarrhea, uncontrollable sugar cravings, as well as the potential for Crohn's disease and irritable bowel syndrome. I had most of these conditions for a good portion of my life because I had a nasty overgrowth of yeast from eating too much sugar, which I saw with my own two eyes on my first live blood cell test. When you get off your sugar, you starve out candida, restore balance to your gut flora, and all these things resolve themselves.

Candida Overgrowth: Symptoms, Assessment, and Treatment

Here are some common symptoms:

- Chronic abdominal gas
- Headaches/migraines
- Excessive fatigue and brain fog
- Intense sugar and alcohol cravings
- Mood swings
- Rectal itching
- Itchy skin
- Acne
- Low sex drive
- Nail fungus
- Hyperactivity
- Anxiety or nervousness
- Being strongly reactive to cigarette smoke
- Belly fat

Chances are, you have some level of excess candida. This at-home test can help you see for yourself.

1. First thing in the morning, before you put anything in your mouth, fill a clear glass with room-temperature filtered water.

2. Work up a bit of saliva, and spit it into the glass of water.

3. Wait for at least 15 minutes and up to one hour.

4. If you see strings (fibers) traveling from the saliva floating on the top down into the water, cloudy specks (particles suspended in the water), or cloudy saliva that sinks to the bottom of the glass, you have a candida problem.

DIY CANDIDA PROTOCOL

It's important that you take steps to reduce candida overgrowth before following the Get Off Your Sugar program. Otherwise, your candida will keep your cravings strong, and your leaky gut will keep your inflammation levels high. Although you can get a prescription for antifungal medication from a doctor, candida overgrowth can often be treated on your own, at home, with this protocol that relies on bioactive silver hydrosol—a safe, nontoxic, natural remedy that has antibacterial, antiviral, and antifungal properties.

I got this protocol from my good friend and colleague Robert Scott Bell, DA, Hom (host of *The Robert Scott Bell Radio Show* and one of the doctors featured in the documentary *The Truth About Cancer*), who suggests pairing bioactive silver (a naturally occurring component of all mammalian milk, many whole grains, and mushrooms that the body excretes safely through the colon[5]) with aloe vera liquid, which helps heal and seal the gut, and probiotic replenishment supplement to repopulate your friendly bacterial population. (*Note:* I recommend the Sovereign Silver brand, which is available to consumers, or Argentyn 23, for health professionals. For the liquid aloe vera, I recommend George's Aloe or Lily of the Desert Organic Aloe Vera. For probiotic supplement recommendations, refer to Chapter 11.)

Three times a day, on an empty stomach, take:

* 1 tablespoon **bioactive silver hydrosol***
* 1 tablespoon **pure aloe vera liquid***

And then in the early evening, take a probiotic supplement. Continue for one to two weeks.

* If you weigh less than 120 pounds, take half this dosage.

Also note: Dr. Bell says the only contraindication to this protocol is if you are taking a sulfonamide antibiotic, such as Bactrim; not because of danger, but because the sulfur binds with the silver, preventing the silver from benefiting the body.

In addition to the DIY candida protocol that I share here, the most important thing you can do to kick a candida overgrowth and bring your bacterial population back into balance is to eat a low-sugar diet. (There are also two foods that could be contributing to your candida overgrowth if you're eating them regularly—nutritional yeast and mushrooms; see page 121 for more information.) You've got to stop ingesting the poison that's causing the damage in the first place. You simply can't be truly healthy until you do. Remember, I'm going to walk you through the seven-step process that makes getting off your sugar easy and effective, so don't panic!

SUGAR AND THE AGE-ING PROCESS

One of the widespread dangers of sugar is that it contributes to a process called **glycation**, which happens throughout the body when a glucose molecule attaches to a protein or fat molecule.

Glycation creates damaging free radicals known as advanced glycation end-products (AGEs). Like most free radicals, AGEs are destructive; they drive up inflammation, and they rot and rust your tissues in a process known as oxidation. Damage by glycation results in stiffening of the collagen in the blood vessel walls,

THE LINK BETWEEN SUGAR AND INFLAMMATION

There are two primary ways sugar leads to inflammation:

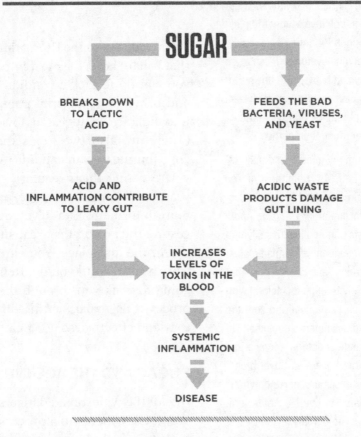

SUGAR-INFLAMMATION PATHWAY

SUGAR

BREAKS DOWN TO LACTIC ACID

FEEDS THE BAD BACTERIA, VIRUSES, AND YEAST

ACID AND INFLAMMATION CONTRIBUTE TO LEAKY GUT

ACIDIC WASTE PRODUCTS DAMAGE GUT LINING

INCREASES LEVELS OF TOXINS IN THE BLOOD

SYSTEMIC INFLAMMATION

DISEASE

leading to high blood pressure, especially in people who also have diabetes. Glycation also causes weakening of the collagen in the blood vessel walls, which can lead to strokes and aneurisms, and even age spots and wrinkly skin. Thanks to glycation, sugar makes you age faster and look older.

In the brain, it's even worse; that's where glycation contributes to the forma-tion of plaques that can lead to Alzheimer's disease (otherwise known as type 3 diabetes) and dementia. (More on this in just a moment.)

The best way to measure how much glycation you may be experiencing is the hemoglobin A1c (HbA1c) blood test, which sheds light on your average blood sugar levels for the past four months by measuring how much glucose (blood sugar) is bound to hemoglobin (a protein found in red blood cells that carries oxygen and gives blood its red color). Because your red blood cells have a life span of 120 days, this test gives you a picture of your glucose levels over the past four months; not just the last few hours (like the glucose tests you can administer yourself with an at-home glucose monitor). This test is used to diagnose and monitor diabetes, but it's useful for everyone as a measure of how much glycation they're experiencing.

||||||||||||||||||||||||||||||||||||||||||||||||||||||||||||||||||||||||

DECIPHERING YOUR HBA1C LEVEL

Below 5.7 percent	Normal
5.7 to 6.4 percent	Prediabetes
6.5 percent or higher	Diabetes

Studies have shown that the higher your HbA1c number is—even if it is still within the prediabetic range and not in full-blown diabetes territory—the higher your risk for cancer[6] and heart disease[7]. That's how important that number is.

||||||||||||||||||

YOUR BRAIN HAS BEEN HIJACKED BY SUGAR

There are no two ways about it: sugar changes your brain chemistry, and it does it through the following mechanisms:

- **Dopamine.** As I discussed in Chapter 1, the sugar you eat is turned into glucose in your blood, which prompts the release of insulin, which lights up the dopamine receptors in your brain associated with feelings of pleasure, which makes sugar eight times as addictive as cocaine.

- **Cortisol.** As I also went over in Chapter 1, when the brain senses it's running out of glucose, it will go into panic mode because it's forgotten how to burn fat and thinks that you must have more glucose now to be able to survive. That's when it cues the adrenal glands to release the stress hormone cortisol, and once you're in a state of physiological stress, you are more likely to reach for sugar to ensure you have the fast-burning energy you might need for fight or flight.

- **Insulin.** The insulin your body releases after you eat sugar can interfere with the healthy functioning of your brain, especially if you chronically overeat sugar and the insulin receptors in your brain start to lose their sensitivity, in what's known as insulin resistance. Insulin resistance in brain cells is associated with Alzheimer's (also known as type 3 diabetes), brain fog, difficulty focusing, and ADD or ADHD in kids and adults.

- **Leptin.** Because insulin influences other hormones in your body, eating sugar also affects your levels of leptin, which regulates hunger and feeling full. More insulin in the brain cues the fat cells to secrete more leptin. When leptin levels go up, it signals the hypothalamus in your brain that you're full and should stop eating. When they go down, it tells your brain you're hungry and you need fuel. The problem is that when leptin levels are perpetually high because insulin levels are perpetually high, your cells lose the ability to hear leptin's signals and everything goes haywire: you're always hungry and never feel full. You start to constantly crave sweet foods as you also become desensitized to sugar, so you need more of it. It's a vicious cycle: eating sugar leads to craving sugar, and craving sugar leads to eating more sugar.

- **Lactic acid.** Remember, a by-product of sugar metabolism is lactic acid, and lactic acid is acidic. Just as it can chew holes in your gut lining and promote inflammation in your digestive tract, it also promotes neuroinflammation, which can manifest as ADD, ADHD, behavior problems, aggression, brain fog, dementia, and Parkinson's. Why have we seen such a staggering rise in ADD and ADHD? I think it's that sugar (and the glycation it triggers) is the number one cause of inflammation of the brain. Most doctors are treating these children with hard-core psychotropic drugs, such as Ritalin and Adderall, when they should be going further upstream to address the *cause*, which is lowering inflammation from a highly acidic and carb-rich diet. The medications are just masking the true problem, and are making our children even more sick and toxic down the road as these drugs bioaccumulate in the liver and the body.

Sugar and Alzheimer's, a.k.a. Diabetes of the Brain

A study by Alzheimer's researchers at UCLA found that in 2017, 6 million Americans had either mild cognitive impairment from Alzheimer's or clinical Alzheimer's, and that number would go up to 15 million by 2060—an increase of 250 percent. It also showed that nearly 47 million Americans had preclinical Alzheimer's in 2017; they predict that in 2060, the number will be almost 76 million.[8]

The link between Alzheimer's and sugar consumption is so strong that the disease is often called *type 3 diabetes*.

It's an accepted fact that people with type 2 diabetes have a higher risk of developing Alzheimer's disease and other forms of dementia; in fact, one meta-analysis in the *Journal of Diabetes Investigation* of all of the research out there through 2012 found that people with type 2 diabetes had:

- 73 percent increased risk of any dementia
- 56 percent increased risk of Alzheimer's disease
- 127 percent increased risk of vascular dementia[9]

Researchers are also saying the higher the blood sugar levels, the faster the cognitive decline.

A big reason why sugar and Alzheimer's are linked is because of glycation, the process I covered in the previous section. When glycation happens in the brain, it promotes the formation of the plaques that are a hallmark of Alzheimer's. These plaques start forming up to twenty years before the disease progresses far enough to be diagnosed, and once the plaques are formed, you can't undo them, the same way you can't unboil an egg. You have to stop new plaques from forming before they start, and reducing insulin and glucose levels in the brain and lowering neuroinflammation is the way to do that. And how do you do that? Get off your sugar!

Science backs this simple dietary strategy: a study published in the *Journal of Alzheimer's Disease* by researchers at the Mayo Clinic followed 937 seniors over nearly four years and tracked what foods they ate most frequently. The risk of mild cognitive impairme... highest—89 percent... group with a high intak... and most reduced—44... those with high fat intake...

SEVEN WAYS TO NEUROPROTECT YOUR BRAIN

1. **Reduce sugar and CRAP-py carbs.** This is a crucial step in protecting your brain as you age. While there are many other things you can do to take care of your brain, reducing your sugar intake is priority number one.

2. **Consume more omega-3 essential fatty acids.** You need essential fatty acids, but your body can't manufacture them. Omega-3 fatty acids (from fatty fish, such as salmon, nuts, seeds, and purified fish oil supplements) are anti-inflammatory in general and particularly important for reducing neuroinflammation. For this reason, they are vital for proper brain function. Research funded by the National Institutes of Health found that people with a higher intake of omega-3s actually have more grey matter in the hippocampus—the area of the brain associated with memory.[11] Higher omega-3 levels have also been found to reduce anxiety[12] and prevent the formation of amyloids, the buildup of proteins that are associated with Alzheimer's.[13] It's even been found that women who have higher omega-3 levels when they are pregnant give birth to children with a higher IQ.[14] Sadly, most Americans are highly deficient in omega-3s; that's why I recommend that everyone take a purified fish oil supplement (for more on omega-3s, see Chapter 6; for supplement specifics, see Chapter 11).

3. **Take brain-supporting supplements.** The supplements that protect your brain health include:

   ❖ **Vitamin D.** People with low levels of vitamin D have a higher risk of later cognitive impairment and dementia,[15] and most Americans are deficient.

   ❖ **Magnesium.** You'll hear me talk more about magnesium in chapters 4 and 6, but for now, know that it's a primary supplement to protect your brain from risk of dementia, cognitive impairment, and Alzheimer's. Researchers have even found that you can reverse brain aging by up to fourteen years with magnesium supplementation![16]

   ❖ **B complex.** The B vitamins reduce oxidative stress and inflammatory reactions in the brain, and they also facilitate the production of neurotransmitters (chemicals that deliver messages between the brain and the body).

* **Antioxidants.** Antioxidants help lower both inflammation and oxidative stress, both of which contribute to cognitive decline. My favorite antioxidants are black seed oil and molecular hydrogen.

4. **Put coconut oil on everything.** Medium-chain triglycerides (MCT) are shorter than most other fatty acids, and thus, are metabolized differently. Instead of being broken down by the gut, MCTs go straight to the liver, where they are turned into ketones and then either used right away or sent to the brain for fuel. Your brain can use either glucose or ketones for fuel, but science suggests that certain parts of Alzheimer's patients' brains have a harder time using glucose; in fact, a 2004 study found that Alzheimer's patients who ingested a drink that contained MCTs performed better on memory tests than those who received a placebo.[17] Coconut oil contains about 66 percent MCTs. While it takes about 2 tablespoons of coconut oil to get the amount of MCTs that is considered therapeutic for the brain, you have to build up your tolerance or else it will upset your stomach. My recommendation is to start with 1 teaspoon, taken with food in the mornings. Gradually add more coconut oil every few days until you are able to tolerate 2 tablespoons.

5. **Exercise daily.** When you move your body, you raise your heart and respiration rates, which delivers more oxygen to tissues throughout the body. In the brain, this extra oxygen spurs neurogenesis—the formation of new brain cells—which then protects against later cognitive decline.[18] Exercise also promotes the formation of neurotrophins, which are proteins that protect brain cells and help them form new connections to one another.[19] In one study of people with a genetic modification that makes them more susceptible to early-onset Alzheimer's, those who exercise at least 150 minutes a week had better cognitive outcomes than those who exercised less or not at all, and that exercise could delay the onset of dementia by as many as 15 years.[20] (I cover exercise in depth in Chapter 12.)

6. **Reduce copper levels.** Copper is a mineral that's often found bound to other molecules in the plaques that form in the brain of Alzheimer's patients, who typically have excessively high levels of copper. Copper in and of itself isn't bad—it's naturally present in food, where it is bound to other organic materials and therefore not available to form these plaques. It's when we ingest copper either through supplements or via drinking water (which typically passes through copper pipes) that we are subjected to free copper, meaning it is single and looking to mingle with other molecules, potentially leading to plaque-like formations in the brain. To make sure that levels of copper in your brain aren't too high, make sure to drink filtered water (preferably from a reverse-osmosis filter or a molecular hydrogen filter) and that any multivitamins or supplements you take either *don't* contain it or don't have more than 100 micrograms (mcg). Copper is also plentiful in red meat; yet another reason to reduce your consumption of it.

7. **Make space for stress relief.** You know it's hard to think straight when you're experiencing a stressful situation (and studies have shown that memory is impaired in those instances). But chronic stress can actually shrink the volume of the prefrontal cortex, a section of the brain that regulates emotions and self-control,[21] and impairs your ability to form and retrieve memories.[22] And we are all subjected to low and high levels of stress all day, every day. To combat the effects of stress on the brain, be sure to regularly give yourself the opportunity for your brain to enter a relaxed state. I love the **BrainTap app**, which guides you through a series of visualizations that calm your mind and was started by my good friend Dr. Patrick Porter. (I talk more about stress relief in Chapter 13, but you can get a free fifteen-day trial of the app and a special visualization for getting off sugar at getoffyourstress.com.)

Sugar and Your Liver: Alcohol Without the Buzz

Did you know that sugar can pose as much of a risk to your liver as alcohol does? That's because your liver metabolizes large amounts of sugar, especially fructose, the same way it does alcohol—as a toxin.

Your liver breaks the fructose down into carbohydrates, which then cues your body to release more insulin, which then triggers fat storage. This doesn't necessarily happen when the fructose comes inside of an apple, because all that chewing and breaking down of fiber means the fructose makes its way to your liver only slowly. But when you *drink* large amounts of fructose—say, in soda, or orange juice, which has even more fructose per cup than soda—throughout the day, the liver gets overwhelmed and so converts most of it into fat.

There are only so many places fat can be stored; the liver is one of them. Your liver is your major organ of detoxification,

and when it gets riddled with fatty deposits, it has to work that much harder to regenerate itself, detoxify your blood, and pull excess glucose out of the bloodstream. This can lead to nonalcoholic fatty liver disease (NAFLD), which can progress into nonalcoholic steatohepatitis (NASH), which adds inflammation and scarring to the list of liver ailments. About 25 percent of people who develop NASH will then go on to develop nonalcoholic liver cirrhosis,[23] which requires a liver transplant.

The rates of NAFLD and NASH have doubled since the 1980s, with approximately six million people (about 31 percent of the US adult population and 13 percent of American kids) having NAFLD and 600,000 with NASH-related cirrhosis.

Sugar and Your Hormones

Sugar doesn't just impact your organs; it also has a pervasive effect on your endocrine system, which consists of the glands in your body that secrete those powerful chemical messengers known as hormones.

Insulin resistance. Insulin is a critical hormone that is responsible for maintaining your blood levels of glucose, among other things. When you constantly eat low-fiber carbohydrates and sugars, glucose is continuously metabolized from these foods and released into your blood. Your pancreas will then secrete insulin to move the glucose out of your bloodstream and into your cells—it's truly a nutrient-transport hormone. The problem is that over time, the insulin receptor sites on your cells can get dulled because insulin is always present—glucose keeps knocking on the door, but it's as if the insulin receptors' ears are clogged and they can't hear the knock. The result? Cellular mayhem.

When your full cells reject the extra glucose, your blood sugar rises, producing more insulin, making those receptors even more clogged and your insulin levels ever more elevated. It's not actually the blood sugar that's the issue, it's the high levels of insulin that leads to so many problems. This is known as insulin resistance, which is a commonly accepted precursor to type 2 diabetes and metabolic syndrome—a family of conditions that include high blood pressure, excess belly fat, and low HDL (the "good" kind of cholesterol) levels.

Insulin resistance can happen all over the body—in the brain, it manifests as Alzheimer's, also known as type 3 diabetes. In the kidneys, it promotes chronic renal disease. In the liver, it leads to type 2 diabetes.

Throughout this chapter, you'll also see how insulin resistance plays a role in many common conditions and diseases.

The worst part is that 80 percent—8 in 10—of Americans are insulin-resistant, and they don't even realize it.

Thyroid hormone. Excess sugar impairs the function of your thyroid, which secretes the hormones that rule everything about your metabolism. The leaky gut that sugar is a direct contributor to raises levels of toxins in your bloodstream, and your thyroid is ultrasusceptible to toxins. It's also highly influenced by insulin, and both the insulin spikes that eating sugar causes and the round-the-clock high insulin levels caused by insulin resistance slowly destroys the thyroid gland. Once its function is impaired, a compromised thyroid slows the body's ability to remove insulin from the blood. It's a downward spiral that can lead to a thyroid dysfunction, including hypothyroidism (where levels of thyroid hormone are too low), hyperthyroidism (when they are too high), and even Hashimoto's disease—an autoimmune illness where the immune system attacks the thyroid gland and levels of thyroid hormone drop to dangerously low levels.

Insulin resistance has also been identified as a risk factor for developing thyroid cancer.[24] Because thyroid hormones rule so many different functions of the body—your weight, your energy levels, your sleep/wake cycles—if you are one of the estimated twenty million Americans with some form of thyroid dysfunction, getting off your sugar will help you feel like yourself again.

Estrogen. Estrogen and sugar share a relationship mostly through fat. Eating excess sugar cues the body to store fat. And the leaky gut that sugar contributes to also encourages the formation of fat cells because that's where the body stores toxins that it can't excrete. The more sugar you eat, the more fat cells you create, and as a result, the more estrogen is produced. This fat-produced estrogen then adds to the estrogen your endocrine system produces and the estrogen-like chemicals (known as xenoestrogens) that we are exposed to via the environment, our water supply, and our food.

This sets you up for estrogen dominance, progesterone deficiency, and hormonal imbalance. This hormonal imbalance is a root cause of such common issues as PMS, premenstrual dysphoric disorder (PMDD), painful cramps, irregular cycles, acne, along with more serious issues, such as polycystic ovarian syndrome (PCOS), endometriosis, and infertility. The hormonal disruption that sugar causes is also a root reason that girls are hitting puberty and women are experiencing menopause at ever younger ages.

PCOS, the most common hormonal disorder of women in America, affecting up to 10 percent of women aged eighteen to forty-four, is directly associated with insulin resistance; high levels of insulin cue the ovaries to pump out more androgens, or what are considered to be male hormones, including testosterone, upsetting the delicate hormonal balance of the reproductive system.

High sugar consumption has also been linked to a significantly increased risk of developing endometrial cancer—a 2013 study that evaluated the diets of 23,039 postmenopausal women over a period of fourteen years found that women who had the highest intake of sugar-sweetened beverages had a 78 percent higher risk than those women who drank the least amount of sugary drinks.[25]

If you go to the doctor because of your painful periods, PCOS, or infertility, they will likely put you on hormones without looking further upstream to determine why your hormones are out of whack in the first place. Eliminating sugar removes a major source of excess estrogen and helps bring your reproductive hormones back into balance naturally. This is especially important if you are trying to become pregnant, as eating a high-glycemic diet (which is a high-sugar, low-fiber diet) was shown by the Nurses Study, which followed more than eighteen thousand nurses over the course of eight years, to nearly double a woman's chances of having infertility (raising the odds by 92 percent) that was related to difficulty with ovulation.[26]

THE LINK BETWEEN SUGAR AND CANCER

Cancer is the number two cause of death in the United States, right behind heart disease. Cancer kills 600,000 every year; that is 1,643 people every day. I remember flying out to speak at Fran Drescher's Cancer Schmancer Masterclass Health Summit, and I started my talk by telling the audience, imagine seven jumbo jets falling out of the sky every day and killing everyone on board—that's how many die from cancer on a daily basis.

You may have heard the saying "Cancer loves sugar." But do you know why people say it? Because cancer requires sugar to stay alive!

Unlike nearly all the other cells in your body, cancer can't use fat for fuel; it can exist only on sugar. That's because cancer cells rely on fermentation to produce their energy (in what's known as an anaerobic—"without oxygen"—process), instead of the oxygen healthy cells use. And only sugar will ferment; not fat.

Our understanding of the true mechanisms behind the development and growth of cancer are still evolving, but what we understand today is that when healthy cells use oxygen for energy, one glucose (sugar) molecule can create as many as thirty-six molecules of adenosine triphosphate (the units of energy manufactured by your mitochondria). On the other hand, the process of anaerobic respiration creates only two molecules of ATP! In other words, for a cancer cell to create the same amount of energy as one normal cell, it must metabolize eighteen times more glucose (sugar).

So, cancer doesn't just need sugar to exist; it needs *a lot* of it. Remove sugar from your diet, and it's like cutting off a terrorist's supply of money; you will make it an awful lot harder for it to inflict widespread damage.

Here's what I take away from this discussion: sugar is not your friend; sugar is cancer's friend.

A PRIME SUSPECT IN HEART DISEASE

Every ninety seconds, someone suffers a heart attack. In that same time, two people will have a stroke, and one person will die of a cardiovascular disease. Heart disease is the number one most popular cause of death in the United States for women and for men.[27]

Sugar has a lot to do with why heart disease is so common. First, sugar is a direct contributor to the previously mentioned metabolic syndrome, a cluster of conditions—increased blood pressure, high blood sugar, excess body fat around the waist, and abnormal cholesterol or triglyceride levels—that occur together, increasing your risk of heart disease, stroke, and diabetes. It creates a perfect storm for cardiovascular disease!

In addition, as we've covered, sugar is highly acidic, and that acidity can cause damage to your blood vessels and gut lining that then cues the body to raise inflammation in an attempt to heal those damaged areas. Sugar consumption is also associated with higher levels of blood pressure. Of course, sugar causes weight gain, too, and being overweight is another major risk factor for heart disease.

A 2014 study published in *JAMA Internal Medicine* analyzed the diets of thirty-one thousand Americans for fifteen years and found that the higher the percentage of daily calories from added sugars, the higher the risk of dying from cardiovascular disease. Study participants who got 25 percent or more of their daily calories from added sugar were more than twice as likely to die from heart disease as those whose diets got less than 10 percent of their calories from added sugars. And this association was true whether the rest of the diet was fairly healthy (following the federal nutrition guidelines) or not.[28] The authors of the study wrote, "We observed a significant relationship between added sugar consumption and increased risk for cardiovascular disease mortality."

Another link between sugar and heart health is that sugar, especially fructose, increases uric acid. Like lactic acid, uric acid nicks up the blood vessel walls, which then requires cholesterol and inflammation to repair. There are thousands of articles showing a strong relationship between increased levels of uric acid and diabetes, high blood pressure, and stroke—all hallmarks of heart disease.

PRIORITY NUMBER ONE: GET OFF YOUR SUGAR

As you can see, when you eat sugar, your gut, brain, liver, biological clock, hormones, and heart all pay the price. If you want the inside of your body to be a healthy environment for every part of you (as well as the friendly bacteria that play such a vital role in your vitality), you've got to get off the sweet stuff. When you do, all these organs and systems can rebound, and that's when you start experiencing more energy and well-being than you thought possible!

Now you know *why* getting off sugar is so important. It's time to start talking about the *how*. In the next chapter, I'll walk you through the elements of my Get Off Your Sugar program so you can see how each step builds on the last and is carefully designed to get you off your sugar *without* cravings or a sense of deprivation.

CHAPTER 2 ACTION STEPS

* Give yourself an at-home candida test (page 24).

* If you see evidence of candida in your at-home test, follow the protocol I outline on page 25 *before* progressing with the rest of the Get Off Your Sugar program.

* Go through the "Seven Ways to Neuroprotect Your Brain" checklist (page 29)—and pick one item on the list to get started on now.

I was in a very high-stress job and working many hours. I was also largely consuming a diet of highly processed foods, including anything with sugar that crossed my path. Constantly exhausted, I was also overweight, with joint pain, high triglycerides, high cholesterol, high blood pressure, and suffering from digestive issues. The final straw was when I developed a fungal infection in one of my toenails, which my doctor wanted to treat with medication that was potentially toxic to the liver. Not really looking forward to taking that medication and trying to find relief for my symptoms, I discovered Dr. Daryl's website.

That's where I learned that every one of my issues were a symptom of an overload of sugar and other acidic, processed foods. I performed the test for candida as described by Dr. Daryl and was surprised to see that it was positive. As I read more about candida overgrowth, it all began to make sense, including the red, scaly rash that had developed on my abdomen. I signed up for the next cleanse.

Within a few days of starting the cleanse, I already felt better, with more energy and clarity than I had experienced in years. I continued following Dr. Daryl's sensible 80 percent approach; after three months, the rash, fungal infection, digestive issues, exhaustion, and 18 pounds were gone. Within six months, my triglycerides and cholesterol were back within normal range.

I have been following his approach for almost three years now. It is a very common sense, realistic approach that I can adhere to, even with my extensive travel schedule. Thank you Dr. Daryl for helping me kick sugar to the curb!   —Sally D., OD, EdD

three

The Get Off Your Sugar Program

BY NOW, YOU KNOW A LOT MORE ABOUT JUST HOW BAD SUGAR IS FOR YOU. BUT I don't want you closing this book after the first two chapters and telling yourself it's too hard to get free from sugar. When you follow my program, it's not hard. I've helped literally thousands of people wean themselves off sugar and transform into fat-burning machines. I've done it for myself. I'm constantly learning everything new that I can about sugar and health, and with this program, I've distilled and organized all of this information and experience into a program that's fully mapped out and designed to give you everything you need to demolish your cravings, heal your gut, remove the number one source of inflammation, gain levels of energy you can only imagine now, lose weight, and feel like you are invincible.

In this chapter, I'll give you both the bird's-eye view and a behind-the-scenes look at just what makes this program so unique and so successful.

THE THREE NUMBERS
THAT WILL SET YOU FREE

There are three numbers that are essential to creating any new habit and to finding success on the Get Off Your Sugar program. They are 7, 21, and 90: numbers that are time-tested and proven to be crucial components of behavioral changes. Let's look at them one by one:

- 7 is the number of days my program gives you to cleanse and detoxify your mind, your body, and your pantry *before* you start to skyrocket your outcome and results. This is how you set yourself up for success. During the first week of the program, you prepare the soil, so that when you start making changes to your daily diet, your body is ready to soak up the goodness that you'll be feeding it, and you will soar. To get off your sugar, you *must* address your mindset as much as your physical body.

- 21 is the number of days it takes to build a habit. That's three weeks of your life— not so long that you'll give up before you start, but not so short that you won't gain some serious momentum and face some trials that will help strengthen your resolve.

- And 90 is how many days it takes to make a new habit an ingrained part of your life. And that's precisely what this program is—it's a lifestyle, not a diet, because a diet is something you do until you lose the weight and then you go back to your previous way of eating. (It also contains the word *die* within it—just sayin'.) The Get Off Your Sugar program is

just how you live your life. It doesn't mean you'll never ever eat sugar again, but because this way of eating both abolishes cravings and helps evolve your taste buds away from loving sugar, and because it takes into account the need for variety in your diet, you will be able to eat sweet stuff occasionally if you choose to (although it's likely true that your definition of delicious sweet stuff will evolve right along with your taste buds).

During the first seven days, you may feel a little bit as if you're on a roller coaster as you're balancing physical cravings with the mental challenge of figuring out how to shop and what to eat. Sugar is a powerful force, in your brain, in your body, in our daily lives, and in our culture at large. It's completely reasonable to assume that beginning to change your relationship to it will have its dramatic ups and downs. At any given time during the first seven and twenty-one days, all you ever have to do is focus on making today the best it can be, and make progress, not perfection, your goal. Our lives here are controlled by one force—*decisions*. When you make the best decision you can in the moment again and again, you're going to grow. And when you're making progress and growing, you're going to have more energy, vitality, and strength in every aspect of your life.

I promise, it does get easier. As you continue through the program and you rectify your nutritional deficiencies and reprogram your taste buds, you'll feel more as if you're in a car with an automatic pilot function. You have to plot your course, but you don't have to stress over every little twist and turn.

THREE GUIDING PRINCIPLES

There's a lot more to this program than mere tactics; a ton of strategy is baked in too. I've done a *lot* of thinking about which step you take first, second, third, and so on, and these strategies have been tested by me and by the more than 120,000 patients I've had the ultimate privilege to serve over the last twenty years. This program works, and it works not simply because it's a list of steps in a specific order, but also because it is built on the following principles:

Add, Don't Take Away. Deprivation doesn't work. Or if it does, it doesn't work for long. I tried to quit sugar multiple times in my life before I figured out the steps that I share here, and none of them stuck. Many times I'd get excited about a new program, only to completely give up two weeks later. It's the same reason why gym attendance spikes at the beginning of January and is back to normal by the time February gets going. Maintaining willpower over the long haul is exhausting. Some people can simply decide to completely give up a category of foods (or something else they're addicted to) and that's it, they're good. But the vast majority of us can't.

A main reason why willpower doesn't last is that simply cutting something out of your life doesn't address the root causes that got you overdependent in the first place. It was only when I started thinking about how to add the things that would make me healthier all the way down to the cellular level, that I made lasting changes to my diet.

Adding is simply much more compelling than taking away. The more good things you add to your diet, the more you will crowd out the bad stuff, *and* the more you help address the nutrient deficiencies, gut bacteria imbalances, and out-of-whack hormones that have kept you stuck in a cycle of cravings.

Weed, Seed, Feed. Recently I was walking down the street in my Upper East Side neighborhood of Manhattan with my six-year-old son. We walked past a building that had recently been knocked down and was a huge pile of rubble. Because he's obsessed with construction, my son was thrilled to see that there was a bulldozer on-site to remove the pile of bricks and clear space for a new building to take shape. I knew that in a week or two, they'd be digging a hole for a new foundation and then they'd start to construct the new building (because no empty lot stays empty for long in Manhattan).

It's the same with your health. If you're like most people, years of eating CRAP-py (completely refined and processed) carbohydrates and high-sugar processed foods has wrecked your gut, whether you feel it or not; you can't just start adding new foods without first clearing out the toxins, bad bacteria, and excess hormones that your former way of eating has contributed to. You've got to remove the old bricks first. Then, you've got to give yourself a new foundation. And only *then* can you rebuild.

That's why my program has three progressive phases: weed, seed, and feed. In the weed portion, you'll do a seven-day detox to get things out of your body, your pantry, and your life that have been keeping you hooked on sugar. Then, for the next twenty-one days, you'll add the nutrients, such as minerals and fats that can then "seed" the new level of health you're seeking to create. And then, finally, you can "feed" yourself with a strength-eating diet based on dark green alkalizing vegetables, clean ketogenic fats, moderate protein, and low carbs, which is, honestly, more than a diet, it's a lifestyle designed to keep you healthy and full of energy.

Every Step Builds on the Last. Because I don't want you to get overwhelmed and give up, I've divided the weed and seed portions of the program into a series of doable steps. It's no different than running a marathon—you would never set out to run 26.2 miles without training. You need to build up to it.

And because I want to set you up with the highest odds of success, I've carefully chosen the order of those steps so that each one makes the ones that come after more effective. So, all you ever have to focus on is taking one new step, and before you know it, you'll have created a huge stacking effect that makes each little step add up to massive change.

The first steps you'll take are to weed and detox your mind, your pantry, and your body. Then, during the seed portion, you'll add in more minerals, which address the deficiencies that contribute to cravings. And then, we'll move on to eating more healthy fats, which will keep you full and help you make the transition to burning fat, and so on, until you are naturally ready to feed yourself the things you need to stay free from the cravings, energy swings, weight gain, inflammation, and brain fog that sugar causes.

FIRE UP YOUR FAT-BURNING ENGINES

In addition to helping you get free of your dependence on sugar, these dietary strategies aim to get you to burn fat instead of sugar as your primary source of energy. Burning fat offers the following amazing benefits:

- **Optimizes cell function**
- **Reduces overall oxidative stress and inflammation**
- **Stimulates autophagy and mitophagy**, which are the body's abilities to clean house and rid itself of damaged cells and mitochondria that aren't functioning properly

Overall, making the switch from sugar burning to fat burning empowers your body to maintain homeostasis, which is the scientific word for "balance." When it's in homeostasis, your body can heal itself, which is what it is innately programmed to do. Think about it: if you get a cut, the Band-Aid and the bacitracin don't heal it; the body does. When you start burning fat, you free up your energy to heal from the inside out.

The basic principles behind making the switch to burning fat are:

- Carbs down

- Fats and minerals up

- Proteins, mostly plant-based, eaten in only moderate amounts

When you eat this way (and remember, I will walk you through how to adopt this strategy step by step), your daily food choices will look like the following. Keep in mind that healthy fats pack a lot of calories in a small amount of space, so while they make up a large portion of your daily calories, they won't take up much room at all on your plate. (See pages 186–187 for a visual breakdown of what your plate should look like, represented two ways: the caloric breakdown and a visual representation.)

50 Percent of Daily Calories from Healthy Fats

- **Healthy oils:** coconut oil, MCT oil, avocado oil, extra-virgin olive oil, macadamia nut oil, black seed oil

- **Raw nuts:** almonds, macadamia nuts, walnuts, pecans, Brazil nuts, cashews, pistachios (last two in moderation because they can accumulate mold)

- **Raw seeds:** chia, flax, hemp

- **Raw nut butters:** almond, coconut, cacao, macadamia nut, tahini

- **Avocados**

20 Percent of Daily Calories from Mineral-Rich, Nonstarchy Vegetables (Greens)

- **Dark green leafy vegetables:** spinach, kale, watercress, romaine lettuce, etc.

- **Cruciferous vegetables:** broccoli, cauliflower, bok choy, etc.

- **Sulfur-based vegetables:** onions, radishes, cabbage, etc.

20 Percent of Daily Calories from Protein

- **Vegetable proteins:** hemp seeds, chia seeds, flaxseeds, hummus, beans

- **Wild-caught omega-3 fish, and noninflammatory grass-fed animal proteins**

10 Percent of Daily Calories from Fiber-Rich, Slow-Burning Carbs and Low-Sugar Fruit

- **Fiber-rich, slow-burning carbs:** quinoa, sweet potatoes, purple potatoes, wild rice, squash, etc.

- **Fruit:** blueberries, grapefruit, strawberries, apples, watermelon, etc.

VARIETY IS KEY TO YOUR HEALTH AND LONGEVITY

In addition to changing *what* you eat, another important thing you're going to switch up on this program is *when* you eat. You won't necessarily eat less in terms of calories, but you will certainly eat less often. Particularly when you consider that the average American eats an average of seventeen times per day!

This constant grazing steadily dumps insulin into your blood, which cues fat storage, creates inflammation, and has a knock-on effect to leptin, your hunger hormone, leaving you constantly hungry and looking for carbs. Ironically, eating less often helps you feel fuller, longer, because it resets your hormones and eliminates insulin and leptin resistance.

On this program, you'll start by aiming to have three meals a day and swap out your unhealthy snacks for healthy ones. The next step is to switch to three meals with no snacks in between. Eventually, once you have weeded and seeded your physiology so that it's ready for this step, you'll work your way to having two meals a day, in a practice known as intermittent fasting, which typically means skipping breakfast and eating only lunch and dinner.

TRACK YOUR TRANSITION TO FAT BURNING

The state of being able to burn fat for fuel is called ketosis. It's named after ketones, or ketone bodies, which are the fatty acids that your body creates when it is burning fat. And the way you start burning fat is by consuming a diet that is high in healthy fats and nonstarchy fiber-filled vegetables, with moderate protein, and low in carbohydrates. The very low-carb intake forces the body to use fat for energy instead of glucose, which produces a high level of ketones in the blood, hence the name.

As you begin to implement this program, you'll want to keep an eye on how you're doing on your transition to ketosis. And there are two ways to do that:

- Use the "Are You a Sugar Burner or a Fat Burner?" chart on the next page.
- Measure the levels of ketones in either your blood or your breath.

To measure the ketones in your blood or your breath, you'll need to purchase an at-home ketone meter. I like KetoMojo, which uses a finger prick of blood to measure ketones as well as glucose. Measuring the ketones in your blood is the most accurate way to monitor your transition to ketosis. Alternatively, you can save yourself the finger prick and measure the ketones present in your breath by using a meter, such as Ketonix.

The least expensive option is to use urine ketone strips, which measure the ketones excreted in your urine, although they are the least accurate of all the monitoring options. As your body gets more efficient at using ketones, fewer of them will come out through your urine, so it can seem as though you're headed out of ketosis when in actuality, you're just getting better at it.

No matter which method you use, choose one and use it to take a baseline measurement now, before you've started doing anything differently. You'll probably see very low or even no levels of ketones and a somewhat high fasting glucose level. But when you see these numbers change over time, it will motivate you to keep going. What you inspect, you respect.

KETONE LEVELS DURING KETOSIS

If you have ketone levels anywhere between 0.5 and 3 mmol/L, you are in ketosis.

These numbers can go as high as 8 or 9 if you are fasting (abstaining from food for about twenty-four or more hours—the length of time it takes varies from person to person and situation to situation).

~~~~~~~~~~

THE DIFFERENCE BETWEEN KETOSIS AND KETOACIDOSIS

It's important to know that ketosis, or the metabolic state of burning fat for fuel, is different from diabetic ketoacidosis, which is a potentially life-threatening condition that people with diabetes (most commonly type 1 diabetes) are vulnerable to. In ketosis, your blood ketone levels can go as high as 8 or 9 mmol/L. In ketoacidosis, they are between 15 and 25 mmol/L. The other piece of ketoacidosis that is dangerous is that blood glucose levels skyrocket to somewhere between 250 and 400 mg/dl. Those with type 1 are vulnerable to developing ketoacidosis because their body doesn't produce enough insulin on its own to lower glucose or to slow the production of ketones. So, glucose and ketones pile up to a dangerous level, creating a highly acidic, and highly dangerous

state. Unless you have type 1 diabetes, you aren't at risk of developing ketoacidosis because the insulin your body produces will lower glucose, and your brain will burn the ketones you produce.

~~~~~~~~~~

Self-Assessment: Are You a Sugar Burner or Fat Burner?

To get a quick glimpse of whether you've got habits of a sugar burner or a fat burner, ask yourself the following ten questions and put a checkmark in the column that best represents your answer. (Use a pencil, because you can erase your answers and retake this assessment as you move through the program and track your progress.) The more checkmarks you have in the "no" column, the better the chances that you're burning sugar for fuel, and you're in fat-storage mode.

Ideally, you'll be able to answer no to at least eight of the ten—the sweet spot for fat-burning.

HABIT	YES	NO
Have you had more than 2 alcoholic beverages in the past 48 hours?		
Have you eaten 1 serving or more of refined carbs, sugar, or grains, such as white bread, cakes, or cookies, in the last 24 hours?		
Have you had any soda (including diet soda), sweetened coffee drinks, sweetened teas, energy drinks, enhanced water, or fruit juice in the last 24 hours?		
Have you had any cravings for sugary foods (including bread, potatoes, and dairy) in the last 24 hours?		
Have you eaten any snacks (food in between meals) in the past 24 hours?		

continues

continued

HABIT	YES	NO
Have you gone for at least 12 hours without food in the last 48 hours?		
Are you an emotional eater (e.g., you overeat when stressed; keep eating, even after you feel full; and reach for food when you're tired, angry, or sad)?		
Do you feel like you need food every 2 hours and struggle to go 3 to 4 hours between meals without feeling shaky or light headed?		
Do you often get stressed? (Stress causes an increase in the hormone cortisol, which triggers sugar cravings and fat storage.)		
Do you have poor sleeping habits? (If your body is not well rested, your metabolism is reduced and your adrenals are stimulated; this puts you into a fat-storage mode.)		
TOTAL YESSES AND NOS		

So, how did you fare?

1–4 Nos:

You are a sugarholic, and sugar is your primary source of fuel.

5–7 Nos:

You are burning sugar as your primary source of fuel, but with a few tweaks, you should be able to transition to burning fat in just two to four weeks.

8–10 Nos:

You are a fat-burning machine.

Your goal by the end of this program is to move at least eight of your answers over to the No column.

Other Sugar-Related Numbers You Need to Know

In addition to measuring your ketones, it's also helpful to keep your eye on blood glucose levels to see how much sugar is impacting your health. These two blood tests are the best for doing that—one, you can do at home; the other, you can get done at your doctor's office.

- **Fasting glucose:** This at-home test requires a finger prick and either a glucose monitor or the KetoMojo device, which measures glucose as well as ketones. You want to take this reading first thing in the morning, before you've had anything to eat or drink.

  Ideal: 70 or below
  Healthy: 70 to 99
  Prediabetic: 100 to 124
  Diabetic: 125 or higher

- **Hemoglobin A1C:** Typically used to diagnose diabetes and part of the bloodwork your physician will order at your annual physical, this test measures your average blood sugar levels for the past 120 days (refer back to pages 26–27 for information on exactly how it does this). Ideally, your levels will be below 5.7; the higher the number, the more likely you are to be burning sugar and experiencing glycation. Prediabetes is 5.7 to 6.4 percent—an estimated 84 million American adults, or about 1 in 3, fit in this category, although most have no idea. Anything higher than 6.5 percent is diabetes.

Other helpful blood tests for monitoring your overall health include:

- **Homocysteine.** An amino acid that is a marker of inflammation. You want your levels to be less than 8 umol/L, although an ideal level is under 6 umol/L.

- **High-sensitivity C-reactive protein.** This marker of inflammation is ideally less than 1 mg/L. From 1 to 3 mg/L is considered a moderate risk of heart disease, and above 3 mg/L is high risk.

- **Vitamin D.** Vitamin D is crucial for immunity and bone health. Ideal levels of this important vitamin are 50 to 70 ng/ml. Anything under 30 ng/ml is a state of insufficiency.

- **Omega-6/omega-3 ratio**. Most doctors will test for omega-3 levels, but not for this ratio of omega-6 to omega-3. The ideal ratio is 1:1 and not more than 3:1. The average American has 20:1. See the Resources section for information about

the blood test I offer that tests this all-important ratio.

- **RBC magnesium.** Ideally 6.0 mg/dl to 6.5. It's important that you don't test the level of magnesium circulating in your serum blood; rather, how much magnesium is in your red blood cells. (Because this test typically requires a doctor's prescription, see Resources for a company that can help you request one.)

Cholesterol Markers

- **Fractionated lipid panel.** Measures the particle size of your LDL cholesterol, as only the smaller LDL particles contribute to arterial damage.

- **Levels of HDL ("good" cholesterol) vs. LDL ("bad" cholesterol).** Ideally, HDL should be greater than 60 mg/dl.

- **Triglycerides.** Ideally less than 100 mg/dl.

- **Ratio of triglycerides to HDL.** Ideally less than 1:1 or 2:1.

- **Ratio of total cholesterol to HDL.** Ideally less than 3:1.

||||||||||||||||||||||||||||||||||||||||||||||||||||||||||||||||||||||||||

YOU'RE NOT IN THIS ALONE

Anytime you're seeking to make a positive change in your life, it's crucial to have support. Come connect with me on Facebook and Instagram (my handle is @drdarylgioffre in both places), where I share my best tips, recipes, and most cutting-edge research to help you kick acid and get off your sugar. It's also a way to communicate directly with me, ask questions, and get feedback right from the source!

\\\\\\\\\\\\\\\\\\

❖ Determine how you'll track your transition to fat burning—will you buy a meter, or use the tracker on page 43, or both?

❖ Assess how many sugar-burner habits you have (pages 43–44) and record your total—it will be motivating to see this number come down over time.

❖ Keep reading. In the next chapter, we'll talk about how to overcome sugar cravings so that you won't be as likely to fall prey to them as you move through the program.

I was desperate to change but was stuck in a routine that day by day was making me sicker. I felt ashamed, embarrassed, and uncomfortable in my body. I had no energy and was depressed. I hated the feeling of loss of control. I did not realize that the culprit of all of my pain and suffering was sugar.

When I visited Dr. Daryl's office for a simple chiropractic visit, he shared with me how he overcame a serious sugar addiction. I finally felt there was hope for me. He taught me just how toxic sugar is and how to get off my sugar. The physical transformation was incredible, but even more astounding was the mental one. In taking back control of my health and life, I felt empowered and capable of achieving any goal I set my sights on. I owe so much of my success and happiness to Dr. Daryl and his powerful program.   —Rebecca G.

four

Outsmart Cravings

EVERY SINGLE DAY, I SEE A PATIENT IN MY OFFICE WHO TELLS ME SOME VARIATION on the following: "I can't live without my chocolate frozen yogurt; I eat almost a whole container every night." Or "Once they bring the bread basket at dinner, I have to eat the entire loaf, I just love bread so much." So many people have some type of food that they can't resist, and then once they have a little of it, they feel like they have to have a lot of it. Once they start, they can't stop.

Trust me, I know all about cravings. I spent decades at their mercy. My sugar cravings were so bad that in the middle of the night, I'd sneak into the kitchen to eat my candy bars so that Chelsea, my now wife who was my fiancée at the time, wouldn't hear the *crinkle-crinkle-crinkle* of the wrappers. This was in addition to the bowl of M&M's I kept on my bedside table. Once, I stocked that bowl with gummy bears instead of M&M's and woke up the next morning with gummy bears stuck to my shirt—talk about leaving a trail of evidence!

My cravings were literally uncontrollable. I always said I'd stop eating candy on Monday, or on New Year's, but nothing could keep me from the sweet stuff when the cravings came. That's another thing I hear from patients all the time: "I'm going to stop eating the sweet stuff tomorrow." This kind of bargaining is a hallmark of addiction.

A lot of my patients don't even realize they're addicted to sugar because their cravings are for pasta or bread. Until I point it out to them, they don't understand that, to your body, grains and carbs are the same thing as sugar because, just like candy, they get metabolized into glucose and result in a big insulin spike. Even if what you crave is steak or hamburgers, when you eat too much protein, your liver will convert the excess into glucose in a process known as gluconeogenesis. If you have any cravings of any type, the odds are high that sugar addiction is at the root.

The good news is that it is possible to overcome cravings. In this chapter, you'll learn the science behind cravings and how to identify the root causes of them, so that you can prevent them from happening in the first place. You'll also discover some snacking strategies that will help you resist the next craving that strikes without feeling deprived.

THE HORMONES BEHIND YOUR CRAVINGS

Something else I hear all the time is, "I'm fine during the day, I eat a healthy breakfast and lunch, but at night I can't help myself." During the day, you're busy. Maybe even too busy to have a proper meal. So, you grab the protein bar or the flavored yogurt or the fruit smoothie and power through your day. Or maybe you're having a bagel at your breakfast meeting and then working through lunch or skipping breakfast but taking a sandwich and

a cookie off the food tray at your working lunch. Either way, you're feeding yourself just enough sugar and carbs to get through the day, and then at night, when you have time to sit and realize how hungry you are, you realize you're actually famished.

By then, it's too late; your body thinks it's starving and has cued the stress response. That's when the adrenal glands release cortisol, which shuts down your immune system and your digestion and turns down the volume on insulin. The body thinks it needs more glucose to prepare to either stay and fight or flee from the impending stress and so cues cravings for sugar and carbs because glucose is such a quick-burning fuel. The next thing you know, you've emptied the bread basket or finished the entire container of ice cream.

As I covered in Chapter 1, when you eat the sweets or the carbs, dopamine is released in your brain, which feeds your addiction because you want to repeat experiences that increase dopamine. At the same time, your blood sugar spikes, causing your pancreas to release a massive secretion of insulin in an effort to get those blood glucose levels down, typically by storing the glucose as fat. Once the glucose is moved out of your bloodstream and into your fat cells (it really does happen that quickly), your body will think it needs more glucose to stay functioning.

Fat cells release leptin, the hormone that tells the brain you're full and don't need any more food. But when you're regularly flooding your bloodstream with glucose and insulin, which triggers more fat stores, the higher your leptin levels get.

Leptin becomes so prevalent that the receptors for it in your brain become desensitized—what's known as leptin resistance. And then you never get the message that it's time to stop eating.

Dr. Robert Lustig wrote in his book *Fat Chance* that healing leptin resistance is "the key to weight loss and the obesity epidemic" and that when your brain can't see your leptin, it will think you're starving; your brain will cue you to eat more so that you can increase energy storage and make you feel lethargic so that you can conserve energy.

For anybody who's looking to suppress hunger, lose weight, and overcome the cravings, you have to regulate your leptin levels. Otherwise, you'll want to keep eating and eating the foods that trigger a dopamine release well beyond your body's need for calories. This cycle of eating purely for pleasure is so common that it's recently been given a new scientific name—hedonic hunger. That's what cravings are; they're not a need for sustenance. They're an addiction to pleasure.

Leptin resistance is why people who are addicted to sugar are craving sweets all the time. And the key way to restore leptin sensitivity is adding healthy fats, plant-based fiber, and more minerals to your diet; by doing so, you'll also naturally crowd out sugar and carbs. We'll talk much more about both of these topics in the chapters to come, but for right now, know that while there are unhealthy fats that can lead to obesity and heart disease, there are also healthy fats that heal your hormones and help you burn fat for fuel. Fat can be your best friend or your worst

enemy, and in this chapter you'll learn how to use it to conquer your cravings.

And trust me: as you get off your sugar, your taste buds will acclimate and the healthy stuff will start to taste just as good as—or better than!—the sweets and the CRAP-py carbs ever did.

YOUR TASTE BUDS CAN CHANGE

Just as your cells can become desensitized to insulin and leptin, so can your taste buds become immune to sweetness. Have you noticed that you need to eat more and more sugar to satisfy your cravings? That's because your taste buds have become desensitized to sweets, and so you've needed to eat more and more of it to register that sweet taste you're craving. It can even get to the point where you never truly feel that your craving is satisfied, but your belly is simply too full to allow you to eat any more.

Normally an apple, a banana, or some blueberries should be enough to satisfy your sweet tooth. But someone who's addicted to sugar and whose taste buds have become desensitized to sweetness will need an entire box of Lucky Charms, a whole pint of ice cream, or a box of cookies.

The good news is that the cells in your body are constantly renewing themselves. For instance, your red blood cells recreate themselves every 120 days, and your skin cells turn over approximately every 27 days. Your taste buds are no exception, and they have an even shorter timeline—they renew themselves every 14 days.

Once that sensitivity is restored, your taste buds will taste things differently.

The bad stuff won't taste as good and good stuff will taste much better. When I was addicted to sugar, I drank three Cokes a day, and they tasted great, but if you gave me broccoli, I'd want to vomit. Now it's the opposite. Coke hasn't changed its recipe; it's my taste buds that have changed.

When you add more of the healthy fats and minerals that suppress the sweetness, as you'll start to do in this chapter and will do even more as you move through the program, your taste buds will change too. Once you wean off the foods that are keeping you trapped in a vicious craving cycle, you'll want to have a piece of fruit—something that tastes fresh and nourishing—instead of a box of cookies. You'll fall in love with my Avocado Chocolate Mousse (which is Kelly Ripa's favorite recipe—see page 263). With these delicious and healthy alternatives, you will still have sweetness in your life; it just won't be taking years off your life when you eat it.

SMART SNACKING WILL HELP YOU TRANSITION

When you know the primary reasons for why cravings happen, you also know how to give your body what it needs to ward off those cravings from occurring in the first place. And what it needs is a well-chosen snack that provides the healthy fats and minerals that will help flip your switch to fat-burning and get you off the roller coaster of rising and falling blood glucose, insulin, and leptin levels and insulin and leptin resistance.

And on a more practical level, at this point in the program, a snack will prevent you from getting hungry, because no matter how strong your willpower is, if you're hungry and having a craving, you will eat the thing you're craving.

Right now, your goal is to go from unhealthy snacks to healthy snacks. You need snacks that are high in healthy fats to fill you up and help you make the switch to fat burning, and minerals to help ward off cravings in the first place. Bonus points if they also have a decent amount of fiber in them to keep you full. Make sure you have supplies for at least three of the following snacks on hand at home, at the office, and wherever you may travel.

CRAVING-SMASHING SNACKS

* ⅓ cup of mashed sweet potato with cinnamon and coconut oil

* 2 to 4 celery sticks with raw almond, cacao, coconut, or macadamia nut butter and hemp seeds

* 2 or 3 green apple slices with raw nut butter and a sprinkle of cinnamon

* A small handful of raw nuts, such as almonds, macadamia nuts, walnuts, Brazil nuts, or pecans

* A small handful of pumpkin seeds

* ½ Hass avocado with 1 tablespoon of extra-virgin olive oil, 1 tablespoon of chia seeds, and a pinch each of cumin, Himalayan pink salt, and black pepper

* Vegetable sticks with hummus or guacamole

❋ A tablespoon of coconut oil with a pinch of Himalayan pink salt, eaten right off the spoon

\\\\\\\\\\\\\\\\\\\\\

WHAT ARE YOUR CRAVINGS TRYING TO TELL YOU?

Beyond the general interactions of cortisol, glucose, insulin, and leptin, every particular craving carries an insight that reveals an imbalance your body is seeking to address. Take a look at the list of common craveable foods for a deeper look at what your body is truly signaling a need for:

1. **If you're craving sweet**

   (cookies, chocolate, cake, candy, pastries, sweetened coffee drinks, etc.)

   What you're actually craving: happiness, energy, sugar

   Nutrient(s) you are most likely deficient in: minerals, such as magnesium (especially), potassium, sodium bicarbonate, and trace minerals; healthy fats

   What it means: Magnesium deficiency (as chocolate is actually high in magnesium). Common causes of mineral deficiency are eating lots of sugar and/or leaky gut. If it's chocolate in particular you're craving, you could also be having feelings of loneliness or sadness, as chocolate is high in polyphenols that boost mood,[1] and just the sight and smell of chocolate can stimulate the pleasure center of the brain.[2] If you are a woman, you could also be in your premenstrual week, when your body naturally needs more carbs to manufacture progesterone, which is spiking

now. You could also be stressed (the vast majority of us are), and the cortisol your adrenal glands are secreting is making you crave sweets for the quick-burning sugar they provide.

What to have instead: green leafy vegetables, which are high in magnesium and other minerals; half an avocado with Himalayan pink salt; a 1-ounce serving of dark chocolate (80 percent cacao or greater); a smoothie made with cacao powder (see page 215 for a recipe); whole-food (yet relatively low-sugar) starches, such as sweet potatoes or roasted squash. You can also try an Epsom salts bath, as Epsom salts are magnesium sulfate and absorb through the skin; a warm bath also takes the edge off stress.

2. **If you're craving salty**

   (chips, pretzels, pizza, fries, actual salt applied to other foods)

   What you're actually craving: minerals. It's not that your body is craving the table salt that these snacks are doused in, it's craving the trace minerals that typically accompany natural salts (which standard table salt—or sodium chloride—has been stripped of). Also, water.

   Nutrient(s) you are most likely deficient in: mineral salts, such as magnesium, potassium, sodium bicarbonate, and trace minerals

   What it means: Natural salt is a delivery mechanism for minerals and trace minerals—if you're craving it, you're likely deficient in these essential nutrients. In addition, the crunch of most salty snacks can be a stress reliever in and of itself—you've got to really chomp down on them, which gives your frustration somewhere to go. And finally, craving salty foods could, paradoxically, mean you're dehydrated, because salt causes the body to retain water.

What to have instead: a tablespoon of coconut oil with a pinch of Himalayan pink salt (a mineral-rich salt); and/or, add a pinch of Himalayan pink salt to a liter of water and drink it. Also try kale chips (recipe on page 255), and crunch on veggie sticks, such as celery, red pepper slices, fennel, jicama, and carrot—dip them into hummus if you feel the urge for chips and dip coming on!

3. **If you're craving white bread, rice, or pasta**

(bread, crackers, rice, muffins)

What you're actually craving: energy, calmness, sugar

Nutrient(s) you are most likely deficient in: mineral salts, such as magnesium, potassium, sodium bicarbonate, and trace minerals

What it means: because these refined grains get metabolized into glucose, craving them indicates you are addicted to sugar. As a result, you are likely mineral deficient, too, since the body uses such minerals as magnesium to neutralize glucose molecules. We also crave these carb-rich foods for all the same reasons we crave sweets (see above).

What to have instead: re-create the textures you crave: try cauliflower rice, or zoodles with pesto; and incorporate whole, unrefined carbs, such as quinoa, sweet potatoes, and squash into your diet. To boost your mineral intake, eat more green leafy vegetables and switch to a mineral-rich salt, such as Himalayan pink salt. And to reduce cravings in the first place, eat more healthy fats.

4. **If you're craving meat**

(steak, burgers, pot roast, chicken wings)

What you're actually craving: protein, fat, or sugar

Nutrient(s) you are most likely deficient in: iron, vitamin B_{12}, healthy fats

What it means: craving these fatty meats indicate a lack of healthy fats. Because they are also high in iron and vitamin B_{12}, the craving suggests a deficiency in one or both of these two nutrients. Also, since excess protein is metabolized into glucose, these cravings could indicate an addiction to sugar.

What to have instead: green juices or greens powders, as chlorophyll, which gives vegetables their green color, serves a similar function as iron in building red blood cells, without the increased cancer risk of supplementing only with iron. Also, up your intake of healthy fats (which I cover in depth in Chapter 7).

5. **If you're craving dairy**

(milk, cheese, ice cream, yogurt)

What you're actually craving: relaxation, sugar, fat

Nutrient(s) you are most likely deficient in: mineral salts, such as magnesium, potassium, sodium bicarbonate, and trace minerals, healthy fats, vitamin A, vitamin D

What it means: All on its own, milk is fairly high in lactose, a naturally occurring sugar. Then, many dairy products have loads of sugars added to them, including flavored yogurts, frozen yogurt, yogurt drinks, and ice cream. So, craving dairy is often a sugar craving in disguise. In addition to indicating that you are trapped in the cycle of being addicted to sugar, craving dairy indicates a need for fat (since whole milk, cheese, and ice cream are all high in fat). Also, many doctors and nutritionists consider dairy cravings to be a sign of deficiencies in vitamin A and/or D, both of which dairy is a good source of.

What to have instead: When you crave dairy, you may just be after that creamy texture. Reach for an avocado to get the rich smoothness you crave, plus a natural energy and mood boost. Try my Avocado Chocolate Mousse (see recipe on page 263)—you'll think you're cheating! Also, canned coconut milk can be a great stand-in for full-fat dairy: try it in a low-sugar smoothie or in a curry.

|||||||||||||||||||||||||||||||||||||||||||||||||||||||||||||||||||||||||||||||||||

FOUR GUT BIOHACKS TO CRUSH CRAVINGS

1. **Take probiotics.** Several strains of *Bifidobacterium* and *Lactobacillus* have been shown to improve anxiety and depression-like behavior, which tend to alter our eating behaviors. Additionally, supplementing with probiotics has demonstrated a significant decrease in sugar cravings. By flooding your gut with beneficial bacteria, you crowd out the harmful bacteria, parasites, and yeast; all of which feed on sugar and contribute to cravings. (For more information on supplementing with probiotics, refer to Chapter 11.)

2. **Eat prebiotics.** Prebiotics are specific types of food that nourish your beneficial microbes. They also support you directly by increasing a protein called brain-derived neurotrophic factor (BDNF),[3] which Dr. Joseph Mercola, author of *Fat for Fuel*, calls "MiracleGro for your brain," reducing levels of the stress hormone cortisol (less stress, which means less emotional eating),[4] and releasing satiety hormones (so you know when to stop eating).[5] Try fiber-rich prebiotic foods, such as onions, garlic, sweet potatoes, chia seeds, leeks, asparagus, dandelion greens, and Jerusalem artichokes.

3. **Create a nutrient-dense environment.** Many people find that their cravings subside substantially a few weeks after adopting a nutrient-dense diet ("nutrient-dense" foods are those that are high in nutrients—vitamins, minerals, the good stuff—and lower in calories). By adding greens, minerals, and healthy fats to your diet—which you will do over the next four weeks—you will mediate a shift in your microbiome away from the pathogenic bacteria that thrive on sugar and thus cause cravings for the sweet stuff.

4. **Stop eating two yeast-promoting "healthy" foods.** I'll talk more about this in Chapter 8, but two foods that many people hail for their health benefits actually promote the growth of candida: nutritional yeast and nearly all mushrooms. When you eat these foods, because they contribute to candida, you are unwittingly making your own cravings stronger (since your gut bugs are the source of so many cravings). I know that

many vegetarians and vegans say that nutritional yeast has been deactivated, so it can't feed yeast. But yeast (deactivated or not) almost always contains high levels of mold toxins, which then encourage candida to grow in your gut. Turn to page 121 for more information (and to learn the **one and only mushroom** I recommend anyone consume—one that boosts immunity, fights yeast, and crushes cravings).

SUGAR SWAPS

To start immediately cutting down on the amount of sugar and carbs in your diet and start outrunning your cravings, swap out the following foods for the low-sugar alternatives listed below.

TYPICAL FOOD	LOW-SUGAR ALTERNATIVE
Yogurt	Chocolate Chia Pudding (see recipe on page 260)
Juice or soda	Water infused with highly concentrated plant-based flavored extracts or (low sugar) fruit pieces
Premade salad dressing	Extra-virgin olive oil with lemon
Chips/crackers	Veggie sticks with hummus or guacamole
Ice cream	A bowl of berries with coconut butter and chopped mint
Milk chocolate	One ounce of dark chocolate or a smoothie made with raw cacao powder
White sugar, coconut sugar, brown sugar	Monk fruit (also known as lo han guo) or stevia
Maple syrup, processed honey, or agave	A small amount of manuka honey, chicory syrup, blackstrap molasses, or ChocZero (a maple syrup with only 1 gram of net carbs per serving) (see info on natural sweeteners on page 60)
Splenda, NutraSweet, or Sweet'N Low	Stevia
BBQ sauce	Dry spice rub
Ketchup	Fresh salsa
Balsamic vinegar	Red wine vinegar, Champagne vinegar, white wine vinegar, apple cider vinegar, or lemon juice
Chili sauce	No-sugar-added salsa

TYPICAL FOOD	LOW-SUGAR ALTERNATIVE
Hoisin sauce, sweet-and-sour sauce, or teriyaki sauce	Homemade Asian stir-fry sauce made with coconut aminos
Cream cheese	Avocado
Whipped cream	Whipped full-fat coconut milk
Sweetened coffee creamer	Unsweetened coconut milk creamer, Acid-Kicking Coffee Alkalizer (see Resources for more information)
Pasta, bread, rice	Quinoa, wild rice, sweet potatoes, purple potatoes, squash

The Three-Step Snack Rule

While I do suggest that you use smart snacks to help you ride out cravings or even avoid them altogether, I prefer that you eat one only after you follow these three steps:

Step one: Drink a big glass of water. Because hunger and thirst are regulated by the same region of the brain, what you perceive as hunger might actually be dehydration. So, the first thing you should do when you notice your appetite starting to rise is to drink a glass of filtered water. To make this step even more potent, squeeze a slice of organic lemon or lime and/or add a pinch of Himalayan pink salt to deliver some trace minerals along with your hydration. Then, wait ten to fifteen minutes.

Step two: If you're still hungry, and you are able, go for a brisk walk. You'll be helping your hormones regulate themselves, oxygenating your blood, and making yourself feel better and healthier in general. And when you feel healthy, you'll be less likely to reach for the unhealthy stuff. Walking also lifts your mood, so if your cravings have an emotional trigger, movement will help remedy that. It doesn't have to be a long walk; just go around the block, or even around the office, if that's all the time you have. Or do 25 jumping jacks. Remember—motion *is* emotion!

Step three: If you're still hungry, have a healthy snack. (For ideas, refer to the list I provided on page 50.)

THE MOST DANGEROUS FORM OF SUGAR

There are two main categories of sugar: monosaccharides (that have one sugar molecule) and disaccharides (that have two sugar molecules). The two primary monosaccharides are glucose and fructose, and the main disaccharides are sucrose (which is what white sugar is; it's made up of glucose and fructose—the fructose is what makes table sugar so sweet), lactose (which is found in milk and is composed of galactose and glucose), and maltose (which is composed of different forms of glucose and is found in beer). Each type of sugar has its own properties, upsides, and downsides. Of these, fructose is the most destructive to your body.

For starters, fructose is one and a half times sweeter than sucrose. The more fructose a food has, the sweeter it becomes. That's why so many food manufacturers use fructose, most often in the form of high-fructose corn syrup.

Unlike glucose or sucrose, fructose is metabolized by the liver, where it can overburden this already hard-working organ of detoxification. The liver will either convert fructose into triglycerides—the fatty acids associated with heart disease—or store the fructose as fat within the liver, where it can lead to fatty liver disease.

Fructose has been shown to impair insulin sensitivity, which leads to higher insulin levels, increased fat storage, and thus higher levels of circulating leptin, all of which leads to cravings, weight gain, and increased risk of type 2 diabetes and insulin resistance in the brain (in other words, dementia). In addition, it takes 56 molecules of magnesium to neutralize one molecule of fructose (as opposed to 28 molecules of magnesium for every one molecule of glucose), and fructose is up to thirty times more glycating than glucose. (Remember from Chapter 3 that glycation is the process of sugar binding with a protein associated with aging in general and neurodegenerative diseases, such as Alzheimer's in particular.)

Worst of all, the number one dietary source of calories in America is high-fructose corn syrup, which is found in soda and all manner of processed foods. The food industry uses it because it's cheap to produce, thanks to farm subsidies for corn, and easy to store and transport.

Your body processes high-fructose corn syrup differently than it does ordinary sugar. The burden falls on your liver, which is not capable of keeping up with how quickly corn syrup breaks down. As a result, blood sugar spikes quicker and then gets stored as fat, so you can become obese and develop other health problems, such as diabetes, much faster than with other types of sugar.

The danger to growing children is even greater as their bodies cannot handle the amount of sugar and fructose they get from candy, processed foods, fruit juices, and other sugary drinks. Because they start young, they bioaccumulate more damage, and as a result, they damage their mitochondria and cellular metabolism, and become fatter and their toxic load becomes higher.

Unless you are paying attention to what you are eating, it is very hard to avoid fructose, and that's another way we get stuck in the cravings trap—we don't even have to seek out the foods that put us on the never-ending treadmill of hedonic hunger. They are hiding in plain sight on nearly every shelf in the grocery store—even in the produce section.

BIOHACKS TO HELP
CRUSH CRAVINGS

If your sugar cravings really have a hold on you—the way mine did on me—there are some bio-hacks that can help diminish your surges of that "gotta have sugar *now*" feeling. (Specific product recommendations for each of these in the Resources section, pages 267–270.)

Chromium. Chromium improves blood glucose control, helps balance blood sugar, and kicks cravings by enhancing the action of insulin and reducing insulin resistance. And our chromium levels reduce as we age. The form you want to look for is 100 percent whole food GTF chromium.

Dosage: Follow package instructions.

Gymnema. This Ayurvedic herb is known as the "sugar destroyer" for its ability to inhibit the taste of sweetness. It also helps regulate blood sugar, nourishes the kidneys, and supports carbohydrate metabolism.

Dosage: Take two 100 mg tablets daily—one at your first meal of the day, one at your last meal of the day.

Sugar-Craving Fat Bomb. This shot cleanses the liver and gall bladder, which will help you lose weight, especially in the belly area.

Dosage: Mix 1 tablespoon of extra virgin olive oil with the juice of ½ organic lemon and drink on an empty stomach whenever the craving monster shows itself. Or better yet, drink in the a.m. to anticipate and prevent cravings.

Apple Cider Vinegar and Ceylon Cinnamon: Ceylon cinnamon regulates blood sugar, and apple cider vinegar can improve insulin function and insulin resistance and reduce fasting blood sugar and HbA1c levels.

Dosage: Mix 1 teaspoon of Ceylon cinnamon and a pinch of Himalayan pink salt into 1 tablespoon of apple cider vinegar and a few ounces of filtered water. Drink it as a shot at any time of day to ward off cravings.

Note: Before starting any supplement regimen, please check with your health-care provider for any contraindications.

IT'S OKAY TO EAT FRUIT
(BUT AVOID DRINKING IT)

Fruit contains sugar, and to your body, all sugar produces a similar result. And most fruits contain fructose, albeit in varying amounts. That being said, the sugar in fruit comes packaged with other things, such as fiber, chromium, water, and other nutrients that all slow the absorption of sugar into your bloodstream and offer health benefits of their own. So, you don't have to completely say good-bye to the entire fruit category. But you do have to educate yourself about the sugar and fructose levels in your favorite foods and then make choices accordingly.

A general rule of thumb is to eat fruit only when it's in season (berries and melons in the summer, apples and squashes—yes, they are technically fruits—in the fall, citrus and pomegranate in the winter). You either want to eat fruit on its own away from a meal, or I like to pair moderate-sugar fruit with a healthy fat so the impact on your blood glucose and insulin levels is moderated. For example, eat berries with a little coconut butter and mint, or apple slices with some raw nut butter. The fat will slow down your metabolization of the sugar in the fruit, resulting in a lower insulin spike.

You don't want to eat fruit as part of or after a larger meal because fruit digests very quickly and can make it all the way through the digestive tract in twenty to thirty minutes. If you eat fruit with a big meal, or even worse, for dessert, the fruit will sit on top of all the other food and start to rot. It's a traffic jam. Melons in particular should always be eaten alone. Whenever possible, wait an hour after eating fruit before having anything else.

To be clear, I'm talking about actual fruit here, not fruit juice. Unless we're talking about a squeeze of lemon, lime, or grapefruit to a glass of water, fruit juice is basically no better than soda and is something that's best avoided entirely.

The problem with fruit juice is that all the things that nature put into the fruit to slow down the metabolization of the natural sugars—namely fiber, vitamin C, and chromium—is stripped away. You're basically just getting the sugar water, which causes a tsunami of fructose to dump into your body. Fruit juice also contains as many calories as soda, although calorie for calorie, orange juice is *worse* for you than soda—it has 18 grams of fructose per ounce compared to soda's 1.7 grams of fructose per ounce.[6] When it comes to fruit juice, just say no.

THE FRUIT INDEX

The following list shows the total sugar and fructose levels of common fruits. The fruits in the low range are fine to eat by themselves. Those in the middle range you should limit to one serving per day and eat with some form of healthy fat (such as coconut oil, coconut cream, or raw nut butters), and those in the upper range should be eaten only sparingly and always with a healthy fat.

FRUIT (100-GRAM SERVING)	TOTAL SUGARS (IN GRAMS)	TOTAL FRUCTOSE (IN GRAMS)
Low-Sugar Fruits (fine to eat alone)		
Lime	0.4	0.2
Avocado	0.9	0.2
Lemon	2.5	0.8
Tomato	2.8	1.4

Moderate-Sugar Fruits (limit to one serving per day and eat with some form of healthy fat)		
Strawberries	5.8	2.5
Papaya	5.9	2.7
Grapefruit	6.2	1.2
Figs (fresh)	6.9	2.8
Starfruit	7.1	3.2
Blueberries	7.3	3.6
Plum	7.5	1.8
Tangerine	7.7	0
Blackberries	8.1	4.1
Cherries, sour	8.1	3.3
Honeydew	8.2	0
Nectarine	8.5	0
Cantaloupe	8.7	1.8
Peach	8.7	1.3
Granny Smith apple	9	5
Watermelon	9	3.3
High-Sugar Fruits (eat sparingly, no more than one per day, and always with a healthy fat)		
Orange	9.2	2.5
Apricot (fresh)	9.3	0.7
Raspberries	9.5	3.2
Pomegranate	10.1	4.7
Kiwi	10.5	4.3
Pear	10.5	6.4
Pineapple	11.9	2.1
Honeycrisp apple	13.3	7.6
Cherries, sweet	14.6	6.2
Mango	14.8	2.9
Banana	15.6	2.7
Dates	66	19.56

ADDING MORE FIBER HELPS BEAT CRAVINGS BEFORE THEY BEGIN

Fiber is important as it slows down the emptying of the stomach, which keeps you feeling fuller longer. And while mineral-rich greens are decent sources of fiber, you ultimately want to consume 30 to 50 grams of fiber a day, and you need more than mineral-rich greens to get that amount.

That's where fiber-rich, slow-burning carbs come in. These complex carbs won't spike your blood sugar, or insulin, for that matter. In fact, they help to balance your blood sugar by slowing the absorption of glucose into your bloodstream, thanks to all the fiber they contain. Fiber also feeds the friendly flora in your gut and scrubs your intestines, thus supporting a healthy digestive tract. They're your allies when it comes to crushing cravings and burning fat.

My favorite fiber-rich, slow-burning carbs include: quinoa, wild rice, sweet potatoes, butternut squash, lentils, chickpeas and hummus, green beans, pumpkin, winter squash, purple potatoes, yams, and chia seeds. Aim to get 10 percent of your daily calories from these foods, or one to two servings a day (a serving of these is ½ cup).

ARE NATURAL SWEETENERS BETTER?

There's a lot of misconception about "natural" sugars and whether they are better for you or not. Just as with fruit, any sugar, no matter its source, is going to keep you stuck in sugar-burning mode and negatively impact your body in some way. Also, some natural sweeteners are even worse than table sugar; for example, agave syrup, which is up to 90 percent fructose! That being said, there are some sweeteners that contain no fructose at all:

SWEETENER PERCENTAGE OF FRUCTOSE

Sweetener	Percentage of Fructose
Stevia	0 percent
Xylitol	0 percent
Monk fruit (lo han guo)	0 percent
Yacón syrup	7 percent
Dates	20 percent
Coconut sugar	38 percent
Honey	40 percent
Maple syrup	40 percent
White sugar	50 percent
High-fructose corn syrup	55 percent
Agave nectar	90 percent

My two favorite sweeteners are monk fruit and stevia. Monk fruit is the sweetener we use in our Alkamind Acid-Kicking Greens and Acid-Kicking Minerals powders. It is a traditional Chinese berry that won't spike insulin. Stevia is derived from the leaves of a plant of the same name and also won't spike insulin. The only problem with stevia is that it can be a little bitter, so I like "unbitterized" stevia (look for this word on the label).

XYLITOL WILL KILL YOUR GUT, AND YOUR DOG!

Xylitol is a sugar alcohol that is as sweet as sucrose but with only two-thirds the calories and only a minimal impact on blood sugar levels. It's less expensive than other sugar substitutes, tastes better, and causes little if any insulin release in humans.

For all these reasons, some people say xylitol is a safe sugar substitute—you can find it in a wide range of foods, from gum to cookies, as well as such products as toothpaste and supplements.

However, I stay away from xylitol and believe you should too. I interviewed my good friend, biological dental expert Dr. Gerry Curatola, for my Get Off Your Sugar Summit, and he says xylitol is pure poison! It is a synthetic chemical made mostly from GMO corncobs and hydrogenation that is very disruptive to the friendly bacterial population in your mouth and your gut.

On top of that, xylitol can be fatal when ingested by dogs. The *Wall Street Journal* did a story in May 2016 about the FDA warnings that xylitol can kill your dog. Just because xylitol isn't strong enough to kill humans, doesn't mean this ingredient is good for us—it can give you bad intestinal gas and diarrhea. That's because humans absorb xylitol slowly. In dogs, xylitol is rapidly and completely absorbed within about thirty minutes. Just a small amount of xylitol can cause a dangerous insulin surge and a rapid drop in blood sugar. I say stick to monk fruit and stevia.

THE TRUTH ABOUT ARTIFICIAL SWEETENERS

Many people think that eating artificial sweeteners offers the best of both worlds—the sweetness without the harmful effects of sugar. Unfortunately, that is not the case. In fact, artificial sweeteners are even worse than naturally derived sugars. They give your body the sensation of sweetness without getting the actual sugar—your cravings aren't satisfied, and as a result, you end up eating many more carbs in an effort to fulfill that promise.

Artificial sweeteners trick your brain and body; when you eat sugar, the body knows how to determine how much sugar it's received because the level of glucose in the blood goes up. With artificial sweeteners, the body is waiting for the calories to come, but they never do, so your sensation of hunger is still there. Your cravings for carbs go up because you are seeking to satisfy the desire for sweetness. Research has shown that artificial sweeteners increase appetite in general, cravings for carbs in particular, and kick off a metabolic cascade that cues the body to store more fat.[7] The San Antonio Heart Study followed people for twenty-five years and found that for every one diet soda a participant drank a day, they were 65 percent more likely to become overweight and 41 percent more likely to become obese.[8] For diabetics, who turn to artificial sweeteners in an attempt to reduce their sugar intake and thus, their need for insulin, it's particularly brutal because the extra carbs it spurs you to eat will only worsen your insulin sensitivity. You think you're doing good by not having sugar, but it's digging you deeper down the hole.

There are three basic types of artificial sweeteners:

- **Aspartame** (Equal) is two hundred times sweeter than sugar and is used in more than six thousand products, including sugarless chewing gum, diet soda, vitamins, and flavored yogurts. Aspartame is primarily made up (90 percent) of two amino acids, **phenylalanine** and **aspartic acid**. These amino acids trigger a rapid release of leptin and insulin into your blood. Phenylalanine lowers neurotransmitters, including serotonin (the happy hormone), and reduces your feelings of satiation, which can lead to overeating. The remaining 10 percent is **methanol**, which is the same thing as wood alcohol. It's a neurotoxin. As if that weren't bad enough, methanol gets broken down in your body into **formaldehyde**, the same substance they use to embalm dead bodies. Formaldehyde increases acidity in blood and can cause kidney issues and impairment of eyesight and organ function. On top of all this, aspartame has repeatedly been shown to increase appetite and caloric consumption.[9]

- **Sucralose** (Splenda) was the subject of a study that found it could reduce gut bacteria by up to 50 percent[10]—that's because it isn't broken down during the digestion process, so it arrives in your large intestine fully intact; your gut bacteria feast on it and die. It also accumulates in your fat cells.[11] Additionally, it has been linked to liver and kidney damage in rats.[12] And despite the fact that people with type 2 diabetes often turn to sucralose to help reduce their blood glucose and insulin levels, it has been found that obese patients who ingest sucralose have greater increases in glucose and insulin, and a slower clearing of insulin, than controls.[13] And when insulin is present, your body cannot burn fat for fuel.[14]

- **Saccharin** (Sweet'N Low) was first discovered in 1876 by a scientist experimenting with derivatives of coal tar in the labs at Johns Hopkins University. One day, the researcher rushed home without washing his hands, then noticed that his dinner tasted unusually sweet. He licked his finger, and saccharin was born. Saccharin and aspartame have both been shown to cause greater weight gain than sugar, unrelated to caloric intake. It is also proven to cause the biggest and most widespread damage to cells and the DNA contained within cells of all the artificial sugars deemed safe by the FDA.[15]

If you've been drinking diet soda thinking that you are trying to lose weight, you've been unwittingly making yourself more dependent on carbs, making your internal environment highly acidic, and cueing your body to store the toxins in the artificial sweeteners in fat so that they won't harm your blood and your organs.

All in all, artificial sweeteners are yet another example of how counting calories is useless for weight loss, because calories are not created equal. Even though artificial sweeteners are technically no or very low calorie, they result in your eating more and having the glucose and insulin reactions as if you had eaten the calories from sugar.

When I see clients who have a diet soda addiction, I start them off by telling them they can still drink it, but they have to have a green juice immediately before they have it. The green juice will decrease your affinity for the sweet taste, just as brushing your teeth makes anything sweet you have right after, taste "off." Green juice is also high in minerals and will give your body what it needs to escort toxins out of the body, without the buffer system of insulin release and fat storage has to kick in.

By advising them to *add* a green juice instead of immediately *taking away* the diet soda—and I know that doing so will help change their taste buds over the next two weeks—my hope is that my clients will naturally stop on their own. Having ownership over their choices and stopping on their own accord is way more powerful than stopping because I told them to.

CHAPTER 4 ACTION STEPS

* Purchase some of the ingredients for the smart snacks listed on page 50.

* Implement the three-step snacking strategy on page 55 before you have a snack.

* Begin modifying your fruit intake now to follow the guidelines in the chart on page 58.

* When you get a craving, use one of the sugar swaps on page 54.

* Just say no to fructose—that includes fruit juice and soda—and diet soda. You can have fructose if it has fiber and vitamin C to slow down the metabolization of the sugars and prevent a big blood sugar spike—in other words, if it's a whole fruit. If you absolutely have to have something with asparatame, sucralose, or saccharin in it, have a green juice first.

For as long as I can remember, I have been addicted to Diet Coke. It's not like I set out to be an addict. It just happened because I love the taste of the stuff, especially with salty foods. I used to drink a Diet Coke with breakfast, lunch, dinner, and in between meals and still want more later that night!

When I was in my early fifties, I started to feel more aches and pains in my knees. For those of you who have ever suffered any type of knee pain, you know how awful and debilitating it can be. Thankfully, with Dr. Gioffre's help, I started to eat healthier by adding more greens into my diet and more healthy fats, like avocados, which are my new addiction!

By adding healthier foods and beverages to my diet, I started to feel a lot less pain and fewer cravings for Diet Coke, which is absolutely unbelievable! Today, I am fifty-six years old and look and feel forty, which I can honestly say has everything to do with Dr. Gioffre's program and way of life.

—RONI DEUTCH, host of *The Roni Deutch Radio Show* on iHeart Radio

PHASE 1: WEED

7 DAYS

five

The First 7 Days: Detox Your Mind, Your Pantry, and Your Body

THERE IS ONE MAJOR REASON THAT MOST PEOPLE WHO TRY TO GET OFF SUGAR END up failing: they didn't set themselves up for success. That's what these first official seven days of the Get Off Your Sugar program are designed to do.

Remember how in Chapter 3 I explained my weed, seed, feed approach? And just as you wouldn't build a new building on an overgrown vacant lot without first clearing out the trash and all the weeds, you can't create health in a body that is toxic and not working properly? Well, that's exactly what this first stage of the program is all about. We are going to get rid of the weeds in your internal environment that are blocking your health and healing.

These weeds fall into three major categories: physical stress, mental stress, and chemical stress. Stress is a silent killer. It's more acid-producing than anything you could put in your mouth—even sugar! And when you are stressed, your body keeps pumping out the cortisol, which cues the body to eat more sugar since it thinks you need that quick-burning fuel so that you can fight or flee. Your body doesn't know and doesn't care whether the stress is from traffic or from an actual threat on your life; it just thinks, *I'm in danger, give me the sugar so I can get out of here.*

You have to acknowledge that we are all subjected to low levels of constant chronic physical, emotional, and chemical stress, all day, every day. We are literally marinating in our cortisol, and it is draining us of the minerals and nutrients we need to perform, both mentally and physically. And what happens then? You go for the CRAP-py carbs (completely refined and processed), because sugar spikes the dopamine receptors eight times more than cocaine, and it makes you feel better about the stress you are going through. If you don't find another way to handle your stress, your body will keep craving and *needing* sugar.

When you address and alleviate your stress, you get your body into a state where it can easily handle the changes you're about to make to your diet. It makes the process so much more manageable and so much easier. And that's what I want for you—I don't want you to have to dive into deprivation and try to will your way through. If you do, you'll crash and likely will rebound into a physical state and level of addiction that is worse than when you started (you probably know what I am talking about). I want you to have an enjoyable journey with a soft landing. And taking the time to weed unnecessary stress out of your life is how you do it.

I know, I know, we all get the message to reduce our stress, from our doctors and from articles by health experts on the web. The question is always, *but how?* The truth is, maybe it's not possible to reduce your stress in any given moment. Maybe you're going through something inherently stressful. What we need to be talking about is how you can get into a peak state where you naturally handle your stress better, instead of your stress handling you.

During the next seven days, you'll clean out your mind, your pantry, and your body so that you can start with a clean slate and jump-start the process of achieving that peak state. Let's get you set up to win.

TRACK YOUR JOURNEY

So that you can see how your efforts are paying off, today (before you actually start making any changes) and each day of the Get Off Your Sugar program, I want you to give yourself an objective rating of how you're feeling and record it in the chart I created for you as part of the Get Off Your Sugar MAP on page 201 of this book. It will be motivating to see how these change over time, as well as to see which steps make the biggest difference for you.

Days 1–3:
Detox Your Mind

I could give you all the hacks in the world to help you switch from sugar burning to fat burning, but the truth is that strategy is only responsible for 20 percent of your success; the other 80 percent comes from psychology. So, for these next three days, your goal is to get your head fully on board with the changes you're seeking to create. That way, you won't be as vulnerable to talking yourself out of making changes. Because that's typically what happens— you decide to do something new, you get excited, you even take a few steps, and then the doubts start cropping up. Thoughts like, *What's the point of all this effort? This is too hard. I was crazy to think this would work.* So, let's short-circuit that cycle before it can even get started.

Each day, you'll complete one exercise designed to give you absolute clarity on what you're going to do and why you're going to do it. I've also included two bonus exercises you can weave in for even more clarity and an even bigger reduction in your mental stress.

If you're tempted to skip this step, thinking you got this, know that there's a reason I'm asking you to do these things.

Remember, I have coached 120,000 patients in the last twenty years, and I've seen firsthand what helps people succeed, and what often leads to failure.

You ready?

Day 1: Calculate Your Wellness Quotient

You know what's really motivating? Seeing your progress. But it's hard to recognize the gains you've made if you don't capture how you were feeling *before* you started making any changes. That's why today, before you start to change a single thing about how you eat, your mission is to do an honest assessment of your health as it is right now.

To do that, give yourself a score from 1 to 10 on the following ten aspects of health. When you're done, add up all your answers—that's your wellness quotient. As you follow the program, you should see this number come up. And that's how you'll know that you're moving the needle.

Tired

        1   2   3   4   5   6   7   8   9   10
        barely able to   full of energy and
        get out of bed   raring to go

Intensity of sugar cravings

        1   2   3   4   5   6   7   8   9   10
        multiple intense   no sugar cravings
        cravings a day   at all

Lack of libido

        1   2   3   4   5   6   7   8   9   10
        no sex drive to speak of   sex drive is high

continues

continued

Constipation

    1   2   3   4   5   6   7   8   9   10

1 bowel movement
every few days
    2 or more healthy
bowel movements/day

Difficulty sleeping

    1   2   3   4   5   6   7   8   9   10

sleeping 5 or fewer hours
per night regularly
    sleeping 7–9 hours
per night with ease

Brain fog

    1   2   3   4   5   6   7   8   9   10

forgetting things;
thoughts unfocused
    brain firing on all
cylinders

Gas/bloating

    1   2   3   4   5   6   7   8   9   10

uncomfortable levels of
gas or bloating daily
    no gas or bloating

Irritability

    1   2   3   4   5   6   7   8   9   10

hair-trigger temper
    even-keeled

Stressed

    1   2   3   4   5   6   7   8   9   10

stress levels off the charts
    managing stress

Headaches

    1   2   3   4   5   6   7   8   9   10

debilitating headaches
4 or more days/week
    no headaches

ADD UP YOUR TOTAL SCORE AND WRITE IT HERE: _____

1–50 points:
You need to seriously focus on your health.

51–70 points:
You're making progress, but there's still room to grow.

71–90 points:
You've done a lot of work, but it's not quite optimal yet.

91–100 points:
Optimal health—all you need to do is make some subtle changes.

Day 2: Declare Your Desired Outcome and Name Your Why

Although I can give you tactics and strategies, what I can't give you is the commitment to actually implement those tactics and strategies so you can get off your sugar. You need two things to build that commitment: your desired outcome and your why. This is crucial information for you to have, because how and what you think impact everything you do. Let's look at your desired outcome first.

There is one major reason that most people who try to get off sugar end up failing: they didn't think clearly about what success means to them. In other words, they didn't know their desired outcome. It's tempting to just start throwing darts at a dartboard, but you can't hit your target if you don't know what your target is.

Your desired outcome is the *result* you are after, and it needs to be specific. It can't be something general, like "I want to lose weight," because all you have to do is lose half a pound and, boom, outcome accomplished. You won't be inspired to keep going. Your desired outcome needs to have as much detail as possible, be time-based, and require you to dig deep inside yourself to accomplish. For example, "My outcome is to lose 7 pounds over the next 21 days—3 pounds in week 1, 2 pounds in week 2, and 2 pounds in week 3." Remember, a goal without a deadline is only a wish.

Get clear on your desired outcome, declare it and your subconscious will hone in on it and help you do whatever it takes to make it happen. So, take a moment now to think about it: what exact result do you want to achieve? Write it down (I made a space for you to record it on page 203), and make sure that it includes a measurable goal and a specific time frame.

It's not enough to stop there, though. You also want to know *why* you want that desired outcome. Getting in touch with what's driving you to make a change will help you keep going after the initial excitement has worn off and things get hard. In other words, knowing your why will make you fly.

To identify your why, try this short exercise: Imagine that you don't follow this program, and your sugar consumption doesn't change. How will you feel six months from now? How will you look in six months if you don't start making some changes? In one year? In five years? Be very specific. Will you be on medication? Will you have developed a life-threatening disease?

Now answer the question "I want to get off my sugar because . . ." Again, be as specific as possible. Give your why at least three reasons. My answer to this question is: "I want to wake up every day with unstoppable energy, just like I had in my early twenties, so that I can kick ass at work, and have more than enough gas in the tank to be fully present and engaged with my family when I get home. I want to be healthy so that I can enjoy these years with my wife and two children (who are three and six years old as I write this), and I want to be around for as long as possible to watch them grow. My father passed at age seventy-four, and with his cancer, he suffered. There's a saying, when one family member gets sick, the entire family gets sick. I never want my family to have to go through the pain that my brothers and mother and I had to experience. So, I choose health over disease, and I create that every day with the choices I make."

Your why has to be so compelling and so clear that when the cravings come at you and obstacles pop up (I'm going to help you anticipate and maneuver around cravings and obstacles as much as possible . . . but they're still going to happen) you'll remember why you're doing this in the first place. That knowledge will help you stay on track and ride out any bumps you might encounter.

As you write down your why, choose the words you use with care. Language is very powerful—if there's something negative in how you state your why, you will subconsciously resist it. For example, don't say, "I'm doing this because I want to remove sugar from my diet," because that's focused on deprivation, and deprivation is *not* motivating, especially when you're in the throes of a craving. A better way to say it is, "I want to replace the sugar in my diet with other foods that make me feel stronger, have better energy, help me detoxify, and get me on the way to optimal health."

I've made a special spot for you in the back of this book to record your desired outcome and your reasons that you want to get off your sugar: turn to page 203 right now, and fill it in while it's fresh on your mind. Once you've captured it, remember: repetition is the mother of skill, so read your outcome and your why daily.

Another powerful thing you can do to keep your why top of mind is to print out a picture either of yourself when you were at your ideal weight or a picture of someone else with the body you'd like to have, which you've pasted a picture of your face onto and put somewhere you'll see it every day—the kitchen is good place, or a bathroom mirror, or a place you typically go late at night to snack. Seeing is believing.

Day 3: Commit to Your Journey

This is where things start to get really real. It's time to commit to yourself that you are going to do the things you need to do to get off your sugar.

Making this commitment will help you stay motivated, even on crazy busy days. This will help you build trust with yourself and confidence that you can succeed.

For now, just commit to these 7 days of detoxing your mind, pantry, and body. Then, when they are done, commit to the 21 days of the program. When they are done, commit to the 90 days to make these new habits a lifestyle. You can take it one step at a time; as you experience the results and feel the benefits, you will be ready to commit for longer periods of time.

Today, and on the next six mornings, read the commitments on the next page, out loud, the moment you wake up. Do it with passion and certainty. These commitments need to be an incantation, not an affirmation, and here's the difference: if you are merely verbalizing the words without emotion, desire, and feeling, then you're not going to be as committed—you are merely saying the words with a lack of an emotional state. Incantations are about speaking what you want to become and can be used to turn a negative or limiting belief or thought into a positive one. Incantations have the power to rewire your brain and get you to take a positive action. You can literally re-create yourself using **incantations**. Here are your incantations for getting off your sugar:

- I commit to supporting my body and spirit as they have supported me for all these years.
- I commit to being honest with myself.
- I commit to cleansing myself of negative self-talk.
- I commit to having a body that is radiant, energized, clean, and strong.
- I commit to making time for myself and taking care of myself so I can receive the full benefits of this program.
- I commit to focusing on my desired outcome rather than getting caught up in how I will get there.
- I commit to giving my body what it needs to experience sugar freedom.
- I commit to giving 100 percent full effort, all day, every day, and if I veer off course at any point, I will immediately get myself back on track.

Extra Credit: Do a Digital Detox Too

The average American adult checks their phone once every twelve minutes, for an average of eighty times a day, according to a 2017 survey conducted by tech company Asurion. These devices that can keep us connected to the people we care about and the world and make our lives easier in so many ways also ratchet up our stress. Because they make us available around the clock, we rarely get the downtime we need to fully decompress and allow our nervous system to switch out of flight or fight and into the restorative mode of rest and digest. Just like sugar, checking your phone releases a hit of dopamine. Technology is another addiction; one that makes it that much easier to stay addicted to sugar because it keeps us in the stressed-out, anxious, and reactive state that can keep us locked in the cycle of eating, burning, and craving sugar.

On top of that, we've outsourced our brains to our smartphones. If you are older than about thirty, think of how many phone numbers you used to be able to memorize. Now, I'm lucky if I can remember a single one! Having so much of our lives stored in a device that's separate from us really escalates our anxiety—we feel we need to be checked in with it at all times so that we don't miss a notification. And God forbid we misplace our phones. That same survey found that 40 percent of people would rather lose their voice for a day than their phone for a day!

To help reduce your mental stress, it's incredibly helpful to implement a handful of strategies that help you detox technology from having such a prominent place in your life. Implement as many of these as you can during these seven days and throughout the rest of the program too:

- Institute certain parts of your home— such as the dinner table and the bedroom—as "phone-free."

- Turn off your Wi-Fi at night; you can get an automatic timer that you plug your router into and that you program to turn off from 11 p.m. to 6 a.m.

- Move your phone more than 4 feet away from your bed, so that you don't get zapped by the EMFs and you also make it harder to pick up your phone if you wake up in the middle of the night (guilty as charged!).

- Disable as many notifications on your phone as you can, so that it dings and captures your attention less.

- Use the Screentime feature on your iPhone or other app to monitor how many hours a day you spend on your phone and then seek to reduce that number over time. (Have you done this? You may be shocked at what you discover!)

- Disconnect to reconnect—turn off the TV at night and play a game, do a puzzle, or read together as a family.

- Remember to look up and get out. Your eyes need breaks from the screens as much as your mind does—instead of picking up your phone or cracking your laptop, take a few minutes to gaze out the window, it will rest your eyes and help you de-stress. Also, get outside for more walks (with no phones), as being in nature relaxes the brain, decreases cortisol, and helps you see other options. You may think that time away from your devices will hurt your productivity, but you'll be so refreshed that your ability to get things done will actually increase.

REDUCE MENTAL STRESS WITH THE 3:6:5 POWER BREATH

Think about it—when you're stressed, is your breath deep or shallow? You'd be surprised how often you hold your breath, depriving yourself of oxygen, which acidifies your blood and keeps you locked in a stress response.

Flood your body with oxygen, remove toxins that may be lurking in your lungs (such as excess carbon dioxide), and usher yourself into a more mentally and physically relaxed state by using my favorite breathing technique, the 3:6:5 Power Breath.

The inhalation stimulates your sympathetic nervous system, which is your fight or flight (and I like to add a third *f*—freeze), while the exhalation stimulates your parasympathetic nervous system, or rest and digest. That is why we aim to exhale more than we inhale. This breathing exercise can literally take you out of fight or flight in less than three minutes. In that same time, it also has the power to change your pH.

How to do it:

Breathe in through your nose for a count of 3.

Hold your breath for a count of 6.

Exhale out your mouth for a count of 5.

Repeat ten times at least once a day (when you wake up) or anytime you feel stress might be getting the upper hand.

Day 4: Detox Your Pantry

Now that your head is in a clearer space, it's time to prepare your physical environment. The best way to kick off a health and fitness journey is to take a look at everything in your fridge, cupboards, and pantry and get rid of any CRAP-py (completely refined and processed) carbs that are lurking there.

Today your assignment is to purge all the things that will tempt you when your energy dips at three in the afternoon, or you get a little hungry before bed, or you wake up at 2 a.m. in total craving mode (as I used to do).

Do you really have to get rid of it? I highly suggest you do, because if it's in the house, and it's a CRAP-py carbohydrate, chances are you're going to eat it when you're having a craving. It's almost impossible not to succumb. Do yourself a favor and remove the temptation. Remember, this phase of the program is about setting yourself up to win. If it's not there, you can't eat it.

Also, your home is a reflection of what's going on in your mind. When things are clean, you feel clearer. I promise you, you will feel a burst of energy after you detox the WMDs (the wheat, meat, dairy, and sugars) from your kitchen.

So, set aside at least two hours and have a garbage bag (for anything expired or freezer-burned), a recycling bin (for empty containers), and a box or two (for anything unopened that you might want to donate to a food pantry or soup kitchen). Then, pick up every food item in your kitchen and read the label. If there's an ingredient you can't pronounce, you can't digest it. If it's processed, get rid of it.

Something to keep in mind as you decide what stays and what goes: if you are looking to lose weight and cut cravings, you will want to keep your net carbs (total carbs minus fiber) under 50 grams total for the day. Doing so can potentially help you lose a pound a day. (Eating 50 to 100 grams total net carbs/day, on the other hand, can help you lose 1 to 2 pounds per week.) Ultimately, you get to choose what makes up those carbs, so choose wisely in regard to what you toss and what you keep.

The list of items you'll want to purge include:

Sauces (BBQ sauce, hoisin sauce, soy sauce, and tomato sauces)

Cereal

Junk food (e.g., chips, cookies, and most bars)

Refined sugars

White flours (including bread, buns, and pasta)

Soft drinks

All forms of dairy (including cheese and yogurt)

Fruit juices

Anything with artificial sweeteners

Grains (rice, cornmeal, popcorn, oats, and bulgur)

Processed meats (e.g., sausage, bacon, hot dogs, and lunch meats)

If in doubt, throw it out!

SWAP BAD FOR BETTER OR BEST

Refer to this list for the things you should get out of your pantry (the items in the "Swap This Out" column) as well as suggestions on what to replace them with (in the "Better Choice" and "Best Choice" columns).

SWAP THIS OUT	BETTER CHOICE	BEST CHOICE
Brown rice	White rice (not a typo, white is better than brown!)	Quinoa or wild rice
Milk or soy milk	Unsweetened almond milk	Unsweetened coconut milk or homemade almond/hemp milk
Vegetable oils (canola, soybean, sunflower, corn oil)	Sesame oil	Coconut/olive oil/avocado oil
Pasta	Gluten-free pasta	Zucchini noodles/kelp noodles
Balsamic vinegar	Apple cider vinegar	Lemon juice
Coffee or black tea	Green tea	Herbal tea
Milk chocolate	Dark chocolate	Raw cacao
Table salt	Sea salt/kosher salt	Celtic Grey Sea Salt or Himalayan pink salt
Margarine/butter	Ghee/grass-fed butter (e.g., Kerrygold)	Coconut butter/raw nut butters (except peanut butters, which you need to toss)
Soy sauce	Tamari/shoyu/Bragg Liquid Aminos	Coconut aminos
Sugar/agave nectar/brown sugar	Coconut sugar/manuka honey	Stevia/monk fruit (lo han guo)
Peanuts	Cashews	Raw almonds/macadamia nuts/walnuts
Carbonated/bottled/tap water	Filtered water	Filtered water with a pinch of Himalayan pink salt
Fruit juice	Freshly squeezed fruit juice	Cold-pressed green juice
Granola/oatmeal	Gluten-free oats	Quinoa porridge
White bread	Gluten-free bread	Sprouted bread (e.g., Ezekiel)
Conventionally raised meat/farmed fish	Grass-fed animal proteins/wild-caught fish	Plant-based proteins
Beer/cider	Wine	Grain-free vodka (e.g., Chopin or Ciroc)/tequila

"BUT DR. DARYL, I CAN'T GET RID OF THIS STUFF; MY KIDS WILL NEVER GO FOR IT!"

The likely reality is that your kids are even more addicted to sugar than you are. I know you love your children just as much as I love mine. I know it's easy to give into the crying for the sweet stuff and the whining for the processed stuff. I've done it too. But let's raise our standards and our expectations for our kids. After all, these are our children we're talking about.

In 2018, researchers at Columbia University of New York found that elderly people who had 30.3 grams of added sugar a day—roughly as much in a can of soda—had a 33 percent higher risk of developing Alzheimer's than did those who consumed only 5.8 grams of added sugar a day.[1] Another study found that a daily 20-ounce serving of sugar-sweetened soda shortened telomeres—the material that seals the ends of the strands of your DNA and generally regarded as a good indicator of biological age—enough to represent 4.6 years; that's the exact same telomere-length loss experienced by a regular smoking habit.[2] Think of it this way: if you give your kids soda, you may be helping them get Alzheimer's, and you may as well be encouraging them to start smoking. Are you okay with that?

Getting the CRAP-py (completely refined and processed) carbs out of your house is the perfect excuse to follow the adage, *If you "can't," you must.* They will hate you for only two weeks. In that time, their taste buds will change. It will most likely be painful. But it will most definitely be worth it. Remember your outcome.

WHAT TO RESTOCK YOUR PANTRY *WITH*

While it's great to get the bad stuff *out,* if you don't replace it with something good to eat, you'll be too tempted to order takeout or grab something from a vending machine that won't help you get off your sugar. These are the foods Chelsea and I always have on hand; with them, we can make any number of easy, delicious meals for us and the kids.

Fresh herbs/spices: basil, cilantro, parsley, garlic, ginger, turmeric, mint

Dried spices: cinnamon, cayenne pepper, black pepper, turmeric, cumin, Redmond Real Salt, Himalayan pink salt, chipotle chile, garlic, paprika, chili powder, cardamom, oregano, curry

Vegetables and fruits: broccoli, celery, carrot, cauliflower, cucumber, green apple, cabbage, greens (choose from spinach, kale, romaine lettuce, arugula, chard), red/yellow/orange bell pepper, red onion, yellow onion, green onion, sweet potato, squash, lemon, lime, avocado, grapefruit, tomato, dates

Healthy oils and fats (liquid): extra-virgin olive oil, coconut oil, avocado oil, MCT oil, sesame oil, almond milk, coconut milk (carton), full-fat coconut milk (can)

Raw nuts, seeds, and nut butters: hemp seeds, flaxseeds, chia seeds, almonds, macadamia nuts, Brazil nuts, walnuts, pine nuts, pecans, cashews, unsweetened coconut flakes, almond butter, coconut butter, cacao butter, sesame tahini

Others: coconut aminos, Bragg Liquid Aminos, cacao powder, cacao nibs, quinoa, wild rice, red lentils, chickpeas (canned and dried), adzuki beans (canned and dried), cannellini beans (canned)

Days 5, 6, and 7: Detox Your Body with a 3-Day Alkaline Cleanse

Now, you're ready to detox your body and relieve the source of your physical stress. For the next three days, you're jump-starting your weaning off sugar by decreasing the number of carbs you eat to less than 50 grams of net carbs and increasing your mineral intake, which will help reduce cravings.

Your diet for the next three days will be chock-full of whole, plant-based, alkaline foods that are rich in minerals, vitamins, phytonutrients, enzymes, and plenty of plant-based keto fats to curb your cravings, suppress hunger, and start to fire up your fat-burning engine. And you'll be preparing these foods in such a way (or, your blender will) that they are easy to break down and assimilate, which will give your gut a break and allow it to focus on healing from its current inflamed acidic state.

The goals for these three days are to:

- Stop the poisons (a.k.a. the sugar and the carbs) that are inflaming your body
- Calm the fire by creating a more alkaline state
- Give your body plenty of absorbable nutrients to get back to homeostasis with
- Ward off future cravings by starting to flip your taste buds and upping your mineral intake
- Jump-start your metabolism and transition to fat burning (which takes anywhere from two to four weeks to fully achieve, but this will give you a running start)
- All in three days!

Because toxins are stored in fat cells, as you liberate these toxins, you can also expect to lose somewhere between 3 and 7 pounds—and unlike the water weight or muscle loss that can happen on other diets, these are fat pounds you'll lose, meaning they won't come right back on after the three days are through.

If all this sounds like a tall order, just know that all the recipes for the foods on this three-day cleanse are easy and taste great. They take ten minutes at most, and you don't have to be a gourmet chef. All you need are the ingredients and a blender. You can double or even triple each recipe and then store your leftovers in an airtight container for up to forty-eight hours, and then you only have to prepare foods on one of the days—the rest of the time, you can grab and go.

Why an Alkaline Cleanse?

I spent the last twenty years of my professional career investigating the true cause of premature aging, inflammation, and disease, and all the evidence led me to acid.

You see, all foods fall into one of two categories, acidic or alkaline. Acidic foods are things like sugar, grains, dairy, artificial sweeteners, and animal proteins, and they're *horrible* for your body, your immune system, and your overall well-being . . . and here's why: think about what acid does from a commonsense standpoint. Acid is so corrosive, it can burn a hole through metal, so think about what that's doing inside your body, your digestive system, your cardiovascular system, your brain!

Acids corrode your system, drive up inflammation, drain your energy, and make you hold onto fat . . . so these are the foods we will be eliminating in this 3-Day Alkaline Cleanse.

Alkaline foods are the exact opposite: they fuel your body, and they're *amazing* at promoting a healthier, stronger you. These are the foods we will be adding in their nutrient dense, raw state.

CAPTURE YOUR BEFORE

You've already given yourself a Wellness Quotient (page 69). That's a great qualitative measurement of your overall health. But, now it's time to gather some quantitative measurements.

Seeing these changes as you move through the program will be help you continue on through the 21- and 90-day portions.

Record the following measurements:

Weight: _____ pounds

Waist (at belly button): _____ inches

Hips: _____ inches

Thighs: _____ inches

Chest: _____ inches

And then, just to make it official, take a photo of yourself in your underwear from the front, back, and side. Trust me, this may sound like a mild form of torture right now, but in ninety days, you will thank yourself for giving yourself a visual reminder of the improvements you've made in your health.

THREE-DAY ALKALINE CLEANSE MEAL PLAN

The basic plan for what to eat during the detox is the same for each day: a detox tea first thing in the morning, hydration throughout the day, a detox smoothie for breakfast, raw soup for lunch (with a hot soup option if you prefer), and salad for dinner, with an optional (but highly recommended) greens powder in the a.m. and a mineral powder thirty minutes before bed. You do have some flexibility here in that you can decide between a few different smoothies and soups, and you can mix up your own salad each night while following a few basic guidelines.

7–8 a.m.: Hydration (Detox Tea, page 220, or lemon water) and deep breathing

8–9 a.m.: Green drink

A high-quality greens powder mixed with cold water or organic celery juice (try my Alkamind Acid-Kicking Greens; see Resources)

continues

continued

Shot of wheatgrass juice

Organic celery juice

Fresh green juice (with no fruit other than ½ green apple)

9–10 a.m.: Breakfast smoothie; choose from:

Dr. Green Detox Smoothie, page 215

Skinny Mint Green Smoothie, page 217

Coco-Berry Smoothie, page 217

Chocolate Almond Smoothie, page 215

Maca Power Breakfast Shake, page 216

10–11 a.m.: Hydration (lemon water)

11 a.m.–1 p.m.: Lunch soup; choose from:

Chilled Green Detox Soup, page 225

Zucchini, Apple, and Basil-Fennel Soup, page 229

Creamy Spinach Basil Soup, page 226

Chilled Cucumber Avocado Soup, page 227

1–2 p.m.: Hydration (lemon water)

2–3 p.m.: Afternoon smoothie or snack; choose from:

Clean Keto Garlic Dip with veggie sticks, page 251

5-Minute Hummus, page 255

Easy Choose-Your-Own-Flavor Kale Chips, page 255

Crispy Chickpeas, page 252

3–4 p.m.: Hydration (lemon water)

5–7 p.m.: Dinner; choose a salad such as:

Salad with Spicy Salsa Verde, page 230

Avocado, Kale, and Pepita Salad, page 232

Pomegranate and White Bean Salad with Tarragon Dressing, page 231

Perfect Salad in a Jar, page 234

7–8 p.m.: Hydration (lemon water)

30 minutes before bed: Minerals (using a powdered mineral supplement dissolved in 4 ounces of water—see Resources for suggestion, or ⅛ teaspoon of Himalayan pink salt dissolved in 8 ounces of water)

COMMON DETOX SYMPTOMS AND HOW TO AVOID THEM

I walk clients through my 3-Day Alkaline Cleanse all year long. I can tell you that on Day 1, everyone's excited. It's the honeymoon phase. Day 2, it can get a bit more real as your hunger can kick in and your body hasn't had long enough to switch to fat burning, which allows it to tap into the tens of thousands of calories stored in your fat cells. You may also experience some detox symptoms, such as:

- nausea
- fatigue
- headaches
- gas
- bloating

While these detox symptoms certainly aren't enjoyable, they are showing signs of healing (even though you may not feel like it's healing). When it comes to toxins, it's better they be moving out of your body than staying in. This is when you need to pull out your *why* that you created on page 203 and use it to fuel you to keep going. Also, remember that by Day 2, you have only one more day to go.

If you feel tired and fatigued, it's because your body is working to process and release toxins that have been stored in your fat cells. So, please, give yourself extra rest now because it takes energy to heal. If you are currently exercising, you can keep going as is, but be mindful that exercise will increase the detoxification on the body, so be sure to add an extra liter of water on exercise days. If you don't currently exercise, I don't recommend starting now, as it will be too much on your system. However, feel free to go for a walk, or gently bounce on a rebounder for ten to twelve minutes daily.

My motto is the *solution* to *pollution* is *dilution*. In other words, be sure to drink plenty of water. I suggest filling a gallon or a half-gallon jug with filtered water and making sure that you drink the entire thing throughout the day so that you can keep track of how much water you've had to drink and ensure that you're getting ample amounts.

The 3:6:5 Power Breath on page 74 can also help your body purge toxins via your lungs and help revitalize you if you are feeling tired.

WHAT COMES NEXT

Congratulations—during this past week, you've rebooted your body and your mind and prepared your inner terrain for some vitalizing new habits to take root!

From here on out, you're going to follow the 21-day program that will walk you through the seven steps to getting off your sugar for good.

Now that you've detoxed your pantry, resist the urge to go back to your "before" diet of CRAP-py (completely refined and processed) carbs and sugar. Stick to whole foods as much as possible, and refer to the "Swap Bad for Better or Best" chart on page 76 to help you choose which foods to add back into your daily routine now that your cleanse is behind you. You can also keep using the healthy snacks I listed in Chapter 4 for the time being.

In general, from this point on, you want to keep the processed foods out. You don't need to go crazy at this point; just try to make better choices, and I will guide you to specific foods in the days ahead. Over the next twenty-one days, you're going to slowly build up to a strength-eating diet.

CHAPTER 5 ACTION STEPS

* Calculate your wellness quotient.
* Name your why.
* Commit to your journey (every day).
* Do a digital detox.
* Use the 3:6:5 Power Breath once a day.
* Detox your pantry.
* Capture your before.
* Complete the 3-Day Alkaline Cleanse to detox your body.

I had been struggling with arthritis for five years and had been on meds for acid reflux for nine years. I am extremely active and love to compete in triathlons—something that was becoming harder and harder for me to do, which made me sad.

My depression drove me to eat more carbs, comfort food, and sugary treats. I didn't even realize how much I was consuming. The pain in my throat and my joints was becoming unbearable. I was looking for answers, and the doctors I was referred to would not give me any reasonable treatment or advice; they recommended only prescriptions and test after test. I was desperate for guidance. I came across Dr. Daryl's website, and things starting making sense: all this stuff I had been eating to make myself feel better was actually making me worse. Following Dr. Daryl's program changed my life and my future. I immediately felt like a weight lifted off my joints. My throat started feeling better. The greens powder I started drinking sent my energy skyrocketing and stopped the sugar cravings completely. The incredible recipes made it easy to revamp everything I put in my mouth.

Within a few short months I was able to increase my activities. It's been a truly amazing experience to dump the sugar overload and get my life back. I am blown away by how I am now able to push myself—hard enough to get on a podium in most every race I do now (and I am fifty-seven years old). I can't believe the change. I am not ready to give up all the things I love. And since I got off my sugar, I don't have to!   —Darlene G.

PHASE 2: SEED

21 DAYS

six

Step 1 (Days 1–3): Re-Mineralize

It's time to plant seeds for your new way of strength eating. Remember, the Get Off Your Sugar program is designed to build on itself—every step makes all the steps that come after it easier and more effective. It's also based on the principle of adding instead of taking away. So, it's no accident that the first step you're going to take to kick the sugar habit is to start adding more minerals to your diet.

I believe there is nothing more important for your health than having healthy mineral levels. Sadly, most of us are woefully deficient in them, and sugar is a big reason for this: when you eat sugar, your body has to draw on its mineral reserves to help you recover.

Getting more minerals every day helps give your body more of the things it needs to heal itself and run efficiently. Even better, it will help ward off your sugar cravings so that all the other six steps will be that much more doable.

If you *didn't* prioritize your mineral intake before attempting to get off your sugar, your cravings would simply be too strong. This is why giving up sugar cold turkey works for so few people: they don't arm themselves with minerals first. Very few people have enough willpower to outlast the withdrawal. Minerals lend you strength so that you don't have to white-knuckle your way through it.

WHY MINERALS MATTER

Your body is an electrical machine—every heartbeat, thought, and cellular process requires a tiny current of electricity to happen. And minerals conduct that energy. Although most people think that carbs, fats, and proteins are the fuels your body needs to survive, it's really the minerals that make your electrical circuitry function. You truly can't live without them. Here are just some of the things minerals do for you:

- Act as the bricks your body uses to build such essential things as bones, teeth, neurotransmitters, hormones, and hemoglobin (the component of red blood cells that shuttles oxygen throughout the body—pretty important stuff)

- Activate the enzymes that regulate all of the vital processes your body undergoes every moment of every day

- Protect your brain by improving function of the synapses and warding off the development of the plaques that are a hallmark of Alzheimer's disease. In fact, minerals are your brain's top line of defense, or as I like to call them, your number one neuroprotectors.

- Play a vital role in getting glucose out of the bloodstream and into your cells

- Serve as a buffering system for toxins in our severely toxin-overloaded world—your body either binds a toxin to a mineral molecule so as to neutralize it by converting it into a weaker acid salt, or stores it in a fat cell.

It's no exaggeration to say that minerals are the key to life. Yet, mineral deficiencies are the most common ailment I see in my clients, whether they come in for headaches, back pain, digestive ailments, fatigue, or brain fog. There's one common denominator—mineral deficiency. We simply aren't getting enough.

The truth is, very few Americans are consuming anywhere near enough of the foods that have the highest levels of minerals (see page 93 for a list of the top 10, but I'll give you a sneak preview now: many of them are vegetables) because we are eating a diet chock-full of CRAP-py (completely refined and processed) carbs. These foods are so nutrient poor that they often have to have minerals added back in an attempt to "fortify" them!

Yet, even if you have a very high-quality diet, rich in the dark leafy greens, raw nuts and seeds, avocados, and other mineral-dense foods that you'll encounter in this chapter, you are likely still mineral deficient because our food supply provides significantly fewer minerals than it once did. In fact, the mineral depletion of our farmland is probably the single most important reason that most Americans are magnesium deficient.

I had the privilege of interviewing Dr. Carolyn Dean, author of *The Magnesium Miracle*, for the Get Off Your Sugar Summit. I learned so much from her, including the amazing fact that magnesium is required for 80 percent of known metabolic functions. She revealed how today you can obtain about one-third of your mineral needs only from good organic food, and while our great-grandparents could obtain 500 mg a day of magnesium from their diet, that number has diminished to 200 mg today. In addition, the magnesium we do get is quickly depleted— eating sugar, working out too hard, many medications, and caffeine all eat up lots of magnesium.

Because minerals, such as magnesium, play a major role in regulating blood sugar levels, which in turn influences insulin and leptin, when you don't have enough of them, you get trapped in that cycle of always craving food, particularly foods that are quick sources of energy . . . like sugar. Prioritizing eating mineral-rich foods in these first three days will help your body stop depleting its resources and start to heal. Only then can you avoid the cravings that keep you trapped in a vicious sugar cycle.

THE FOUR MIGHTY MINERALS YOU CAN'T LIVE WITHOUT

While there are nineteen major and minor minerals in the blood, for the sake of this program we're going to focus on the top four for helping you kick the sugar habit. They are:

Mighty Mineral #1: Magnesium. Involved in activating seven to eight hundred enzymes in the body, magnesium is one of the most critical—and typically, the most deficient—minerals. Magnesium helps muscles contract and relax, including those in your digestive tract and your

arterial walls, so this mineral plays an important role in digestive and heart health. It also stabilizes blood pressure, calms the nervous system so that your body can sleep deeply enough to have time to heal itself, and helps enzymes do their work. Enzymes facilitate chemical processes, and as we age, we produce fewer of them, so magnesium becomes even more crucial as you get older.

Magnesium helps regulate your blood sugar levels—it takes 84 molecules of magnesium to neutralize one molecule of table sugar (which is a combination of fructose and glucose), 56 molecules to neutralize one molecule of fructose, and 28 molecules to neutralize 1 molecule of glucose, which explains why, if you've been eating too much sugar for too long, your magnesium stores are likely drained. And the more you stabilize your blood sugar, the fewer cravings you'll have.

Magnesium is also your number one neuroprotector. Supplementing with magnesium has been shown to reduce the number of plaques in the brain of mice with Alzheimer's disease,[1] dramatically increase long-term spatial memory in rats, and strengthen the connection between synapses in the brain so that it functions better.[2]

And magnesium has been shown to help headaches: those subject to migraines often have low levels of magnesium,[3] and a 1996 study showed that migraine sufferers who took a magnesium supplement every day for twelve weeks reduced incidences of migraines by 41.6 percent (compared to 15.8 percent in the group who took a placebo).[4]

Magnesium is so important that it's one of the top five supplements I recommend everyone take (we'll cover it in Chapter 11). But for this first step of the program, we're going to focus on upping your levels of it by consuming more foods that contain it.

Mighty Mineral #2: Calcium. Like magnesium, calcium also activates enzymes, tones the nervous system, and plays a role in your muscular contractions. Calcium is the most abundant mineral in the body, and because of that, it steals all the attention, especially within the osteoporosis world.

You probably think you've got calcium under control—after all, most of us have been told at least a hundred different times, whether by a doctor or an article on a health website, to make sure you get enough calcium for strong bones. But there are a few problems with how most of us go about getting our calcium needs met:

- Calcium needs to be in a 1:1 ratio with magnesium, and most people are deficient in magnesium already, so taking calcium supplements only pushes you more out of balance. The average American has ten times the amount of calcium that they should. In fact, one of the *major* causes of inflammation in our body is too much calcium. Luckily, this excess can be dramatically reduced by increasing our magnesium levels, which then also reduces systemic inflammation levels.

- Many of the typical American foods provide calcium in all the wrong ratios to magnesium. Dairy has a 10:1 ratio of calcium to magnesium; for orange juice, it's 27:1! On top of that, many Americans take calcium supplements in a misguided effort to ward off osteoporosis—not only do most calcium supplements contain the cheapest, most poorly absorbable form, calcium carbonate, but also taking those supplements only pushes their calcium to magnesium ratio further out of whack.

- Another huge problem is that when we have too much calcium, it doesn't get excreted; it gets stored. That sounds like a good thing until you learn that it is typically stored in all the wrong places. Calcium gets absorbed through the large intestine with the help of vitamin D and magnesium, and then once it's absorbed, vitamin K_2 tells the calcium where to go. Without sufficient amounts of these three vitamins and minerals, excess calcium will get deposited in arterial walls (leading to hardening of the arteries and cardiovascular disease) and joints (contributing to arthritis). That's why calcium supplements rarely make it to the bones.

- If you're taking a statin drug to lower cholesterol, it's even worse, as vitamin K_2 is synthesized by an enzyme that is blocked by the statins. So, even though you're taking the medication to help with heart health (by reducing cholesterol), you are unknowingly accelerating the buildup of arterial plaque.

- If you're seeking to get calcium by consuming more dairy, you're inadvertently creating an acidic environment that forces your body to leach calcium from your bones. I know this sounds counterintuitive and as if it couldn't possibly be true, but even researchers at Harvard found, after following women for twelve years, that those who consumed a higher amount of dairy had more hip fractures than women who ate less dairy.[5] It's for this reason that I say, "Dairy is scary."

For all these reasons, calcium is actually a mineral that I *don't* recommend you take as a supplement (more on this in Chapter 11), because you're much more likely to keep your calcium and magnesium ratio in line when you get your calcium from the mineral-rich foods I cover in this chapter, as nature is great at providing nutrients in balance to each other (whereas many supplements are not).

Mighty Mineral #3: Potassium. There are many reasons to love potassium: it helps regulate your heartbeat and reduces both blood pressure and the risk of stroke. It also decreases muscle cramping—whether that's during exercise, in the middle of the night, or when you are menstruating. It helps build strong muscles and bones. As a bonus, it can even reduce the appearance of cellulite!

The recommended daily intake of potassium is 4,700 mg, which only about 2 percent of Americans manage to get. Most of us are getting closer to 2,500 mg a day. This is a problem not just because it means we aren't getting enough potassium; it means we also have a poor potassium-to-sodium ratio. Like calcium and magnesium, potassium and sodium need to be in proper proportions to each other. Our ancestors, with their diet of fruits, vegetables, seeds, and other plants, typically ate about

11,000 mg of potassium per day and only 700 mg of sodium, or a potassium-sodium ratio of 16:1. Now, with our heavy reliance on sodium-heavy processed foods (of the wrong kind of salt; see the box on page 91 for more info) and our low intake of vegetables, the typical potassium-sodium ratio is more like 1:1.3 (2,500 mg of potassium to 3,400 mg of sodium).[6]

The good news here is that by adding more sources of potassium to your diet—which you will start to do for these first three days in the form of dark leafy greens, spinach, and broccoli—you'll rectify both the overall deficiency and the skewed ratio to sodium, and you won't need to take a supplement to do it.

Mighty Mineral #4: Sodium bicarbonate. Also known as baking soda, sodium bicarbonate is a whiz at neutralizing acid and promoting alkalinity. In fact, when your body is in an acidic state, the stomach, pancreas, and kidneys will create bicarbonate to help neutralize acid and help you maintain a balanced blood pH of 7.4.

You may be thinking, "But didn't Dr. Daryl just say that most of us are getting way too much sodium?" Sodium *is* an important, health-promoting mineral. In fact, it's essential for life.

Also, sodium bicarbonate is a completely different animal from the sodium chloride (otherwise known as table salt) that's in processed foods and most salt shakers. For starters, sodium bicarbonate has less sodium than sodium chloride—28 percent versus nearly 40 percent, respectively. Even more important, sodium bicarbonate is alkalizing, whereas sodium chloride is not (it is neither acidic nor alkaline). Deficiencies in sodium bicarbonate have been linked to hypertension, kidney stones, stroke, and osteoporosis. You can get it through leavened foods, such as breads, thanks to the presence of baking soda (which is 100 percent sodium bicarbonate), but since these foods are high in carbs and sugar, I recommend taking it in a supplement (see the Resources section for a recommendation).

IMPORTANT TRACE MINERALS

Mighty, but Mini, Mineral #1: Chromium. Chromium is a trace mineral, meaning you need only a tiny bit of it (as opposed to say, calcium, which makes up about 2 percent of your total body weight). Even though you don't need a lot of it, it's still superimportant to your health, primarily because it helps regulate your blood sugar levels. Chromium is like a taxi for glucose—it binds with glucose and shuttles it out of the blood and into your cells and then brings it back out of the cells when you need it. When you've got plenty of chromium on hand, your body has to release less insulin in an effort to keep blood sugar stable. If you have either form of diabetes, insulin resistance, or a history of eating too much sugar, chromium is extra important to you. True deficiency in chromium is rare, but many people have suboptimal levels, in part because there's less of it in the soil used to grow our food. That's why broccoli is on the list of foods that you want to prioritize eating these

next three days, because it's a great source of chromium.

Mighty, but Mini, Mineral #2: Zinc. Trace mineral zinc is an important player in immunity, as it helps your body form the white blood cells that fight infection. It's also a protector of your DNA. While these are two great reasons to make sure you're getting enough, zinc also plays a role in how your body uses glucose and insulin, and a deficiency can trigger sugar cravings. Pumpkin seeds, one of the top ten foods you'll be eating more of in these next three days and as we progress, is a fabulous source of zinc, as are spinach (another top ten food), chickpeas, and Brazil nuts.

HOW DO YOU KNOW YOU ARE MINERAL DEFICIENT?

Here are nine signs you need some more minerals in your diet:

1. **You can't sleep.** Minerals are calming to the nervous system—you can't get into rest-and-digest mode without them. So, if your mineral levels are low, your system will be too stimulated to sleep soundly or for long periods of time. You may fall asleep just fine, but then wake up in the middle of the night (when your minerals are being recruited by the liver for detoxing), or you may have difficulty falling asleep in the first place (because you don't have mineral levels sufficient enough to quiet the nervous system). This is why I tell my patients to take their mineral supplement thirty minutes before bed (more about that on page 99).

2. **You are constipated.** Magnesium helps relax muscles throughout your body, including in the digestive tract. You may not realize it, but muscles are responsible for moving food waste out of your body, so if those muscles aren't functioning properly, your digestion can slow to a crawl.

3. **You experience frequent cramps and muscle spasms.** Remember, your body uses minerals to neutralize toxins. People often experience leg cramps in the middle of the night because that's the peak time for your liver to process metabolic toxins out of the body. If your mineral levels are already low, when most of your minerals are being used to bind toxins, there won't be enough to relax your muscles and you'll get a cramp.

4. **You get frequent headaches.** All headaches originate in the neck—you can't have a headache without pressure on one of the nerves in the neck, which control blood flow to the brain. When you are mineral deficient, muscles contract and spasm, which will pull your spine out of alignment, putting pressure on the nerves that are causing your headaches. A chiropractic adjustment will remove the pressure causing the headache, but taking minerals will remove the underlying cause. Inflammation contributes to headaches, too, and low levels of minerals promote inflammation as well.

5. **You have ADD, brain fog, depression and/or anxiety.** Minerals play so many vital roles in your brain health that mineral deficiencies can show up as a lot of different mental health challenges. Some of this is related to the workings of the brain itself—magnesium has been shown to help regulate receptors in the brain necessary for learning and memory[7] as well as those associated with depression and anxiety[8]—and some of it is related to their role in the stress response—low levels of magnesium have also been linked to higher levels of cortisol and adrenocorticotropin hormone, which are excreted by the adrenal glands in response to stress. So, mineral deficiencies make you more susceptible to stress and then less able to deal with it when you encounter it.

6. **You crave sugar.** Minerals are involved in the production of insulin, which regulates your blood sugar levels, so if you don't have enough, your insulin could be contributing to your cravings in an effort to stabilize blood sugar. They also play a role in how your brain regulates your levels of dopamine, the neurotransmitter that's involved in pleasure, so if you're craving the rush that sugar brings, it could signal an insufficiency in minerals. Also, chocolate is high in magnesium; craving it can indicate a mineral deficiency.

||||||||||||||||||||||||||||||||||||||||||||||||||||||||||||||||||||||||||||||

TO SALT OR NOT TO SALT?

I can't tell you how many clients come in to my office and tell me that their doctor has them on a strict no-salt, no-fat diet. I tell them they may as well walk to the graveyard; going without salt completely is literally a prescription for death. What would happen if you put all the fish in the ocean on a no-salt diet? They would die, and you're no different! Doctors simply don't know about the distinctions between salts because they get very little nutrition training, so they lump all salts in together in a category labeled "bad." But the right kind of salt is absolutely crucial for health. Salt is responsible for . . .

* Carrying nutrients into and out of cells

* Being an essential component in blood plasma, lymphatic fluid, and even amniotic fluid

* Maintaining and regulating blood pressure

* Helping your brain communicate with your muscles so you can move

There are salts that kill and salts that heal.
Table salt is sodium chloride, which raises blood pressure and promotes inflammation. It has been entirely stripped of all accompanying minerals that are found in naturally occurring salt. In addition, it is loaded with synthetic ingredients, such as anticaking agents, bleach, and fluoride. Truly, table salt is no one's friend. But that doesn't mean you should avoid all salt altogether.

The salts that heal are life-giving, because in addition to sodium, they contain many trace minerals that your body needs but are less and less present in our food supply. Using them to season your food (or even mixed in to a glass of water) is an easy and effective way to get those trace minerals into your body. The salts I recommend you add to your food every day are:

* Celtic Grey Sea Salt

* Himalayan pink salt

* Salt from the Great Salt Lake (Redmond Real Salt)

I used to recommend clients use any old sea salt, but there is evidence now that a lot of sea salt is contaminated with plastics, so I'm sticking with the above recommendations. And I don't expect this to change anytime soon—by the year 2050, it is anticipated that there will be more plastic in the ocean than fish.

You can also absorb the trace minerals in salt through your skin. My favorite way to do just that is to take a hot bath in which you've dissolved Epsom salts (which are a form of magnesium) and baking soda (sodium bicarbonate). The minerals will penetrate the skin and get absorbed directly into your bloodstream. The warmth of the bath and the calming minerals make it deeply relaxing and the perfect thing to do to get ready for bed. Throw in a few drops of your favorite essential oil and you are in for a real treat.

The recipe for the bath is:

  2 cups Epsom salts

  1 cup baking soda

  10 drops essential oil, such as lavender, eucalyptus, or lemon

A BONUS: FIBER

All the foods that are high in minerals are also high in another health-promoting substance—fiber. When you eat fiber, it slows down the metabolization of sugar, which prevents your blood sugar from spiking. This, in turn, lowers your insulin levels.

It also:

- Helps you feel fuller, longer, which in turn wards off cravings, hunger, and getting "hangry"

- Promotes elimination so your toxic load is decreased, freeing up more of the minerals in your body to support daily bodily functions and the integrity of your bones, muscles, joints, and functioning of your brain

- Feeds the healthy bacteria in your gut, which helps boost immunity, promotes healthy levels of neurotransmitters responsible for mood, and advances absorption

- Provides antioxidants, which promotes cellular and, in turn, whole-body health

TOP TEN MINERAL-RICH FOODS

Nature is a genius at making sure that nutrients come packaged in a balanced way, with the right blend of components that your body can easily use. Here are the top mineral-rich foods you should try to eat daily:

Mineral-Rich Food #1:
Broccoli Sprouts

Calcium: 78 mg (6% of RDI)
Iron: 720 mcg (4% of RDI)
(per cup, raw)

Sprouts are baby versions of the vegetables they grow into, and they are undeniable superfoods. Just as seeds contain extra nutrition to fuel growth, sprouts are also jam-packed with nutrients, particularly sulforaphane and isothiocyanate—two compounds that have demonstrated anticancer properties. In fact, my friend Liana Werner-Gray, author of *Cancer-Free with Food*, calls broccoli sprouts the number one cancer-fighting food.

A general rule of thumb is that sprouts have thirty times the nutrition of the

fully grown version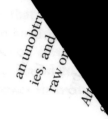
Whereas mature br
els of minerals th
sprouts the mine
tein molecules,
bioavailable.

How to eat them: Pile spr
top of a salad or use them in lieu of ic
altogether. You can also add them to a juice or smoothie. Only one note of caution: sprouts are susceptible to mold and, very rarely, *E. coli* contamination. Always keep your sprouts refrigerated, and if you're pregnant, avoid them.

Alternatives: Sunflower seed sprouts, pea sprouts, watercress sprouts

Mineral-Rich Food #2:
Spinach

Magnesium: 23.6 mg (6% of RDI)
Manganese: 0.3 mg (13% of RDI)
Potassium: 167 mg (5% of RDI)
(per cup, raw)

All dark leafy greens are incredible sources of minerals, vitamins, and fiber; but, call me Popeye, spinach is my favorite. In addition to being a great source of magnesium, potassium, and manganese, it's also sky high in vitamin K, which your body converts to K_2 to help direct calcium to your bones instead of your blood vessel walls, kidneys, or brain, where it can cause dangerous plaques.

How to eat it: Spinach's delicate texture and mild flavor makes it super versatile—

...sive addition to juices, smooth-
... soups—and tasty whether eaten
... sautéed.

*...ernatives: Swiss chard, kale, mustard
...reens, collard greens, beet greens*

Mineral-Rich Food #3:
Red Bell Pepper

Iron: 0.6 mg (4% of RDI)
Manganese: 0.2 mg (8% of RDI)
Potassium: 314 mg (9% of RDI)
(per cup, raw)

To be sure, all bell peppers, no matter their color—and all types of peppers, for that matter—are full of beneficial nutrients. But red bells pack a big mineral punch because they're left to ripen on the vine the longest. They're a good source of iron, as well as vitamin C. In fact, 1 cup of chopped red bell pepper provides a whopping 317 percent of the RDI for this vitamin. And that's important, because vitamin C enhances the body's ability to absorb iron. Red bell peppers are also especially high in the carotenoid antioxidant capsanthin (which contributes to their bright red color), as well as good sources of the carotenoids beta-carotene and lutein, both of which play important roles in eye health. Sweet red bell peppers are also rich in the nutrient lycopene, which has antioxidant properties and may help boost heart health, as well as protect against certain cancers.

How to eat it: Red bell peppers are sweet, not spicy, and are extremely versatile. En-joy them raw as crudités with dip or on top of salads. Toss them into a stir-fry or veggie sauté, or try stuffing them with quinoa and baking them. They also hold up to roasting and light grilling.

Alternatives: Yellow or orange bell peppers (green are too acidic); chile peppers

Mineral-Rich Food #4:
Brussels Sprouts

Iron: 1.2 mg (7% RDI)
Magnesium: 20.2 mg (5% RDI)
Manganese: 0.3 mg (15% RDI)
Potassium: 342 mg (10% RDI)
(per cup, raw)

Like red bell peppers, Brussels sprouts contain the beneficial synergistic pairing of iron and vitamin C. Low in calories, at less than 40 per cup, Brussels sprouts are also low-carb, with just 8 grams per cup. They're a nutrient powerhouse, with great levels of vitamins, minerals, antioxidants, and fiber, which is crucial for normal gut function. And they may provide cancer protection, thanks to their content of compounds called glucosinolates and such antioxidants as kaempferol. What's more, they're also one of the best plant sources of the omega-3 alpha-linolenic acid (ALA), which is important for driving down inflammation in your cells and body.

How to eat it: Take care to avoid over-cooking Brussels, especially if you're boiling them, as it will only intensify their bitter flavor. Proper cooking renders them almost sweet: try them roasted or sautéed, simply with just a little olive oil, salt, and pepper. You can even enjoy them raw and thinly sliced in salads.

Alternatives: Broccoli, cauliflower, cabbage, kale, collard greens

Mineral-Rich Food #5: Broccoli

Potassium: 457 mg (10% of RDI)
Magnesium: 32 mg (8% of RDI)
Chromium: 18.55 mcg (53% of RDI)
Phosphorus: 104.5 mg (15% of RDI)
Iron: 1 mg (6% of RDI)
Calcium: 62 mg (6% of RDI)
(per cup, raw)

Broccoli is versatile, tasty, full of fiber, and a great delivery system for sulforaphane, which has been shown to have powerful anticancer properties; antioxidants, which can cool the inflammation that plays a role in nearly every chronic disease; and isothiocyanates, which improves detoxification by preparing toxic compounds for elimination. Speaking of elimination, broccoli's high fiber content helps keep you regular. On top of all this, broccoli also contains a lot of different minerals.

How to eat it: How can't you eat broccoli? It is tasty eaten raw, lightly steamed (which may increase the sulforaphane content), sautéed, or blended into soups. This is definitely a vegetable you'll want to add to

your basket every time you go to the grocery store, so that you always have some on hand.

Alternatives: Brussels sprouts, cabbage, cauliflower

Mineral-Rich Food #6: Watercress

Calcium: 40.8 mg (4% RDI)
Manganese: 0.1 mg (4% RDI)
Potassium: 112 mg (3% RDI)
(per cup, raw)

The term *nutrient density* refers to the quantity of nutrients a food contains in proportion to how many calories it provides. Because watercress is an extremely low-calorie yet vitamin- and mineral-rich food, it is highly nutrient dense. Indeed, it ranks as the most nutrient-dense food on the CDC's Powerhouse Fruits and Vegetables list, in part thanks to its concentration of minerals, including calcium, manganese, and potassium, along with vitamins A, C, and K. Like the other cruciferous veggies mentioned earlier, it's rich in free radical–neutralizing antioxidants and glucosinolates (which get broken down into isothiocyanates). It's also a good source of dietary nitrates, which benefit heart health by reducing inflammation and stiffness in blood vessels and lowering blood pressure.

How to eat it: Watercress packs a slight, perhaps unexpected, peppery kick, a lot like arugula. Use it as you would any leafy green—in salads, sandwiches, smoothies, sautés, and the list goes on. Just keep in mind that it will cook up and wilt much faster than tougher, hardier greens, such as kale. You can also use it in place of basil for an exciting twist on pesto!

Alternatives: Arugula, spinach, endive, dandelion greens, beet greens, radicchio, radish sprouts

Mineral-Rich Food #7: Cucumber

Manganese: 0.2 mg (12% RDI)
Potassium: 442 mg (13% RDI)
Magnesium: 39.1 mg (10% RDI)
Phosphorus: 72. 2 mg (7% RDI)
Copper: 0.1 mg (6% RDI)
(1 average-size, with peel, raw)

Cucumbers really are "cool": not only can they help calm and soothe irritated, inflamed skin when applied externally, but they're packed with vitamins and minerals, including copper, which I've yet to discuss here. Copper plays a role in everything from bone health to immune system function, and it also helps the body absorb iron. Not to mention, cucumbers are a great choice for hydration, as they're 95 percent water and also contain the electrolyte minerals potassium and magnesium, which help balance the amount of water in your body. Cucumbers are also rich in the anticancer compound cucurbitacin, as well as anti-inflammatory and antioxidant phytonutrients. Of note is the flavonoid fisetin, which may improve cognition and memory.

How to eat it: Consume cucumbers raw, as crudités or in salads. They're also a great ingredient for chilled soups, such as gazpacho. When fermented as pickles, cucumbers provide even more nutritional benefits.

Alternatives: There are an incredible number of types of cucumbers out there, each with a slightly different taste profile; experiment with these varieties. If you're looking to mimic the coolness and crunch of cucumber, try jicama or celery.

Mineral-Rich Food #8: Kale

Manganese: 0.5 mg (26% RDI)
Copper: 0.2 mg (10% RDI)
Potassium: 299 mg (9% RDI)
Calcium: 90.5 mg (9% RDI)
(per cup, raw)

Hands down, kale is one of the most nutrient-dense foods out there. Not only is it rich in the minerals listed above, it's low in oxalate, a substance found in some plant foods that can prevent your body from absorbing the minerals found in them. It's a win-win! It's also one of the best sources of vitamin K there is, and a good source of B vitamins, too, including vitamin B_6, along with vitamins A and C. More specifically, it's abundant in the antioxidant beta-carotene, which the body converts into vitamin A. Vitamin A is important for skin and hair health, as well as immune and reproductive function. Kale is one of the best sources of lutein, which, as I briefly mentioned earlier, is involved in eye health;

lutein may help reduce the risk of macular degeneration and cataracts.

How to eat it: Enjoy it raw in salads or steamed, sautéed, and added to your favorite soup or casserole recipes. When making a raw kale salad, massage the leaves with your hands to soften them and release their nutrients. You might also try baking it to make kale chips: remove the stems from the kale, chop or rip the leaves into bite-size pieces, toss with olive oil and seasonings, and bake until crispy—or see the recipe on page 255 for some flavoring ideas.

Alternatives: Collard greens, cabbage, Brussels sprouts

Mineral-Rich Food #9:
Celery

Potassium: 286 mg (8% RDI)
Manganese: 0.1 mg (6% RDI)
Calcium: 40.4 mg (4% RDI)
(per cup, raw)

Similar to cucumbers, celery is mostly water and incredibly hydrating, yet high in soluble and insoluble fiber and mineral content. Indeed, it contains an array of minerals essential to bodily functions, a mixture that may also help neutralize acidic foods and aid in digestion. But it's not just fiber and minerals that make celery an excellent digestive aid and intestinal healer: the veggie contains the anti-inflammatory compound apiuman, which has been shown to decrease risk of stomach ulcer and improve the integrity of the stomach lining. Actually, celery contains

upward of twenty-five anti-inflammatory compounds that can help dampen that internal fire throughout the body, thus reducing risk of disease.

How to eat it: Celery is best enjoyed as fresh as possible. Of course, it can be eaten raw with a salad, as crudités with dip, or topped with almond butter with a sprinkle of Himalayan pink salt and hemp seeds. But it's also delicious steamed, braised, or added to stir-fries or juices. And don't discard the leaves: they contain more potassium and calcium than the stalks. Add the leaves to salads or sautés, and use them along with the stalks in soups and stews.

Alternatives: Cucumbers, jicama, fennel, bok choy

Mineral-Rich Food #10:
Spaghetti Squash

Manganese: 0.1 mg (6% RDI)
Potassium: 109 mg (3% RDI)
Iron: 0.3 mg (2% RDI)
Zinc: 0.2 mg (1% RDI)
(per cup, raw)

Spaghetti squash contains a mix of nine minerals that play important roles in bone health, most notably manganese. This particular mineral may help prevent osteoporosis by boosting bone structure and metabolism. Working in combination with other minerals, such as zinc, it helps support bone density. This squash is low in calories and high in fiber, especially when compared to pasta made with refined flour, for which it can easily be substituted. It's also a good source of vitamins A and C, which act as antioxidants in the body, as well as omega-3 fatty acids, which combat inflammation, among other health benefits.

How to eat it: This winter squash variety can be easily prepared a number of ways: steamed, slow cooked, baked, you name it. As I mentioned above, it is often used as a healthier, more nutritious substitute for pasta. That's because when it's cooked, its flesh can be scraped into spaghetti-like strands with a fork. Top with your favorite sauce or use in any recipe you would use noodles. Or try stuffing halves of the squash with your favorite ingredients and baking.

Alternatives: Other winter squash varieties, such as acorn, butternut, and pumpkin; or zucchini

Other Mineral Superstars

Avocado. You are going to hear a lot more about avocados in the next chapter, but you don't have to wait until then to start adding them. In addition to being a great source of fat, an avocado is also a great mineral delivery system, with good amounts of potassium, magnesium, and copper.

Cacao. It's not *all* about the greens—you do get to have fun with your new mineral-rich ways! Cacao is a great source of iron, magnesium, potassium, and calcium. You can have it in Chocolate Chia Pudding (page 260), Avocado Chocolate Mousse (page 263, which you can have for breakfast, lunch, dinner, or snack), and even a 100 percent cacao chocolate bar.

YOUR RE-MINERALIZING ACTION PLAN

Now that you know *why* minerals are so important, it's time to start getting more of them into your body. Here's exactly how I want you to go about doing just that.

Eat your minerals. For the next three days, your primary mission is to have three forms of greens—it could be a green smoothie, green juice, green soup, a salad, or a scoop of greens powder mixed into a glass of water—per day. Definitely prioritize the top ten mineral-rich foods (or their alternatives, if you prefer those) in all your meals and snacks, but your real barometer of whether you are "getting" this challenge is those three doses of greens per day. Don't worry too much about whatever else you're eating on these days; you'll naturally crowd out some of the less healthy things you might otherwise be eating.

Switch out your salt. You already got rid of your table salt during the Detox Your Pantry phase, right? If you didn't then, do it now, and replace it with one of the salts I list on page 92, which contain trace minerals. Using them in your cooking will help up your daily mineral intake.

Give yourself extra doses. Once a day for the next three days, treat yourself to an extra shot of minerals. You can do this by adding ⅛ teaspoon of Himalayan pink salt (or other salt I list on page 92) to a glass of water, or mixing it into a teaspoon of coconut oil, or taking a mineral supplement that combines sodium bicarbonate, calcium, magnesium, and potassium (see the Resources section for a recommendation). I advise taking your minerals thirty minutes before bedtime in a small (4-ounce) glass of water—getting your minerals at night will help your body wind down for sleep. It will also help neutralize the acids and toxins your body processes as you sleep, so that it won't have to rev itself up by doing all that work. You'll sleep better and wake up energized.

Soak in your minerals. Take at least one Epsom salts bath in the next three days. Bonus points for taking one every day (see page 92 for details).

Don't panic. If you don't like the taste of greens or the other mineral-rich foods, stick with it, and don't let yourself believe that you'll never like these foods. You are retraining your taste buds. Two weeks from now, you'll have changed your palate, and you will even start to crave these foods because they provide your body with such vital nutrients. I promise! So, anytime you catch yourself thinking, "I can't do this for the rest of my life," and maybe even feeling sorry for yourself, know that your tastes—and your thoughts—will change quickly if you stick with it.

SERVING SIZES OF MINERAL-RICH GREEN FOODS

To make it simple, I'm suggesting you get *at least* three green-based foods (be they a juice,

a smoothie, a soup, a salad, or a powder) per day. But ultimately, you're seeking to have 7 to 10 servings of mineral-rich green foods per day, broken into 2 or 3 per meal (when you're having three meals a day; you'll need to make this 4 or 5 per meal if and when you get down to two meals a day, as I outline in Step 5). To help you gauge how to hit those targets, here are the serving sizes of different types of greens:

> Green vegetables, raw: 1 cup
>
> Green vegetables, cooked: ½ cup
>
> Green juice, smoothie, or soup: 1 cup

Sample Day of Step 1

First thing in the morning beverage: A scoop of powdered greens or ⅛ teaspoon of Himalayan pink salt mixed into a glass of water

Breakfast: Skinny Mint Green Smoothie (page 217)

Lunch: Perfect Salad in a Jar (page 234)

Optional afternoon pick-me-up: Fresh or powdered green drink (a bonus; more is better)

Dinner: Have a raw green soup as part of your evening meal (choose your favorite from the section starting on page 225)

Before bed: Water with a pinch of Himalayan pink salt or minerals powder

* Eat three servings of greens per day (you'll work up to 7 to 10 servings per day over time, so if you're already eating 3 servings of greens per day, make it your goal for the next three days to eat 2 to 3 servings per *meal*).

* Procure a high-quality sea salt (choose one from the list on page 92).

* Take one extra dose of minerals per day, per the instructions on page 98.

* Take at least one Epsom salts bath.

* Remind yourself that your taste buds are changing.

TRACK YOUR JOURNEY

So that you can assess the immediate impact of getting more minerals, record how you felt on each of these three days in the chart on page 207 of this book.

I was at a low point in my health journey. Work had been very stressful for months, I was getting minimal sleep, and trying to be there for my family too. I gained twenty-five pounds by skipping meals, eating processed food, rewarding myself with snacks at midnight, and sitting in front of a computer most of my day. I needed a change. Following Dr. Daryl's program is the best thing I have ever done for myself. I stopped dairy, gluten, and caffeine first. Within a couple of weeks, I started to feel better. Next I started taking greens powder and mineral powder every day. It was amazing how much better I felt, but I wanted more. I bought a mini trampoline and bounced twice a day. I did Dr. Daryl's cleanse. I am not a cook but his recipes got me into the kitchen. Within a few months, I had lost twenty-six pounds, felt great, and was on the health journey for life. This program was everything I needed and more. My mother fought cancer three different times and it finally won. If only we had this information back then! —LEAH R.

seven

Step 2 (Days 4–6):
Add More Healthy Fats

In this second step, you're going to continue getting your three servings of greens each day, and you'll start adding in plenty of fat with each meal and each snack (although the fat will quickly help you feel fuller, longer, so this is where you'll likely start to notice that you don't *need* snacks the way you once did—go with it).

Every single day, I have a conversation with a patient who, when I tell them they need to start eating more healthy fats, looks at me as if I have two heads and says, "I can't eat more fat! I'll get fat!" For decades we have been brainwashed—often by the sugar industry—to think that fat is the root of all nutritional evil. The truth is that some fats are healthy—and they are crucial for your short- and long-term wellness. You not only want to eat them, you want to eat a *lot* of them. In fact, your target is to consume 50 to 70 percent of your daily calories from healthy fats.

Fat has gotten a bad rap for decades; it really culminated in the low-fat craze that swept America in the 1990s (remember Snackwells fat-free cookies?) and still continues to this day (think of the popularity of the air fryer). I know it's hard to undo that programming. But denying yourself of healthy fat is one of the unhealthiest things you can do; without it, your body is forced to burn sugar for fuel, your glucose and insulin levels remain high, your brain doesn't get the building blocks it needs to function well, and your heart health suffers.

Of course, you can't keep eating CRAP-py (completely refined and processed) carbs and then add a lot of fat on top of that—you will gain weight and you won't get the benefit of burning fat for fuel or lowering blood glucose and insulin levels. That's why the first step in Get Off Your Sugar is to eat more mineral-rich foods—all those greens will give you the nutrients and the fiber you need to make the transition to burning fat and also crowd the carb-rich foods off your plate naturally. Once you start adding in the fats, too, you'll feel full for so much longer that not only won't you have the room for the carb-rich foods, you won't have the appetite for them either.

Before we go into *how* to start eating more healthy fats, let's talk about *why* they're good for you.

BENEFITS OF HEALTHY FATS

Just to make sure you're fully on board with the idea of eating more fat, I want to give you a little tour of the many powerful things eating healthy fats does for you.

- **Regulates weight.** Just as it's true that eating sugar leads to burning sugar leads to craving sugar, eating fat leads to burning fat (and also leads to the eradication of your cravings for sweet stuff!). At any given time, the average person has tens of thousands of calories stored in their fat cells; eating more fat is how to start to unlock those calories, burn body fat, and lose excess weight. Once you start feeding your body good fats, it will think, "Oh, we're getting good calories here; it's okay to release some of this extra fat we've been carrying around because clearly there will be more coming."

  Even if you are slim, the most dangerous fat in the body is the fat that accumulates around your abdominal organs (also called visceral fat or belly fat); eating fat and burning fat will help shed that dangerous-for-you fat too. Just to be clear, if you start consuming a lot more fat *without* also cutting down on carbs, you'll gain weight. You really can't live in both worlds. But because my program is based on adding foods to your diet, you will naturally crowd out the carbs as you progress through the steps. This step is where you'll really start to notice your cravings are lessening; as long as you follow the steps I prescribe in the order I prescribe them, your carb intake will lessen significantly.

- **Protects the brain.** Your brain is 60 percent fat, and ketones are its preferred fuel. The nerve endings in your brain are also lined with fat, which comprises 70 percent of the myelin sheath, the natural coating that forms around nerves that facilitates communication and prevents damage. When you eat more healthy fats, your brain works better; brain fog lifts, mood stabilizes, and the risk of dementia goes down.

- **Improves your cholesterol numbers.** Most cholesterol is actually your friend, as research has found that the lower overall cholesterol levels are, the higher the risk of death. Eating more healthy saturated fats, medium-chain triglycerides, and monounsaturated fats raises your HDL (or "good") cholesterol. LDL is typically labeled "bad," but there are two different types of LDL—a light, dense, fluffy form that is benign; and the smaller, denser form, which is more likely to oxidize and damage arterial walls. Eating more fat also raises levels of the fluffy, benign form of LDL. While conventional medicine will tell you that any total cholesterol level over 200 is bad, research says the sweet spot is between 200 and 240; anything under 180 is problematic and a sign that you need more healthy fats in your diet.

Promotes feelings of fullness and eradicates cravings. Eating more healthy fat keeps you fuller, longer. That alone will help ward off snack attacks. However, eating more healthy fats also dramatically lessens cravings because it helps you become a fat burner, which means your body won't go into freak-out mode after every meal once your blood sugar levels decline. The more you replace carbs, sugars, and excess proteins in your diet with mineral-rich foods and healthy fats, the lower and more stable your blood sugar will be. And that means fewer cravings.

Reduced likelihood of developing cancer. Of course, our understanding of the science behind cancer continues to grow and evolve by the day, but there is a growing school of thought that since cancer cells rely on the fermentation of sugar for their energy (rather than a process that healthy cells use, known as the Krebs cycle, which uses oxygen), reducing carbs and increasing healthy fats deprives cancer of the fuel it needs to grow. This is a theory based on the work of Dr. Otto Warburg, a Nobel Prize–winning German physician who, in the 1920s, discovered that cancer cells derive their energy through fermentation, and Dr. Thomas Seyfried, a professor of biology at my alma mater, Boston College, and author of *Cancer as a Metabolic Disease.*

Improved absorption of nutrients. Many nutrients, including vitamins A, D, E, and K, are fat-soluble, which means they need to be eaten with fat in order for your body to be able to absorb them. This explains why a 2017 study found that people who ate salad with an oil-based dressing absorbed higher amounts of eight micronutrients than did folks who ate the salad with no oil-based dressing.[1]

FATS THAT HEAL, FATS THAT KILL

While it's absolutely true that fat is a vital part of health, it's *also* true that not *all* fat is good for you. There are some that are downright dangerous all on their own—namely **trans fats**, also known as partially hydrogenated fats, which are found in processed foods and fried foods. There are other fats that are okay in moderation but become problematic when you have too much of them—primarily pro-inflammatory **omega-6 fats** from vegetable oils, which you'll learn more about in just a moment, and **saturated fats** from conventionally raised animals, which you'll learn more about in Chapter 8.

The healthy fats you want to start eating more of in this step—and from here on out—are:

Certain polyunsaturated fats. There are two basic kinds of polyunsaturated fats: the "good" omega-3 fatty acids, which are anti-inflammatory, and the "bad" omega-6 fatty acids, which are pro-inflammatory. Now, both omega-3s and omega-6s are what's known as essential fatty acids—essential because you need them to function, and your body can't make them on its own. Omega-6s on their own aren't inherently bad—after all, inflammation in the short term is what helps you heal from injury. So, you do want to consume some omega-6s, which primarily are found in nuts and seeds. It's just that in our modern diet, we tend to eat far too many omega-6s (because they are what's found in vegetable oils, such as corn, soy, sunflower, safflower, cottonseed, peanut, and canola oils, used in nearly all processed foods).

When you eat more omega-6s than omega-3s, you get inflammation everywhere, especially in the brain, where they have to compete for the same enzymes. Inflammation in the short run is how our body heals: if you slam your finger in the door, inflammation is bringing nutrients and oxygen to damaged tissue. But if inflammation is chronic and prolonged, that's creating every degenerative inflammatory disease, heart disease, diabetes, cancer.

There are three different types of omega-3s: **alpha-linolenic acid (ALA)**, which is plant-based (from flax, chia, hemp), and **docosahexaenoic acid (DHA)** and **eicosapentaenoic acid (EPA)**, which are animal-based (from wild-caught salmon, pastured egg yolks and beef, and purified fish oil). DHA supports healthy brain development and cognitive function, whereas EPA fights inflammation. ALA needs to be converted by the body into EPA and DHA, but this is a very inefficient process. For this reason, the best way to insure you're getting enough omega-3s is to get it from purified fish oil supplements.

Together, omega-3s trigger the process of purging damaged cells known as apoptosis, which is a vital way your body rids itself of disease. On the other hand, omega-6s oxidize your cells and can allow cancer to proliferate. They also enhance the risk of depression, shorten your telomeres (the proteins that seal the ends of your DNA strands—the longer they are, the longer you are likely to be healthy and stay alive), and are associated with aging, heart disease, and dementia.

As humans evolved, we were eating primarily foods that are high in omega-3s, such as fish, nuts, meat, eggs, and seeds. Over the last 150 years, we've started eating way more refined, omega-6-rich oils and the processed foods that contain them. Now, omega-3 deficiency contributes to ninety-six thousand preventable deaths per year. (See the box on page 107 for more about how to ensure you get enough omega-3s.)

Monounsaturated fats. These are omega-9 fats, and include avocados, olives, avocado oil, and olive oil, as well as sesame oil, macadamia nuts, pistachios, and almonds. One monounsaturated fat is oleic acid, which is what avocados are high in—77 percent of the calories in an avocado come from oleic acid. This is great news, as oleic acid reduces inflammation and has been shown to be protective against heart disease and cancer.

The right saturated fats. The healthiest saturated fats are medium-chain triglycerides (MCTs), which are found in coconut oil and MCT oil. These fats are anti-inflammatory, antioxidants, buffers of acids, and great at nudging your body into fat-burning because they bypass the digestive tract and go straight to your liver, where they are converted into ketones—the fatty acids the body uses as a preferred source of fuel.

I consider coconut oil to be a perfect food. It's highly alkaline. It's also incredibly versatile—it can be used in sautéing and baking as it can withstand high temperatures without degrading, and can also be eaten raw—either mixed into a smoothie or right off the spoon. It also contains capric, caprylic, and lauric acids, which are antimicrobial, antibacterial, antiviral, and antifungal, meaning it helps you ward off infections. It also helps kill yeast, as yeast is a fungus. Because yeast contributes to cravings, when you give your body more coconut oil, you kill more yeast, and your cravings lessen even more. As a bonus, you can even rub the oil on your skin, as it makes a great moisturizer and makeup remover.

Fats to avoid. Just as important as eating enough healthy fats each day is avoiding the fats that can skew your omega-6 to omega-3 ratio and contribute to disease. They are:

Canola oil

Conventionally raised beef, chicken, eggs, pork

Corn oil

Cottonseed oil

Cured meats (lunch meats, hot dogs, salami)

Farmed fish (including salmon)

Grapeseed oil

Flax, hemp, and chia oils*

Hydrogenated oil

Margarine

Peanuts

Peanut butter

Peanut oil

Safflower oil

Shortening

Soybeans

Soybean oil

Sunflower oil

Trans fats

Walnut oil*

*The whole-food versions of these are healthy; it's just that their oils quickly oxidize and turn rancid.

THE MOST IMPORTANT NUMBER YOU NEED TO KNOW

A primary reason why omega-3s are so important is that they counterbalance the inflammatory effects of omega-6 oils. For this reason, you really want to make sure that you keep your blood levels of omega-6s and omega-3s in close proximity to each other. Anything below a 4:1 ratio of omega-6s to omega-3s is considered healthy. Above that, things start to go downhill. Above 10:1 is very serious, and anything above 15:1 is a critical problem as you have a high potential of developing a chronic degenerative disease. For my previous book, *Get Off Your Acid*, I interviewed Dr. Joseph Hibbeln, who did studies on murderers and people in insane asylums, and he found that on average their ratios were 70:1! They had so much neuro-inflammation that their brains got hijacked, and they couldn't make sane decisions.

Sadly, the average American has a ratio of omega-6 to omega-3 that is as high as 20:1. I have tested the ratios of thousands of patients, and I commonly see numbers ranging from to 25:1 to 50:1. I even tested a high school student who was having severe depression, and her ratio was 88:1, which is extremely dangerous. Knowing and optimizing your ratio matters, and it matters a lot.

You can have your overall omega-3 levels as well as your ratio of omega-6 to omega-3 measured by your doctor, but their method of measurement—a serum blood test—isn't all that accurate. A serum blood test uses blood drawn from your arm, and it reflects only the omega-3s present in your body for the last couple of days. So, if you had salmon for dinner two nights ago, it could look as if your omega-3 levels are fine, when overall they are low.

In my practice, I measure the levels of essential fatty acids of my patients by administering a capillary blood test, which tests the 75 percent of your blood found in the smaller vessels of your body—as opposed to the 25 percent circulating in your veins and arteries. Because the blood in these small vessels doesn't turn over as quickly as your venous blood, a capillary test assesses your average level of omega-3s over the last 120 days.

Recently, one patient came in with many of the hallmarks of omega-3 deficiency: dry skin, hair that was falling out, brittle nails, skin issues, and low energy. According to her doctor (and her serum blood test), this patient had levels of omega-3s that were too high! Even though she ate salmon about once a week, her symptoms were screaming omega-3 deficiency. I suggested she take the capillary test. (I told her if her levels were still high, I wouldn't charge her for the test; that's how confident I was.) The capillary test showed that her ratio of omega-6s to omega-3s was 28:1!

It just goes to show you how many conventional doctors aren't up on the latest research—many have never even heard of this test before, so if they are testing your ratios, they're testing using serum blood instead of capillary blood.

In my practice, we offer the Alkamind Omega-3 Acid Inflammation Test. It's an at-home test kit that uses a painless, needle-less drop of blood from your finger and tells you your overall omega-3 levels as well as your omega-6 to omega-3 ratio. (You can learn more about it in the Resources section.)

THE BEST WAY TO ENSURE YOU GET ENOUGH OMEGA-3S

The best way to rectify any imbalance in your omega-6 to omega-3 ratio is to consume more omega-3s. And while you can get omega-3 fatty acids from foods (including some wild-caught fish—salmon, as well as anchovies, sardines, trout, and herring—pastured egg yolks, and hemp, chia, and flaxseeds) and you should absolutely eat those foods on a regular basis, you have to eat an awful lot of them to get the recommended daily 3 grams of omega-3s. On top of that, most wild-caught fish is contaminated with heavy metals, such as mercury. That's why the best way to ensure you're getting all the omega-3s you need is to take fish oil supplements that have been purified to remove mercury and other contaminants. Ideally you want those omega-3s in a 2:1 ratio of EPA (which reduces inflammation) to DHA (which optimizes brain function); check the label, it should list the amounts of each of these essential fatty acids. The one exception to this ratio is children; because their brains and nervous systems are still developing, they need more DHA than EPA. Also, I recommend pregnant women take extra omega-3s each day, especially in the first trimester (or ideally even before you get pregnant) as the baby's brain forms early, and DHA is a crucial ingredient for healthy brain development. *As always, consult with your health-care provider before beginning a supplement regimen.*

THE SECRET FAT THAT REPAIRS THE DNA DAMAGE CAUSED BY SUGAR

As if you need another reason to get your omega-3s, a 2019 good news/bad news scientific discovery makes it even more vital that you do. First, the bad news: researchers at UCLA found that fructose actually changes the way the DNA in your brain is expressed by altering which genes get turned on and which get turned off. Many diseases, including diabetes, cardiovascular disease, Alzheimer's disease, and ADHD, are linked to genetic changes in brain DNA.

The good news is that these researchers also found that DHA reverses the genetic changes that fructose contributes to. Xia Yang, a senior author of the study and a UCLA assistant professor of integrative biology and physiology, said, "DHA changes not just one or two genes; it seems to push the entire gene pattern back to normal, which is remarkable."[2] When you get off your sugar and up your healthy fats—including DHA—you really are impacting your health for the better, all the way down to the genetic level.

This wasn't the first time sugar has been linked to declines in cognitive function. A 2012 study fed rats a high-fructose corn syrup–sweetened beverage for six weeks, then tested the rats' ability to remember a maze they had learned before the experiment began. The rats were slower and had less activity between the synapses in their brain. The researchers fed a separate group of rats omega-3 fatty acids, including DHA, for the same amount of time; that group got better and faster at the maze.[3]

THE HEALTHY FATS TO START EATING NOW (AND KEEP EATING THROUGH THE REST OF THE PROGRAM)

The following is a list of the healthy fats you want to start eating on a regular basis. I've bolded the very best ones—prioritize eating those, but anything on this list will help you get and stay in a fat-burning zone. You can eat them alone, start cooking with them, or sprinkle them on top of your greens and salads. I think you'll find that they make everything more delicious and filling.

CATEGORY	FOOD	SERVING SIZE
Omega-3s	**Wild-caught salmon**	Size of a checkbook
	Trout	Size of a checkbook
	Herring	Size of a checkbook
	Sardines	¼ cup
	Anchovies	¼ cup
	Pastured, organic egg	1 egg
	Purslane	½ cup
Raw seeds	Black seeds (also called black cumin)	1 tablespoon
	Chia seeds	1 tablespoon
	Flaxseeds	1 tablespoon
	Hemp seeds	1 tablespoon
	Pumpkin seeds	1 tablespoon
	Sesame seeds	1 tablespoon
	Sunflower seeds	1 tablespoon
Raw nuts	Almonds	Small handful (5–10 nuts)
	Baru nuts	Small handful (5–10 nuts)
	Brazil nuts	Small handful (2–3 nuts)
	Hazelnuts	Small handful (5–10 nuts)
	Pecans	Small handful (5–10 nuts)
	Walnuts	Small handful (5–10 nuts)
Raw nut butters	Almond butter	1 tablespoon
	Cacao butter	1 tablespoon

	Coconut butter	1 tablespoon
	Hazelnut butter	1 tablespoon
	Hemp butter	1 tablespoon
	Macadamia nut butter	1 tablespoon
	Tahini	1 tablespoon
Raw oils	Avocado oil	1 tablespoon
	Coconut oil	1 tablespoon
	MCT oil	1 tablespoon
	Extra-virgin olive oil	1 tablespoon
Nut milks	Almond milk, unsweetened	½ cup
	Coconut milk, unsweetened (carton)	½ cup
	Coconut milk (canned)	½ cup
	Hemp milk, unsweetened	½ cup
	Avocado	½ avocado
	Coconut meat (shredded, unsweetened)	1 tablespoon
	Olives, kalamata	5

YOUR ASSIGNMENT: GET THE GOOD FATS YOU NEED

I want to make this very simple for you. Over the next three days, keep your greens intake going *and* make sure you are getting seven to ten servings each day of the healthy fats I just listed. That breaks down to two or three servings per meal, based on three meals a day. If you're ahead of the game and already intermittent fasting (which you'll start doing in Step 5), you can eat them over your two meals a day and have one in the morning without breaking your fast.

Your cravings should be starting to lessen with the minerals you've been taking in; adding these healthy fats will help reduce them further. The only thing to be careful of now is to not eat too many carbs, because if you start eating more healthy fats without reducing your carb intake, you'll end up gaining weight. So, if you're going to have a snack, swap out your carb-heavy snacks (a bag of pretzels, for example) with a serving of one of the healthy fats.

...e it's true that the "eat fewer calo-
...s, lose weight" adage is false—because
not all calories are created equally, and
eating too many calories from sugar,
carbs, and (as you'll learn in the next
chapter) protein will result in storing fat
and gaining weight, it is still helpful to
know approximately how many calories
a day you should eat, because calories
are still a number that is easy to track.
Knowing your daily calorie target will
help you determine how many of those
calories should come from fat, protein,
and carbs.

Average man: 2,000 to 3,000 calories

Average woman: 1,600 to 2,400 calories

There is a range here because your ideal
calorie target depends on your age, size,
activity level, and whether you're pregnant.
Just remember, it's not only about the
quantity of calories you consume, it's about
the quality of those calories.

THE HEALTHIEST NUT IN THE WORLD (YOU'VE NEVER HEARD OF)

Baru nuts grow on 30-foot-tall trees in the savan-
nas of Brazil—trees that have a root system so
deep that they don't need any irrigation to grow.
They are one of the healthiest nuts in the world,
and are brought to the American market in an en-
vironmentally and culturally sustainable way by
the company Barùkas, which was founded by my
friend Darin Olien, a.k.a. the "Superfood Hunter."

A ¼-cup serving of the nuts has 140 calories com-
prising 10 grams of fat, 6 grams of protein, 12
grams of carbs, and 5 grams of fiber (for a total of
7 net carbs), as well as significant amounts of
magnesium, manganese, copper, potassium, calcium, and zinc. That's more fiber than in any nut
and more antioxidants than in the most popular
nuts, with 25 percent fewer calories (that is one
drawback of nuts—calories can add up quickly).
For such a healthy, plant-based source of protein
and fat, baru nuts also taste great—a cross between a cashew, an almond, and a peanut.

BAD/BETTER/BEST SOURCES OF FAT

NEVER	BETTER	BEST
Margarine	Grass-fed butter or ghee	Avocado, coconut butter, or raw nut butters
Commercial whipped cream	Heavy whipping cream, whipped	Full-fat coconut milk, whipped
Cow's milk or soy milk	Raw goat milk, raw camel milk, store-bought coconut*, almond*, or hemp milk* *carrageenan- and cane sugar–free	Homemade coconut, almond, or hemp milk

Milk chocolate	Dark chocolate (at least 80 percent)	Raw cacao or 100 percent dark chocolate (with no added sugar) or raw chocolate
Dairy yogurt	Coconut, almond, or hemp yogurt	Chia pudding or Avocado Chocolate Mousse (page 263)
Dairy cream cheese	Nut-based cream cheese, store bought	Homemade nut-based cream cheese, hummus, or guacamole

IS COCONUT OIL FAKE NEWS?

In 2018, the American Heart Association (AHA) issued a recommendation that people avoid the saturated fats in coconut oil and eat polyunsaturated fats—like those in vegetable oils—instead. And in a YouTube video that went viral, Karin Michels, an adjunct professor of epidemiology at Harvard T. H. Chan School of Public Health, called coconut oil "pure poison." So what's the deal, is coconut oil safe or not?

When you look at what the AHA based its 2018 recommendation on, it's four studies from the 1960s and 1970s that don't even look at the health effects of coconut oil—they used partially hydrogenated coconut oil, which is a different creature entirely from the virgin coconut oil that I and so many other health practitioners recommend. There have been plenty of studies in the last three decades that support a positive association between saturated fat consumption and heart health, including the Women's Health Initiative, which health writer Gary Taubes called "the single largest and most expensive clinical trial ever done."[4]

The conventional medical establishment, which includes the AHA, is still fixated on cholesterol as a cause of heart disease instead of on what it really is—a witness to the crime, but not the perpetrator. It's true that the fat in coconut oil is saturated and that eating coconut can raise overall cholesterol levels. So, when you eat this, you will see an overall increase in your total cholesterol, but this is a *good* thing, as increased total cholesterol (with healthy HDL and LDL markers) increases longevity and lowers cancer rates. Saturated fat, including the MCTs in coconut oil, does raise LDL levels, but the fluffy, benign form of LDL, not the bad, dense, sticky type.

On top of that, by suggesting that people replace saturated fat with polyunsaturated fats in vegetable oils, this health "advice" will only lead to dangerously high ratios of omega-6s to omega-3s and omega-3 deficiency. It's also going to increase inflammation and their potential for chronic inflammatory degenerative disease.

Strategies to Make Sure You're Getting Your 7 to 10 Servings of Healthy Fats

- Add a tablespoon of chia seeds to your powdered or fresh green smoothie that you started drinking in Step 1, or water, or unsweetened almond milk.

- Replace any unhealthy fats you've been eating with healthy fats—if you've been using bottled salad dressing, for example, which probably has omega-6 soybean or sunflower seed oil in it, switch to using a tablespoon of extra-virgin olive oil and freshly squeezed lemon juice.

- Cook with the raw oils listed on page 109.

- Add a tablespoon of one of these raw oils to your green smoothie.

- Blend healthy fat in your coffee or tea—add coconut oil, MCT oil, or Alkamind Acid Kicking Coffee Alkalizer.

- Add raw nuts and seeds to your salads, salmon, wraps, or veggies.

- If you need a snack, snack on raw nuts, raw seeds, olives, or avocado slices.

- Top any dish with a tablespoon of healthy oil.

- Consider a fat bomb for dessert (for recipes, see pages 256–259).

STEP 2: ADD MORE HEALTHY FATS ACTION PLAN

* Start getting at least two or three servings of fat at every meal; supplement with high-fat snacks if needed.

* Keep eating, with the same frequency, the greens that you started consuming in Step 1.

* If you notice that you aren't as hungry for snacks in between meals, it's okay to start skipping them. If you're still wanting a snack, that's fine; just make it a healthy snack with plenty of fat.

TRACK YOUR JOURNEY

Capture how this step is affecting you by filling out the chart on page 207, and compare it to how you felt after Step 1.

eight

Step 3 (Days 7–9): Get Protein Smart

PROTEIN IS A VITAL COMPONENT OF ANY DIET. AFTER ALL, IT'S COMPOSED OF AMINO acids, which your body uses to build and repair your bones, muscles, and hormones—pretty important things to have. As important as protein is, we have put it on a pedestal. And I understand it—fat was vilified for decades, and lately carbs are coming under fire as being public enemy number one. The problem is that when it comes to protein, it is definitely possible to have too much of a good thing.

There are two main issues with protein: (1) your body needs a lot less of it than you probably think it does; and (2) most Americans are getting their protein from animal sources, which are high in pro-inflammatory omega-6 fats and toxic chemical residue, thanks to the soy and corn most animals are fed. Animal protein is also highly acidic and typically contains a lot of antibiotics (more on this in just a moment). You're not what you eat—you are what the animal you eat, eats!

If you are a meat lover, don't start shaking in your shoes just yet. I know people love their sushi or their steak—there's a place for some animal proteins in your diet if you choose. It's just that they should be kept to at most once a day, rather than at every single meal.

This step of the Get Off Your Sugar program is all about recalibrating your protein strategy. First, let's look a little more deeply at why you need to pay more attention to your protein.

THE PERILS OF TOO MUCH ANIMAL PROTEIN

You need a lot less protein for maintenance and repair than you likely think you do. Any protein you consume above the amount that your body needs for maintenance and repair gets converted into glucose by the liver in a process known as gluconeogenesis. This means that when you load up on animal protein, anything that isn't used elevates your blood sugar, which raises your insulin, which triggers fat storage, which explains why high protein consumption is linked to increased body weight.[1] Basically, if you eat a giant porterhouse steak, you're dumping sugar into your bloodstream and inviting extra pounds to settle in. It's important to note that you get into trouble only with animal protein, not from plant-based proteins.

In addition, eating too much animal protein has the following adverse effects:

- **Stresses the kidneys.** When you overconsume protein, you create high levels of blood urea nitrogen (BUN), which is a by-product of protein metabolism. BUN then cues the kidneys to get rid of water and carry along buffering minerals, such as calcium, magnesium, potassium, and sodium bicarbonate, with it. As a result, your kidneys are forced to overwork, you get dehydrated, and you get mineral deficient. High protein consumption has also been linked to kidney stones.[2]

- **Leaches minerals out of bones.** Other by-products of protein metabolism that are excreted by the kidneys are urea; ammonia; and the triple acid threat of nitric, sulfuric, and phosphoric acids. This triggers your bones and muscles to release some of their minerals to help buffer the acids, and then the minerals and the acids are flushed out of the body through the urine. Over time, this mineral depletion results in weakened bones.[3]

- **Feeds the growth of pathogenic bacteria, such as yeast.** Because excess protein is converted into sugar, and bad bacteria thrive on a sugar diet, eating too much protein contributes to high levels of yeast, in particular, candida.

- **Impairs gut function.** It's not just the quantity of protein the typical American eats, it's the poor quality of it too. Eighty percent of antibiotics sold in the United States are purchased by the livestock industry. You may think you haven't had antibiotics in years, but if you had conventionally raised chicken in your dinner last night, you had them yesterday (and likely the day before that and the day before that). And these antibiotics are like a napalm bomb going off in your gut, creating leaky gut that can affect you for years.

Animals raised on concentrated animal feeding operations (CAFOs), as a whopping *99 percent* of farm animals in the United States are,[4] are fed an artificial diet of grains high in omega-6 fats that are genetically modified to be resistant to pesticides, so they are doused in toxic chemicals too. The fats and the toxins get passed directly to you when you eat the meat. The antibiotics and the pesticides wipe out the friendly bacteria in your gut, and the omega-6s trigger inflammation that can lead to leaky gut. Also, when these animals are killed, you're literally eating their fear in the form of the cortisol they secrete in their last moments.

- **Increases your risk of cancer.** Too much protein stimulates an important signaling pathway in your body known as the mammalian target of rapamycin (mTOR) pathway. This is an ancient pathway that exists in virtually all organisms, including bacteria. Under normal circumstances, mTOR plays an important role in regeneration, but when it is overstimulated, it can trigger unwanted growth in the form of the proliferation of cancer cells. Reducing your protein intake has been shown in animal studies to inhibit mTOR,[5] which then lessens the likelihood of cancer growing.

- **Negatively impacts life span.** Within your body is a constant tension between damage (growth) and damage control (repair). One hormone that tilts the scale toward damage is insulin growth factor 1 (IGF-1), and your protein intake dictates how much IGF-1 you produce. IGF-1 is often found in milk that's been treated with bovine growth hormone, which has been linked to early puberty in girls; it's also known to mutate healthy human breast cells to cancerous cells and contribute to colon cancer. When you keep your protein intake low to moderate, you also keep IGF-1 low, which then boosts your life span. Dr. Ron Rosedale, author of *The Rosedale Diet*, says it simply: "Reducing protein extends life."

Really, reducing your carbs and upping your fat *without* also reducing your protein is like driving a Mercedes with one wheel off. Keeping your protein intake, and thus your glucose, insulin, mTOR, and IGF-1, low allows the body to stay pointed toward maintenance and repair and out of breakdown mode. Let's look at how to make sure you're getting just the right amount—and right kind—of protein.

CALCULATE HOW MUCH PROTEIN YOU NEED

The average American gets five times the amount of animal protein they need. As a general rule, you want to be getting somewhere between 40 and 70 grams of protein a day, and this amount should make up fewer than 20 percent of your total caloric intake. The exact amount of protein that's right for you depends on your size, activity level, and stage of life. The first step to calculate your daily protein target probably requires you to get out a calculator (unless you are pretty good at math).

You want to calculate how many grams of protein you need a day based on your *ideal* weight, not your actual weight. Let's say you weigh 150 pounds, but your ideal weight is 130. Take 130 and divide it by 2.2 to convert it to kilograms. In this instance, that answer is 59.09. Round that to the nearest whole number, which gives you 59.

Then, multiply your rounded weight in kilograms by 0.8, which reflects that you want to eat 0.8 grams of protein for every kilogram of weight. That answer is 47.27. Round that to nearest whole number and you get 47—how many grams of protein a person who really ought to weigh 130 pounds should eat in total each day.

If you're pregnant, an athlete, have a very physical job (such as landscaping or moving furniture), or are over seventy,[6] increase that by 25 percent.

At the bottom of this page is a form to help you find your daily protein target. Take the final number at the end of each line and move it to the beginning of the next line.

WHAT "THE RIGHT" AMOUNT OF PROTEIN LOOKS LIKE ON YOUR PLATE

Once you know your daily protein target, you want to spread that total out evenly throughout the day. So, if you're having three meals a day, and your daily protein target is 47 grams, that's 15 to 16 grams of protein at every meal. Once you start intermittent fasting (which we'll cover in Step 5) and eating only two meals a day, that's 23 to 24 grams at each meal.

To give you an idea of what that will look like on your plate, a 3-ounce serving of cooked meat (about the size of a deck of cards) or flat fish (about the size of a checkbook) has, on average, 21 grams of protein in it, or about as much or more than the total amount of protein you should have in one meal. (So, an 8-ounce burger or an 18-ounce steak is way, way too much protein for one sitting!) One egg has 6 grams of protein; likewise, ½ cup of chickpeas has 6 grams. Remember that vegetables have protein in them too—spinach, for example, has 5 grams per cup, and raw kale has 2.5 grams per cup. And hemp seeds, the best vegetarian source of protein, provides 11 grams per three tablespoons. So, you can see how quickly you meet your protein needs; it doesn't take a big steak. If you're going to have animal-based protein, make it your goal to have 2 to 4 ounces of high-quality, pasture-raised animal protein and no more. Make the protein the side show, not the main event, and always pair it up with a salad or green vegetables. From a plate perspective, your mineral-rich vegetables and raw nuts and seeds should still be taking up the most space. Your protein will be your next-largest component, and then the fats will likely be drizzled on top.

CALCULATE YOUR DAILY PROTEIN INTAKE

Ideal weight: _____ pounds / 2.2 = _____ kilograms

_____ kilograms rounded to the nearest number = _____

_____ rounded kilograms x 0.8 = _____ grams

_____ grams rounded to the nearest number = _____ grams of protein you should be eating in a day that so did the vegetarians and vegans—70 percent more, in fact.[7]

QUICK CHECK-IN: HOW MUCH PROTEIN HAVE YOU REALLY BEEN EATING?

Just as it's helpful to look back at your actual food consumption to determine how much sugar you've been eating, it's also illuminating to calculate how much protein you've been consuming. Go back to the forty-eight-hour retrospective food diary you did on page 202 and use either nutritiondata.self.com or cronometer.com to count up how many grams of protein you ate.

I know that most who are reading this are going to skip over this very important exercise. In fact, the research says that number will be 80 percent of my readers. But to start changing your life, you're going to have to start doing things differently than you have in the past. You also cannot change a habit you don't know you have. So, please, illuminate yourself and calculate how much protein you've been eating!

Are you on track? If you're like most Americans, you've been eating three to five times more protein than you should be having, and that excess has been converted into sugar, which has been converted into fat. Bringing your protein consumption into line with the guidelines I'm sharing here will further help you get off your sugar (and lose weight).

It's important to note that **even if you're a vegetarian or a vegan, you're probably still eating way too much protein**! A 2013 study looked at the nutrient intake of over seventy-one thousand meat eaters, vegetarians, and vegans. Not surprisingly, the study showed that nonvegetarians got 80 percent more protein than they truly needed each day. What *was* surprising was that so did the vegetarians and vegans—70 percent more, in fact.[7]

THE UPSIDE OF EATING THE *RIGHT AMOUNT* OF PROTEIN

Although most Americans are eating as much as five times the amount of protein they need, there are a few of us who aren't eating *enough*. And eating too little protein is an invitation for cravings for CRAP-py (completely refined and processed) carbs. When your protein levels are low, your body knows it needs energy. So, it will crave the foods that will give you that energy the quickest—namely, carbs and sugar. Many times when a sugar craving hits, your body is really crying out for protein. If you consume the right amount of protein, and the right quality of protein, you will outsmart your cravings, as the protein only minimally impacts blood sugar and insulin (again, as long as you're not eating more than you need).

If you haven't been getting enough protein, upping your intake to the proper level can work wonders in helping to manage cravings—especially when you eat it regularly throughout the day. For starters, getting enough protein helps your body stay satiated and full, so you're less likely to resort to snacking on sugary foods. Protein also helps to keep blood glucose levels steady and greatly aids in the production of serotonin, the happiness hormone that also plays an essential role in the regulation of our appetite.

MAKE THE ANIMAL PROTEIN YOU EAT THE BEST IT CAN BE

While I am a huge proponent of eating more plant-based proteins, I'm not going to tell you to stop eating meat (except for chicken—see why in the box below). I will tell you to not eat more than you need, to keep the number of times you have it in a week to seven or less (one serving a day), and to make what meat you do eat the best possible quality.

In general, the best type of meat to eat is free-range, cage-free, no hormones or antibiotics added, from organic grasses grown in pasture. *Pastured* means the animals were allowed to forage for their natural diet—grass for cows, and grubs and seeds for chickens. Animals raised for food that aren't pastured are generally fed corn and soy that are naturally high in omega-6 fats and typically doused in pesticides and genetically modified organisms.

If you eat eggs, make sure you eat the yolk as well as the white because that's where the good omega-3 fats (DHA) are. To keep your protein intake in check, you don't need a three-egg omelet—one or two eggs (cooked in coconut or olive oil) and eaten with some avocado or sautéed greens will get you all the protein you need in one meal. Just make sure your eggs are from pastured, organic chickens (see why in the box on this page). I know pastured eggs cost more; they are worth the expense because nothing is more important than your health and your family's health.

Ultimately, eating higher-quality meats means you have to get back in the kitchen, because the more you eat out, the more you lose control of your ingredients. Look at it this way: your top priority is your health. A restaurant's top priority is its bottom line, and very, very few will pay extra for better ingredients—even Michelin five-star restaurants! If you are going to eat meat, eat it at home because it costs restaurants so much more to buy wild-caught or grass-fed animal proteins that if it doesn't say "grass fed" or "wild-caught" on the menu, I can all but guarantee you that it's not. If a restaurant spends the money for healthy animal proteins, you can guarantee it is going to let you know about it. Save meat for your at-home menu, where you can control the quality.

The best way to ensure the quality of your meats and eggs is to buy them at a farmers' market or farm stand where you can talk to the farmer about their practices. There are also many websites where you can buy meat from reputable sources. (For salmon, my favorite source is Vital Choice.com.) And by reducing the quantity of meat you buy, you should be able to spend a similar amount of money for higher-quality meat.

||||||||||||||||||||||||||||||||||||||||||||||||||||||||||||||||||||||||||||||||||

THE #1 MOST INFLAMMATORY ANIMAL PROTEIN (HINT: IT'S NOT RED MEAT)

Red meat is often considered the least healthy form of animal protein, but it's not the most damaging. That honor goes to conventionally raised chicken because it has the highest levels of arachidonic acid, a highly inflammatory omega-6 fatty acid. This is because most chickens are fed corn and soy, both of which are high in omega-6 fats. This is true only for conventionally raised chicken, which has forty times higher levels of arachidonic acid than pastured chicken does. All the more reason to justify the higher cost of pastured meat!

If you choose to eat chicken, pairing it up with bitter green vegetables—such as spinach, chard, watercress, arugula, kale, dandelion greens, broccoli rabe, or endive—will neutralize some of its inflammatory effects.

\\\\\\\\\\\\\\\\\\\\\\\\

THE CASE FOR PLANT-BASED PROTEINS

The evidence is clear: plant-based protein is better for you than animal-based protein. A 2018 study published in the *International Journal of Epidemiology* asked more than eighty thousand participants about their typical diet over the course of a year, and then followed them for six to twelve years. The primary thing the researchers analyzed was how much plant protein versus animal protein the study subjects consumed. They found the more meat people ate, the higher their risk of death from cardiovascular disease, and the more they got their protein from nuts and seeds, the lower that risk fell. The group with the highest meat intake had a 60 percent higher risk than did those with the lowest intake. And the group that ate the most nuts and seeds had 40 percent lower risk than did those who consumed the fewest nuts and seeds.[8] In addition, studies have found that:

- **Meat is high in advanced glycation end products (AGEs)**, the same sticky proteins that form in the brain when you eat excess sugar that I covered in Chapter 2 and that also play a role in cardiovascular damage,[9] and it's worse if you have diabetes.[10]

- **Meat raises levels of IGF-1**, which, as I covered earlier in this chapter, promotes cancer growth as well as fat storage. High intake of red meat and processed meat (sausage, salami, lunch meat) have been linked to colon cancer.[11]

- **Meat is high in iron**, which seems like a good thing, except that the body doesn't have a way to rid itself of excess iron. As people age—especially men, but also postmenopausal women who are no longer shedding blood (and therefore iron) each month—the tendency is for iron levels to get too high. And iron is easily oxidized, which means it is inflammatory and has ties to many diseases associated with aging, including cardiovascular disease and Alzheimer's.[12] Eating just one milligram of the heme iron found in red meat and poultry a day is associated with a 27 percent increase in cardiovascular disease—hamburgers have 2 to 3 milligrams. This is why I recommend everyone over age fifty give blood at least once a year, to alleviate excess iron. Also, the chlorophyll in plants is as effective at building blood cells as iron is.

- **Meat leads to weight gain.** Once you know that excess protein is metabolized into sugar and excess sugar is stored as fat, it's no surprise that meat consumption has been found to be associated with weight gain.[13]

- **Meat increases risk of diabetes.** And it doesn't take a lot of extra meat to do so; eating just an extra half-serving of red meat a day raises the risk for type 2 diabetes by 48 percent.

- **Meat shortens life span.** A Harvard study found that people who ate the highest amount of red meat died the youngest—typically from colon cancer or cardiovascular disease. Those who eliminate or significantly reduce how much meat they ate extended their life span by 20 percent.

||||||||||||||||||||||||||||||||||||||||||||||||||||||||||||||||

JUST SAY NO TO THE SANDWICH

I know, I know, a turkey or ham sandwich is the classic American lunch. But it is terrible for you. So bad, in fact, that I think of it as cancer jammed in between two sugar tsunamis.

Why? Processed meat (sausage, salami, lunch meat) has been linked to colon cancer. And the wheat bread is not only loaded with gluten, but also contains amylopectin A, a carbohydrate that is unusually susceptible to digestion by your salivary and stomach enzymes, which means it raises your blood sugar to sky-high levels. When I interviewed Dr. William Davis, author of *the New York Times* bestseller *Wheat Belly*, for my Get Off Your Sugar Summit, he said, "Two slices of whole wheat bread raise blood sugar higher than six teaspoons of table sugar."

||||||||||||||||||

In addition, meat requires a lot of energy for the body to digest and assimilate, which is kind of a wasteful expenditure when you consider that the protein you get from meat originally came from the protein of a plant; animals are just the middlemen. Also, as we get older, we produce fewer of the enzymes needed to break meat down. So, even if you are eating enough protein, you may not be *assimilating* the nutrients it contains. Remember, you're not what you eat—you're what you *digest, absorb, and assimilate*.

Why go to all that trouble and expose yourself to that much risk, when you can get the same amount of protein from 1 cup of cooked lentils compared to 3 ounces of beef or three large eggs?

This is before even considering the environmental impact of raising animals for meat. A 2017 study found the three largest meat producers—Tyson, Cargill, and JBS—emitted more greenhouse gasses in 2016 than the entire country of France.[14] And a study published in the journal *Science* found that while animals raised for meat provide only 18 percent of the world's total calories, they account for 83 percent of the land used for agriculture.[15] The quality of the animals' lives is also typically terrible. It's a disgrace the way most animals raised for food are treated—they live in cramped, artificial environments, are force-fed food that's not their natural diet, which makes them sick, and then they're killed. It's not just for your own health's sake that you want to eat more plant-based proteins; it's also for the sake of the health of other living creatures and the planet as a whole.

Remember, the Get Off Your Sugar program is based on *adding* new foods, not *taking away* old favorites. I believe that by focusing on eating more plant-based proteins, you'll see (a) how easy it is to meet all your protein needs with plants, and (b) how good you feel when they naturally crowd out some of the meat you have been eating.

MYTH BUSTERS: MEAT IS THE BEST SOURCE OF VITAMIN B$_{12}$

There's a rumor that vegetarians don't get enough vitamin B$_{12}$ because it's found only in meat. Although meat does deliver B$_{12}$, it isn't the original source. B$_{12}$ is made by bacteria that live in the soil and the ground water; the animal eats the food that's been grown in the soil and then passes it on to the human who eats the animal.

The reason many people, not just vegetarians, need to supplement with B$_{12}$ is that our soil quality has been degraded by chemical fertilizers, pesticides, and industrial farming methods. With less B$_{12}$ in the soil, there's also less of it in our food, and therefore, in us. A full 39 percent of people tested, including meat eaters, are low in vitamin B$_{12}$. And that's why everyone—not just vegetarians—should be taking a B$_{12}$ supplement. (See Chapter 11 for my specific supplement recommendations.)

YOUR MISSION: GET PROTEIN SMART

For these three days of the Get Off Your Sugar program, your challenge is twofold:

1. You want to figure out how much protein you're eating versus how much you actually need, so that you can start to bring your quantity into a healthy range for you. It's about being mindful.

2. Then, you want to make the protein you do eat as high-quality, and ideally plant-based, as you can. To do that, you can start incorporating more of the proteins in the list on page 127.

If you're a meat eater, challenge yourself to make at least one of your protein choices a day plant-based, and make the meat you do eat the sideshow and not the main event. If you're vegetarian and vegan make sure you're getting enough variety of higher-quality sources, such as hemp seeds, hummus, chia seeds, and quinoa—and you'll naturally eat fewer carbs as a bonus.

To make it as easy as possible for you to eat more plant-based proteins, I've listed my ten favorite sources beginning on page 122.

TWO VEGAN FOODS I *DON'T* RECOMMEND

There are two foods in particular that many vegans and vegetarians rely on to provide flavor and texture to foods that I consider to be unhealthy:

1. **Nutritional yeast.** Many vegans and vegan food products use nutritional yeast to give food a nutty, cheesy flavor as well as a little extra protein. I advise you stay away from nutritional yeast because, just like its name says, it's *yeast.* It can contribute to candida overgrowth.

2. **Mushrooms.** Many vegans or vegetarians will eat mushrooms as meat substitute. But

mushrooms are fungi, and yeast are fungi. Eating mushrooms that you buy at the store can feed the yeast in your gut and promote an overgrowth. **The one exception** is the *chaga mushroom*, which grows on the trunks of birch trees and is a powerhouse source of antioxidants and a specific type of sugar, known as beta glucan, which research has shown help the immune system function more optimally and protect against autoimmune conditions.[16] Known as the "mushroom of immortality" in Siberia, "diamond of the forest" in Japan, and "king of plants" in China, chaga has antibacterial, anti-inflammatory, and antifungal properties. It is said to have the highest level of antioxidants of any food in the world and also the highest level of superoxide dismutase (one of the body's primary internal antioxidant defenses). As such it's a great way to boost immunity and reduce cravings, because unlike regular mushrooms (and nutritional yeast, for that matter), chaga helps your body heal from candida overgrowth, and candida is a major driver of cravings, as I discussed in Chapter 4. Chaga isn't a mushroom you can buy in the produce section of your grocery store—look for it in capsule form, organic.

MY TOP TEN PLANT-BASED PROTEINS

Why are vegan proteins best? In addition to being loaded with protein (contrary to popular belief), they also double as a great way to get more necessary nutrients, such as fiber, antioxidants, and electrolytes. Animal proteins, on the other hand, often lack these and can also be filled with health-robbing nitrates, sodium, and antibiotics.

There are so many great sources of plant-based proteins that it's hard to know where to start! The following ten are delicious, versatile, and easy to find and store. Make it a goal to have two to three of these foods a day, spread out throughout the day, and you'll be doing great on the protein front.

Plant-Based Protein #1: Hemp Seeds

Protein per 2 tablespoons: 10 grams

Hemp seeds (which will not get you high, although they are a nonpsychotropic cousin of marijuana) are one of my all-time favorites. A full third of their calories come from protein, and they also contain all nine amino acids (meaning they are a complete protein), and more easily digested by your body. They also contain lots of omega-3 fats, and I love a food that multitasks!

How to eat them: Hemp seeds have a delicious, rich, nutty taste, akin to pine nuts. Add them to smoothies; sprinkle them over salads, stir-fries, or sautéed veggies; put them on top of avocado slices or celery boats. Blend them into hummus or stir into your quinoa. You can even have them for breakfast—stir them into coconut yogurt.

Plant-Based Protein #2: Chia Seeds

Protein per 2 tablespoons: 5 grams

Like hemp seeds, chia seeds also contain all nine essential amino acids and are a great source of omega-3s—they are 20 percent protein and 50 percent omega-3 fatty acids. Chia seeds are also 40 percent fiber, making them one of the best sources of fiber in the world. Their fiber content explains why chia seeds can absorb so much water that they form a gel when soaked; it's also what makes them a great thickening agent for smoothies and puddings.

How to eat them: Put them in your smoothies, beverages, or green drinks. Use them to replace an egg in baking by soaking 1 tablespoon of seeds in 2½ tablespoons of water. For constipation, soak 2 tablespoons of chia in 6 ounces of water for ten minutes and drink daily. My Chocolate Chia Pudding (page 260) is a favorite of everyone in my house, including my two young kids, and I think it will become one in your house too!

Plant-Based Protein #3: Beans

Protein per cup: mung (14 grams), adzuki (17 grams), navy (16 grams), black (15 grams), white (17 grams), and kidney (15 grams)

Beans are versatile, inexpensive, and last a long time in your cupboards. Our pantry is stocked with several different kinds of beans at all times; when the Covid-19 pandemic hit, and stores were ransacked, we were ready. They are also alkalizing and good sources of minerals, including zinc, calcium, and selenium, as well as folate.

How to eat them: You can add cooked beans to salads, or toss them with olive oil and a little lemon juice, or use them in soups, stews, and chilis. If you have trouble digesting beans, see the box on page 125 for tips on making them more GI-friendly. And if you're new to eating beans, start with just one small serving (¼ cup) during these three days, and then next week, you can try having them twice in a seven-day period.

Plant-Based Protein #4: Lentils

Protein per cup: 18 grams

A member of the legume family, lentils are made up of more than 25 percent protein. They're also great sources of B vitamins, magnesium, zinc, and potassium. With a few different varieties to try—brown, red, yellow, small green lentils known as Puy for the region in France where they are grown, and small black lentils known as Beluga because they resemble caviar—you'll never get bored of them.

How to eat them: Beyond the classic lentil soup, you can make a salad out of lentils, or eat them on top of a leafy green salad, or even use them to make a hummus-like dip. It's important to at least soak, and, if possible, sprout your lentils to remove the lectins and antinutrients that can cause irritation and inflammation in your gut. (I get more into soaking and sprouting on page 125.)

Plant-Based Protein #5: Avocado

Protein per cup: 10 grams

I told you that you get to eat as many avocados as you want on the Get Off Your

Sugar program! That's because in addition to being high in healthy fat and fiber, avocados also are a significant source of protein. They really are a perfect food.

How to eat them: Eat them sliced and drizzled with olive oil, Himalayan pink salt, lime juice, and hemp seeds; make guacamole and eat with veggie sticks; add them to smoothies; have them on top of Ezekiel bread toast. I also love to do this with my children: hold the avocado by its largest half, peel the top half, and eat it like an apple. It's also great in Avocado Chocolate Mousse (page 263), added to any salad, or with quinoa and some adzuki beans to create a well-balanced meal packed with protein and healthy fat.

Plant-Based Protein #6:
Pumpkin Seeds

Protein per 2 tablespoons: 9 grams

These powerhouse seeds are packed with a crunch and an impressive punch of protein. They are also packed with magnesium, iron, zinc, omega-3 fats, and fiber.

How to eat them: By the handful, sprinkled over salads, add to quinoa dishes—the combinations are endless of how these seeds can easily be incorporated into your daily diet.

Plant-Based Protein #7:
Chickpeas

Protein per cup: 12 grams

Also known as garbanzo beans, chickpeas are a tasty legume that are incorporated into cuisines around the world because they work so well with all different kinds of flavor profiles. They're also great sources of fiber, which is stabilizing for blood sugar and helpful for digestion.

How to eat them: Roasted, they make a great crunchy snack; they're also great in curries, soups, stews, and salads. And, of course, chickpeas are the main ingredient in hummus, something kids and adults love equally.

Plant-Based Protein #8:
Quinoa

Protein per cup: 8 grams

Is there anything quinoa can't do? It's got all nine essential amino acids (and so is a complete protein) and is a great substitute for grains. Funnily enough, quinoa is not a grain—it's the seed of a plant related to spinach, beets, and Swiss chard. The one tricky thing about quinoa is that it should be rinsed before you cook it; it is coated with a naturally occurring phytochemical called saponin that can taste bitter or soapy, so you just want to run it under the tap in a wire mesh strainer (so that all the quinoa doesn't leak out through the holes in your colander) before you cook it.

How to eat it: Quinoa is a go-to in my house—we always make a big pot so that there is some already cooked, ready to for reheating, in the fridge. It's great for breakfast sautéed in coconut oil with some greens and a scrambled egg (of course you can do it sans egg as well); a scoop of it hearties up a green salad; you can use it to make favorites like granola and paella; it's a great substitute for rice in stir-fries; and when you need something to eat but don't feel like cooking, you can combine it with your favorite canned bean and some avocado—sprinkle some pink salt, cumin, and black pepper over it, and boom, you've got dinner. Or, here's another way to prepare it that will blow your mind: sauté uncooked quinoa in coconut oil, and it will actually *pop*, making a quinoa popcorn.

Plant-Based Protein #9: Almonds

Protein per ¼ cup: 7.5 grams

These tasty nuts are high in vitamin E, magnesium, and manganese and also in fiber. The only thing to be aware of is that almonds are required by law to be pasteurized. One method of pasteurizing some companies employ—even on almonds that are labeled "organic," uses propylene oxide (PPO), a chemical that is used in making polyurethane plastics and has been classified by the Environmental Protection Agency as a 2B carcinogen, which means it's officially "possibly carcinogenic."[17] That's why it's best to buy your almonds online (or from a local farm, if you live in California where the vast majority of almonds sold in the US are grown) where you can make sure the almonds are raw and aren't pasteurized using PPO.

How to eat them: By the handful, as homemade nut milks, or as raw almond butter spread—my favorites are from the brands Gopal's (its raw sprouted almond butter is delicious) and JEM (which has amazing flavored raw sprouted almond butters).

Plant-Based Protein #10: Broccoli

Protein per cup: 5 grams

Surprise, vegetables have protein! Broccoli is just one of them—spinach also has 5 grams per cup; kale has 3 grams per cup. But I hope you're already eating more spinach and kale thanks to Step 1; let this step be a nudge to start eating more broccoli. As a cruciferous vegetable, broccoli has anticancer properties. It's also a good source of calcium and antioxidants, particularly vitamin C.

How to eat it: Raw, dipped in hummus, sautéed in stir-fries, pureed into soup, roasted and drizzled with olive oil and lemon juice.

WHAT IF YOU CAN'T DIGEST BEANS?

Humans do not produce the enzymes needed to digest the sugar in beans. Beans are also high in antinutrients such as phytic acid and lectins, which are aggravating to the digestive tract. Those two facts explain why beans have a reputation of being gas-producing. Luckily, there are ways to make them more digestible.

Soaking and sprouting beans reduces the lectin and phytic acid content and adds moisture to dried beans, all of which helps them move through the digestive tract without causing a lot of upset. Here are two ways to soak beans:

The traditional method: Place dried beans in a bowl and add enough water to cover by a few inches. Put the bowl in the fridge overnight. In the morning, drain, rinse, and then your beans are ready for cooking. (If you're soaking in the morning, make sure they're submerged for at least eight hours before cooking.)

The fast method: When you are in a time crunch, pour the dried beans into a large pot and add enough water to cover the beans by a few inches. Add 1 teaspoon of Redmond Real Salt or Himalayan pink salt, and boil for one minute. Turn off the heat, cover the beans, and let them stand for one hour—then they're ready for cooking.

If you don't have time to soak or sprout, or don't have a pressure cooker, the brand Eden Organics soaks, steams, blanches, and rinses its beans before pressure cooking and canning them in a BPA-free can. We always have a few cans of Eden Organics beans in our pantry for those times we need food, fast.

Additionally, try these steps to make beans easier to digest:

Chewing. The first step in digestion is chewing. Make sure you are chewing your beans well and not just wolfing them down. Your teeth and your saliva can do a lot to break down food and make it more digestible, if you use them correctly.

Pressure cooking, such as in an Instant Pot, destroys the lectins and makes beans more digestible.

Adding a strip of dried kombu seaweed, a few coins of fresh ginger, slices of fennel, and/or ground cumin or cumin seeds to the cooking water of beans also makes them easier to break down and less likely to cause gas and bloating.

Start slow, eating only 1 tablespoon a day and gradually work your way up to eating ½ cup.

Take digestive enzymes. If you are over the age of thirty-five, or you have any digestive issues, such as IBS, you should be taking a digestive enzyme (more about this in Chapter 11). If you haven't been taking an enzyme yet, start—it will likely help you move the beans along.

Experiment. Smaller beans, such as adzuki and navy beans, are typically more digestible than larger ones. Experiment with different types of beans and see how your body does with each one. Maybe you're great with cannellini beans but black beans, which are much more acid-forming, really don't agree with you.

WHAT YOU EAT WITH YOUR PROTEIN MATTERS TOO

Proteins are digested in the stomach by acid, whereas starches (carb-rich foods) are broken down in the stomach but *digested* in the small intestine by alkaline compounds. Eating both at the same time essentially shuts down the digestive process because the acids of the stomach and the alkaline chemicals in the small intestine cancel each other out. The result is that the food you've just eaten sits in your gut, slowly putrefying and causing gas and bloating. So, if you are eating any carb-rich foods, please, have them separately from your proteins and pair them up with greens. *All foods* combine well with greens!

GOOD/BETTER/BEST
SOURCES OF PROTEIN

Note: Although I do not eat these animal proteins in column one, *if* you continue to eat meat, focus on the animal proteins in this list in moderation based on parameters laid out earlier, and begin to add variety, with more of the foods in columns two and three.

ACCEPTABLE ANIMAL PROTEINS	BETTER PROTEINS	BEST PROTEINS
Small amount of high-quality, pastured organic meat or eggs. Make sure it's the side show, not the main event. Pasture-raised chicken breast, eggs, grass-fed beef, grass-fed bison, grass-fed lamb	Wild-caught fish high in omega-3s, such as salmon, herring, sardines, anchovies, trout, halibut, scallops, cod	Plant-based proteins, such as raw nuts, seeds, legumes (especially lentils and beans), quinoa, chlorella, wheatgrass, and plant-based protein powders

PROTEIN SWAPS

TYPICAL FOOD	BETTER ALTERNATIVE
Peanut butter	Raw almond butter
Conventional ground beef	Grass-fed ground beef
Conventional eggs	Pastured, organic eggs
Tofu	Chickpeas
Flavored yogurt	Unsweetened coconut yogurt
Whey protein	Hemp seed protein
Cow's milk	Unsweetened almond milk or macadamia nut milk
An 18-ounce porterhouse steak	A 4-ounce fillet (of grass-fed beef, of course, or, even better, wild-caught salmon)
Turkey chili	Lentil chili

HOW TO CHOOSE A PLANT-BASED PROTEIN POWDER

First and foremost, stay away from whey, because whey is dairy, and dairy is acidic. It has a 10:1 ratio of calcium to magnesium, which means most of the calcium is not usable. On top of that, dairy is highly mucus-forming and inflammatory, which leaves you congested with a weakened immune system.

Plant-based protein powders are a great way to ensure that you are getting enough protein, especially if you are vegan or vegetarian. Plus, in addition to being very convenient (just add them to a smoothie or glass of water and you are ready to go), they are cost-effective and convenient. Ideally, you'll choose a plant-based protein that has:

* a variety of protein sources, such as hemp, pea, and sacha inchi (a Peruvian superprotein)

* healthy fats that are also high in protein, such as chia seeds, flaxseeds, or hemp seeds

* high-mineral ingredients, such as sprouts

* MCT or coconut oil

* healthy sweeteners, such as stevia or monk fruit

What you don't want your plant-based protein powder to have is anything genetically modified, gluten, soy, dairy, artificial sweeteners, added sugars (e.g., fructose or high-fructose corn syrup), sugar alcohols (e.g., erythritol or xylitol), or grains (e.g., rice protein).

When making your protein shakes, you can add it to filtered water or coconut/almond/hemp milk. Be sure the nut milks are carrageenan-free and cane sugar–free.

My company, Alkamind, also sells an organic, plant-based protein powder—refer to the Resources section for more information.

STEP 3: PROTEIN SMART ACTION PLAN

* Calculate how much protein you should be getting.

* Calculate how many grams of protein you consumed during the forty-eight-hour retrospective food diary that you filled out on page 202.

* Match your actual protein intake to your targeted intake.

* Eat more high-quality, plant-based protein by eating a variety of the foods listed starting on page 122.

* If you eat animal protein, make sure it is the best quality it can be, and keep it within 2 to 4 ounces in any one meal.

* Continue eating your three servings of greens a day and two to three servings of fat per meal.

TRACK YOUR JOURNEY

Assess how this step is impacting you by filling out the chart for Days 7–9 on page 208.

nine

Step 4 (Days 10–12): Spice Things Up

MOST PEOPLE THINK OF HERBS (THE FRESH, GREEN LEAVES OF PLANTS) AND SPICES (the seed, stem, roots, bark, or buds of plants) as nice-to-haves; the equivalent of flavorful accessories. But they are nutrition powerhouses that deliver health benefits, such as blood sugar regulation, detoxification, digestion support, anti-inflammatory effects, and more.

Herbs and spices are also super stars of the antioxidant world—a mere teaspoon of cinnamon has as many of the anti-inflammatory compounds as ½ cup of blueberries (and blueberries have one of the highest antioxidant scores of any fruit); and just ½ *teaspoon* of oregano has as much antioxidant power as a ½ cup of sweet potatoes. *And* they take the taste, smell, and appearance of your food to another level. What's not to love?

You might be intimidated by using herbs and spices, but by the end of these next three days, you'll be adding them to everything—and experiencing firsthand not only how easy they are to use, but how satisfying and nourishing they are. You'll be massively upping your nutrient intake, and I think you'll be pleasantly surprised by what a nice flavor payoff they bring. Also, because herbs and spices are so flavorful, eating them will help retrain your taste buds away from liking sweets.

Your assignment over the next three days is to keep the previous steps going and then add at least one herb (fresh or dried) or spice to everything you eat or drink. As you'll learn in the next chapter, diet variation is a key component of long-term health, and varying the flavors and nutrient profiles of your food by working an array of different herbs and spices into your diet is how you do that!

TOP TEN HERBS AND SPICES FOR GETTING OFF YOUR SUGAR

The following, listed in order of importance, are the herbs and spices you should be cooking with on the regular to optimize your health and energy.

1. Garlic. Affectionately known as "the stinking rose," garlic adds zing to everything you add it to, unless it's roasted—when it's sweet and spreadable as butter. If you could pick only one food or spice for the health of the cardiovascular system, this would be it! The sulfur compound allicin, the most powerful component in garlic, helps lower blood pressure by increasing nitric oxide in the wall of the arteries. This helps the wall of the artery relax, so your blood pressure is lowered. Allicin also gives garlic its telltale smell, pungent bite, and delivers the health benefits, which include antibacterial, antifungal, antiviral, and anti-inflammatory effects.

How to eat it: If you like it roasted, slice the top off as many heads of garlic as you like, drizzle each head with 2 teaspoons of extra-virgin olive oil and rub the oil in, then place in a covered ceramic dish and roast at 300°F for one hour (turning up to 400°F for the last 10 to 15 minutes for more caramelization, if you like it extra sweet). You can then add the soft cloves to mashed sweet potatoes or any other vegetable. Toast garlic slices in a skillet on your stovetop, then add to sautéed greens for a nutty crunch. Or add very thin slices at the end of cooking sautéed greens. Add raw minced garlic to hummus, pesto, or salad dressings.

2. Ginger. With its myriad uses, this rhizome is the Swiss Army knife of the spice world. It's a potent remedy for nausea (including morning sickness)[1], promotes digestion, and improves circulation. Ginger's so effective at settling upset stomachs that a study from the University of Rochester Medical Center found that chemotherapy patients who took ginger before and after treatment had a 40 percent reduction in nausea.[2]

Ginger is also incredibly warming; it can even make you sweat, which promotes detoxification. It's also a natural expectorant, meaning ginger helps loosen mucus so that you can expel it. As an antioxidant, it's also anti-inflammatory. I find that eating ginger or drinking ginger tea soothes my stomach and raises my energy at the same time; once you start eating it, you won't want to live without it.

How to eat it: Ginger's spicy bite makes it a great addition to green juices and smoothies. A little goes a long way—use about ½ inch of fresh, peeled, minced ginger for one serving. Add it to your stir-fries, quinoa dishes, and soups. Ginger gets less spicy the more it's cooked; add it right at the end if you want more zing. Make a tea with it by adding a few slices of peeled, raw ginger to 2 to 3 cups of water and boil for at least 20 minutes—discard the ginger slices before drinking.

3. Turmeric. You can hardly go to a coffee shop in New York City, where I live, without seeing a turmeric latte (sometimes known as golden milk). This bright yellow spice is having its moment in the culinary sun—no longer relegated to being one of the many spices in curry powder or taken only in capsules for its anti-inflammatory effects. Those effects come from curcumin, a potent compound in turmeric that is so powerful it's used as a treatment for arthritis. It also appears to slow tumor growth and is a powerful antiviral.

Ready to reap these benefits? Aim to consume between ½ and 1 teaspoon of ground turmeric (2.5 to 5 grams) per day with food.

Fresh is best. It is a knobby root that looks similar to ginger; we buy it at the farmers' market in bulk to bring down the cost (it can be expensive) and then freeze it, especially to use for the winter months. I have also seen a pound of organic turmeric on Amazon for seven bucks (if you can't find it at your farmers' market).

How to eat it: Turmeric is a tasty, colorful addition to savory dishes. And although it's a key ingredient in curry powder, it's actually not spicy-hot on its own. Use it in stir-fries, mix it into your quinoa and/or beans, incorporate it into curries and soups, add it to your salad dressings. If you're getting tired of bland roasted veggies, turmeric is a tasty way to add a different flavor to your plate. It goes especially well with cauliflower, squashes, and sweet potato. Sprinkle it on generously, before or after cooking, along with Himalayan pink salt and black pepper. It's also delicious sprinkled on wild-caught fish before you bake, pan-fry, or grill it. Even though I love fresh turmeric, you can absolutely use the powdered form. One teaspoon of the ground, jarred spice equals one inch of fresh turmeric.

One of the biggest hits with our kids is Chelsea's Tofu Scramble—fermented tofu with turmeric to give it an egglike appearance and a dose of anti-inflammation. Whether you use fermented tofu, chickpeas, or pastured eggs, add 1 teaspoon of ground turmeric to the mixture when scrambling—it's an easy way to boost your intake without overpowering your taste buds!

You can also drink it—in golden milk, or make a tea with the fresh root (see the Detox Tea recipe on page 220). Add it to your green smoothie (such as the Dr. Green Detox Smoothie on page 215). However you have it, mix it with a little freshly ground black pepper, which makes it more bioavailable and increases the potency of turmeric by 2,000 percent, to get the biggest health bang out of it. If you are using the fresh root, be sure to peel it first. Also, while its deep yellow color is beautiful, it can stain, so just be aware when you are handling it!

4. Cinnamon. This warming spice is a master blood sugar regulator. It has this effect because it slows the release of food from your stomach, so that high-carb foods don't result in a big glucose spike. In fact, a 2013 review of ten different studies suggest that cinnamon lowers both fasting blood glucose and total cholesterol.[3] It reduces inflammation, supports your immune system, and takes anything that's acidic and makes it a little more alkaline. **One note of caution:** A compound found in cinnamon, called coumarin, is a natural anticoagulant, which makes consuming too much cinnamon a potential concern if you are taking a blood-thinning medication. However, there are two types of cinnamon—Ceylon and cassia. And Ceylon cinnamon has only trace amounts of coumarin, making it a safer and better source. Look for the word "Ceylon" on the label.

How to eat it: Sprinkle it in your coffee (prior to brewing), tea, or smoothies; over berries; on slices of green apple. It also makes a great addition to chia pudding. You can make your own cinnamon tea by stirring a teaspoon of ground cinnamon into a cup of hot water—with its antimicrobial properties, it will help your body fight off a bug if you've caught a cold, and will help your digestion if you've eaten too much. My kids and I eat it sprinkled over a piece of toasted Ezekiel bread (which is made out of sprouted wheat; while I recommend avoiding breads and flour, if you have to have a piece of bread, make it Ezekiel) with raw almond butter and manuka honey, and it essentially cancels out the sugar in the honey.

5. Cilantro. Common in Mexican, Thai, and Vietnamese dishes, cilantro adds a fresh, citrusy flavor to foods. It's one of those flavors that people either love or hate. I *love* it; how about you?

Cilantro has so many health benefits. It's a natural sedative that can help ease anxiety and a great source of antioxidants, particularly quercetin. It's most distinctive benefit and one of its most powerful properties is that cilantro binds heavy metals so they can be excreted through the digestive tract instead of stored in fat cells.

How to eat it: Add to green juices, beans, soups, salsas, salads, slaws, and sauces. Of course, it's a great addition to guacamole. If you're cooking with it, add it at the end of cooking to preserve flavor and nutrients.

6. Basil. This herb shows up in cuisines around the world because its licorice-y flavor is such a universally tasty accompaniment to all manner of foods. Consumption of basil slows the release of sugar in the blood, which helps keep insulin and inflammation levels low, and is essential for diabetics. Basil also helps restore the body's natural pH levels and feeds healthy gut bacteria. A healthy microbiome increases immunity and promotes healthy digestion. And basil is really easy to grow—I have a pot of it growing on my New York City windowsill year-round.

How to eat it: Add it, chopped or julienned, to salads, stir-fries, and wraps. Put it in your green juices and smoothies for an added layer of flavor and aroma. Enjoy it in my Creamy Spinach Basil Soup (page

226). And of course, it makes a great sauce when blended into pesto (see the Raw Zucchini Pesto Pasta on page 237).

7. Curry powder. This tasty blend is a great way to get a lot of spices in one fell swoop. Curry powder gets it signature yellow color from turmeric, but it also typically includes a mix of coriander, cumin, cardamom, bay leaf, ginger, cinnamon, mustard seeds, and fennel seeds. Different blends will have varying levels of heat, depending on which peppers—whether they be black pepper, red chiles, or other hot peppers—are used and in what amounts. It's like one-stop shopping that adds a great depth of flavor to a wide range of dishes. It's really a powerful health booster that also happens to be delicious.

How to eat it: Add it to scrambled eggs and tofu or chickpea scrambles, sautés, curries (naturally), and soups.

8. Oregano. This great-smelling plant that grows wild across the hills that border the Mediterranean Ocean is one of the most powerful antiviral, antibacterial, and antifungal herbs you can get. Oil of oregano has long been taken to help fight infection; why not take it all the time? Oregano is loaded with antioxidants—1 tablespoon of fresh oregano leaves has as much antioxidant activity as a medium-size apple and four times more than blueberries. It's also a powerful antifungal and can help you rid yourself of candida (see pages 24–25 for more on determining whether you have candidiasis). Another great benefit of oregano is that it is ridicu-

lously easy to grow—I also have a pot of it next to the basil on my windowsill. If I can grow it, so can you!

How to eat it: You can eat the leaves fresh or dried. They are great mixed into vinaigrettes, incorporated into any Mexican or Italian dishes you may make, or sprinkled over roasted vegetables (especially cauliflower).

One of the best ways to benefit from this herb is to make oregano tea, as it will reduce bloating, help your digestion, and promote weight loss. To make it, put 1 tablespoon of oregano leaves in the bottom of a coffee cup and fill the cup with boiling water. Let it steep for about 10 minutes, then strain the leaves out and drink.

You can also buy oregano oil at your health food store. This powerful antibiotic and antiviral can help you stay healthy all winter—put ten drops of oregano oil into 2 tablespoons of coconut oil for a hand sanitizer (store in a glass jar). You can also put one drop of oregano oil in a bowl of steaming water and use a towel over your head to make a tent and breathe the steam in to ward off respiratory infections.

9. Rosemary. A member of the mint family, rosemary is prized both for its flavor and its fragrance. Studies show its woodsy scent helps improve concentration and may boost mood. Research suggests that rosemary, even in the small amounts common in cooking, may help prevent cognitive decline in older people.[4]

Rosemary is a rock star of the herb world. This woody, fragrant herb helps your genes express themselves optimally (assisting in turning off bad genes and turning on good ones). It's also anti-inflammatory and antitumor. And it's been shown to boost memory and cognitive performance, reducing seasonal allergy symptoms, and relieve the pain of osteoarthritis. I mean, really, why wouldn't you want to get more of this wonder food into your diet?

How to eat it: You can eat rosemary fresh or dried. Put full dried leaves into a spice grinder and add it powdered to everything—quinoa, salads, beans, soups, stews. Infuse it in some olive oil and then get the benefits of rosemary every time you eat this healthy fat.

10. Fenugreek. Cookbook author Monica Bhide wrote in the *Seattle Times* that dried fenugreek leaves are "often my go-to ingredient when something I am cooking just tastes blah," and that they "smell divine." Fenugreek is a legume grown in North Africa and India; its leaves and seeds are great for adding a sweet flavor that tastes like a mix of celery and maple syrup. Fenugreek has been shown to reduce fasting glucose and hemoglobin A1c (the blood test that measures the average of the last 120 days of blood sugar), stimulate milk production in breastfeeding women (I added fenugreek to all of Chelsea's food after the birth of both our children), and increase testosterone and libido.

Men and women alike will appreciate this: fenugreek has been found to stimulate hair growth and make it less vulnerable to shedding. Fenugreek seeds have vitamin C, potassium, iron, protein, and compounds known as steroid saponins that, again, help to promote hair growth.[5]

How to eat it: Use the leaves to flavor steamed peas, stews, soups, salads, or curries. If you opt for using the seeds, it's best to soak them overnight to remove the lectins—inflammatory compounds in the hulls of many seeds that are self-protective mechanisms for the seeds—and the bitterness. Once they are dry again, you can toast them in a hot pan on the stovetop for a few minutes until they release their aroma. Use dried and powdered seeds in smoothies, curries, chia pudding, or to add a unique element to a tomato sauce.

Other Excellent Herbs and Spices

Of course, you don't have to—nor should you—limit yourself to these herbs and spices. There are so many other options that are tasty as well as health-promoting too. As you continue through the Get Off Your Sugar program and lifestyle, work the following herbs and spices into your regular rotation; think of them as tasty supplements!

Allspice	Horseradish
Anise	Lavender
Bay leaf	Lemon balm
Cardamom	Mint
Celery seeds	Mustard seeds
Coriander	Nutmeg
Cloves	Parsley
Cumin	Sage
Dill	Sesame seeds
Fennel	Vanilla bean

If you buy fresh herbs, here's a way to make them last longer: wash them when you get home and lay them out on a towel to dry on the counter. Then either keep them in a glass in the fridge with their stems immersed in water, or wrap the stems in a damp paper towel and put the whole bundle in a plastic bag that you store in the produce drawer.

* Add fresh herbs to a pitcher of water and keep in the fridge; we always have a big glass jar in ours—cucumber and mint is a great combo, and our kids go crazy for watermelon-and-basil-infused water. It's a great way to get everyone off sodas and seltzers (which add acidity to the body) and delight the taste buds while also delivering extra nutrients.

SPICE UP YOUR BEVERAGES

Drinks are fabulous ways to get more herbs and spices into your body. There's a reason that trendy bars are incorporating more herbs and herb-based bitters into their cocktails—they taste great and really take the taste factor of your beverage to the next level. Some of my favorite ways to drink my herbs and spices include:

* Turmeric ginger tea (see Detox Tea, page 220),
* Herb-infused ice cubes—freeze sprigs of fresh basil, oregano, or rosemary in water and then add them to your beverage of choice,
* Use bitters to make a festive mocktail for yourself,
* Steep fresh herbs—cilantro, basil, rosemary, oregano, or a blend of your favorites—in hot water to make a tasty tea,

QUICK SPICE HACKS

Want more spice in your life? Add spices to your:

    Morning tea or coffee

    Vinaigrettes

    Salads

    Water

    Beans

    Quinoa

    Guacamole

    Hummus

    Avocado slices

    Mayo (make sure it's olive oil or avocado oil, to cut down on omega-6s)

    Special-occasion cocktail

TRACK YOUR JOURNEY

Keep tabs on your progress by filling out the chart for Days 10–12 on page 208.

STEP 4: SPICE THINGS UP ACTION PLAN

* Buy at least two different fresh herbs to have on hand—ginger and rosemary, for example, or garlic and cilantro. If you're inspired, get three and make the third something you haven't tried before (see the list on page 134 for suggestions).

* Incorporate at least one herb or spice into everything you eat or drink these three days.

* If you're new to using herbs and spices, stick to trying one at a time so that you can see which tastes you prefer before you start blending them.

* Consider growing your favorite herb or herbs on your windowsill. It's a low-cost experiment that can pay long-term dividends.

* Continue eating your two to three servings of greens per day, two to three servings of healthy fats per meal, and keeping your protein consumption moderate and high-quality.

ten

Step 5 (Days 13–15): Time Your Meals

INDUSTRIAL FARMING, REFRIGERATION, AND MODERN TRANSPORTATION MEANS THAT we can eat anything, anytime, anywhere, and we don't have to do any hunting or gathering—that is, physical exercise—to do it. We just have to open the cabinet or the fridge (as I mentioned in Chapter 3, the average American does that seventeen times per day!). While this type of grazing can stimulate the body's metabolism, there are more downside effects than upside.

First and foremost, during the Paleolithic period, when the human genetic makeup was forged, our ancestors had to hunt and forage for their food. They had to eat according to the seasons, and in variable amounts—after a big hunt, they would feast; other times, they would eat whatever they could find; and sometimes, there was no food readily available, and they didn't eat. We were meant to adapt to an ever-changing food supply and to be flexible in how we metabolized the foods we ate. Our ancient ancestors were forced to adapt. Now, we've lost that flexibility.

When you eat constantly, you are also constantly dumping insulin into your blood, which cues the body to store fat, creates inflammation, and has a knock-on effect to your hunger hormones, such as leptin and ghrelin. Therefore, you are always hungry, never full, and constantly looking for carbs over more healthy foods.

As important as it is to make better choices about the foods you eat—as we have done in the first four steps of the Get Off Your Sugar program—another vitally important tool is to increase and vary the periods of time when you *don't* eat—in other words, when you fast for different lengths of time in what's known as intermittent fasting. Intermittent fasting has become en vogue, but people don't even understand what it really does. Most people think of it as a weight loss tool, period, the end. But the true power and purpose of intermittent fasting is to move the body away from burning sugar as the primary source of fuel to burning fat. Yes, it helps you lose weight, but there's so much more to it than that. Fasting helps you in so many ways— and the beauty is that once you regain the ability to burn fat, which you have been working on since Step 1 of this program, you won't even feel hungry during the times when you're not eating. The goal is not to eat less, but to eat less often.

VARIETY IS EVERYTHING

Changing your patterns of when and how often you eat is called *diet variation*, a strategy that mimics the way our ancient ancestors, who regularly experienced unpredictable cycles of feast and famine, ate.

When you regularly switch up your eating times, you force your body to adapt. It's a very similar strategy to the one you want to take with exercise—exercise, like fasting, is a beneficial stressor. It breaks your muscles down so that they will rebuild and be stronger than before. If you only ever do the same exercise, at the same time, at the same intensity, your body will quickly stop responding. But when you work different muscle groups in different ways, your body is forced to grow stronger and more agile.

When you incorporate diet variation, your body responds favorably in multiple different ways, including:

- **Weight loss:** Think about it—if you want to lose fat, you have to be able to burn fat. Fasting nudges your body into fat burning by forcing it to go without any potential sources of glucose (whether they be from carbs or from excessive protein) so that it has no choice but to burn fat for fuel. And when you are fasting, guess where that fat comes from? From your own fat stores.

- **Visceral fat loss:** Visceral fat, a.k.a. belly fat, forms inside the abdominal cavity around the organs. It is the most dangerous kind of fat. And research shows that intermittent fasting is equally as effective at reducing belly fat as consistent caloric restriction (defined as eating only 45 percent of a regular caloric intake).[1]

- **Reduced "muffin top" and "bleg":** The other type of fat that develops in the torso is subcutaneous fat, which, as its name suggests, develops under the skin and is very difficult to get rid of. You probably know this type of fat as a muffin top (the fat that's stored under the skin in the belly) or the bleg (the fat that collects in the hips and upper thigh, or where the butt meets the leg). The reason this subcutaneous fat is so stubborn is that cells contain two different types of receptors for adrenaline and noradrenaline—alpha receptors, which hinder a fat cell's ability to be burned, and beta receptors, which make fat cells easy to mobilize and be burned for energy. (You can remember it this way: alpha receptors stand for "antiburn" and beta receptors stand for "burn.") Subcutaneous fat cells have more alpha than beta receptors.

The good news is that when you go for longer than about twelve hours without eating, the resulting drop in insulin levels activates more beta receptors in the subcutaneous fat, and thus some of the fat that your body will burn for energy will come from these troublesome areas.[2]

- **Improved microbiome:** When you go without food, you also deprive the unhealthy bacteria in your gut—the kind that thrives on sugar, such as yeast—of food. As the bad guys dwindle, your good gut bugs can thrive because they don't have to compete for space or resources, and they are getting their favorite foods in the hours that you are eating, including lots of fiber (known as prebiotics) and healthy fats. It's an important *reset* for your microbiome.

- **Prevention and/or reversal of type 2 diabetes:** When you fast, you lower both glucose and insulin levels. This helps heal insulin resistance, which is a primary precursor of type 2 diabetes. In

addition, several studies have found that intermittent fasting is capable of cueing the body to increase the number of islet beta cells in the pancreas—the cells that produce insulin and that are damaged in both type 1 and the late stages of type 2 diabetes.[3] A 2019 study also found that, even when they didn't make any other changes to their diet, men at risk of developing type 2 diabetes improved their glucose levels and lowered their risk by eating all their meals within a nine-hour time frame. That translates to finishing dinner by 7:30 p.m. and having breakfast at 10:30 the next morning.[4] And that's without also reducing their carbs!

- **Improved cellular regeneration:** When you go longer than fifteen or so hours without food, your body kicks off a process called *autophagy*, which translates to "self-eating." It's a very beneficial process of your body destroying all damaged or dead cells. At the same time as this is happening, your body also begins to generate *new* stem cells— the baby cells that can be used wherever the body needs them most. Autophagy is only for the bad guys, not the good guys. As Dr. Dan Pompa, the expert in cellular detoxification whom I first mentioned in Chapter 1, says, during a fast, the body will use bad cells and debris for energy and nutrition. Your cells are getting nourished without the consumption of any new food. During a fast, the body is literally "eating without eating," using your old, abused, oxidized, inflamed cellular debris as fuel for creating new, healthier, stronger cells. Giving your body a break allows it to get to work, eating the stuff it needs to get rid of.[5]

- **Improved mitochondrial health:** When you fast, you increase what Dr. Pompa calls *metabolic mitochondrial fitness*. By increasing the interval of time between your meals you force your mitochondria—the organelles within your cells that convert the food you eat into energy—to switch from using sugar to using fat for fuel. This forces your mitochondria to become what's called metabolically flexible; you're essentially cross training your mitochondria. And because fat is such a cleaner burning fuel than sugar, your mitochondria are subjected to fewer free radicals and oxidative damage when they burn fat instead of sugar. So, your mitochondria get fitter, and they are also subject to less damage.

- **Benefits your genes:** While your DNA doesn't change, the way your genes are expressed—what's known as epigenetics, a process that controls which genes are turned on and which are turned off—is influenced by many things, including diet, stress, and toxin exposure. Fasting improves epigenetic expression, which cleans up your DNA, turns off the bad genes, and turns on the good ones. Fasting also lengthens telomeres—the bits of genetic material that seal the ends of the strands of DNA and protect them from fraying or getting tangled with one another. Longer telomeres are associated with a younger biological age, so in this sense, fasting can help turn back the clock.

- **Contributes to a longer life:** In addition to lengthening your telomeres, fasting helps bring down blood glucose and insulin levels, and as Dr. Ron Rosedale said, the lower your insulin levels over the course of your life, the longer you'll live. In fact, a 2018 study published in *Cell Metabolism* found that mice who ate only once a day lived 40 percent longer than the ones that had access to food around the clock.[6] If that's not a powerful incentive to eat less often, I don't know what is!

- **Downregulates inflammation:** We don't die of infection or old age, we die of inflammation! And burning sugar promotes inflammation because it's a dirty-burning fuel. Fasting helps you make the switch to burning fat and creating ketones, which have been shown to protect against the effects of oxidative stress that triggers inflammation.[7]

So, let's talk about how to start reaping the benefits of fasting. Don't worry, I'm not going to tell you that you have to go seven days drinking only lemon water or anything extreme like that. Like everything else in the Get Off Your Sugar program, we're going to make a gradual shift that's appropriate for you and your body. I'll talk more about exactly how to do that in just a minute, but first I want to cover the step that everyone should take at this point: stop eating at least three hours before you go to bed.

WHY YOU *SHOULD* GO TO BED HUNGRY (OR AT LEAST NOT FULL)

One of the most important things you can do to start eating less often is to stop eating at least three hours before bedtime. That means if you go to bed at 10 p.m., you want your dinner to be over by 7 p.m. Why? Your body doesn't need energy at that hour of the day—since the glucose won't be needed by your muscles, any excess will be stored as fat. Forcing your mitochondria to metabolize your food at such a low-energy time of day will also create more free radicals and subject them to more damage. Your stomach can also take several hours to empty completely; if you go and lie down for a night's rest with a full belly, you're more prone to acid reflux. And finally, focusing on digestion during sleep will divert energy and attention away from what the body is designed to be doing during that time, which is repairing and detoxing itself.

When you finish your last meal at least three hours before you go to bed, you naturally fast a minimum of ten to eleven hours, eight of which are spent sleeping, so you won't even have a chance to miss eating.

A 2018 study published in the *International Journal of Cancer* found that for people who ate dinner at least two hours before bedtime, the women had a 16 percent lower risk of breast cancer and the men had a 26 percent lower risk of developing prostate cancer.[8]

In addition to setting the stage for restful sleep, telling yourself that the kitchen is closed in the hours before bedtime is helpful because nighttime is hardest for people who struggle with sugar addiction. When I was hooked on sugar, I could eat well during the day while I was busy at work, but once I was home and things got quieter, all my plans to eat healthy got derailed. Does this sound familiar? It is something I hear again and again from clients as well. Cutting out all eating after dinnertime can remove an opportunity to

start eating and not be able to stop. All the things you've been doing in the steps leading up to this point will help you avoid nighttime eating—the **minerals** will reduce your cravings and the **healthy fats** will keep you full, as will the **fiber** from your **plant-based proteins**. Make sure you have all of these types of foods in the last meal of your day, to keep you satiated and curb cravings.

If you're doing all these things, try drinking a glass of water, as thirst can come hidden as hunger. According to a study at the University of Washington, drinking 8 ounces of water at bedtime can shut down your evening hangry pains.[9]

I think I know what you're thinking right now: *He wants me to drink water before bed? I'll have to pee!* Maybe in the beginning . . . think of a dry sponge under a water faucet—the water bounces right off. But after a few days, as you become more hydrated, that dry sponge begins to soak up the water, so you won't have to get up and go pee. Your sleep and your cravings will get better too. Bonus: add some trace minerals, either a pinch of Himalayan pink salt or a pinch of a mineral powder (see the Resources section for a recommendation).

To fall asleep and stay asleep, your body and brain need to relax. Minerals, especially magnesium, facilitate this process by activating the parasympathetic nervous system, which is responsible for the rest and digest functions of the body, including getting you calm and relaxed. Plus, the body is most acidic between 1 and 3 a.m., so these minerals will help your body calibrate its pH, neutralizing these acids so your body doesn't need to spend its own energy doing so, another major reason that people can't stay asleep at night.

And if you tried everything and are still feeling the urge to eat close to bedtime, eat a tablespoon of coconut oil with a sprinkle of Himalayan pink salt; it will help tide you over until you fall asleep without impacting your blood glucose or insulin levels.

THREE HACKS TO WARD OFF NIGHTTIME SNACKING

If you have a hard time resisting eating at night, try these three simple solutions:

1. **Check in with yourself.** Often, nighttime eating has more to do with boredom, habit, or stress than it does with hunger. Before you start eating anything, ask yourself: *What am I really feeling?* If you don't stop to ask, you may never realize that you're really feeling tired, lonely, or bored.

2. **Turn off the screens.** It's so easy to polish off a couple of servings of anything when you're zoned out and interacting with a screen, whether it's a TV, computer, tablet, or other device, because you're not fully present to what you're doing or how you're feeling. Break the association between watching and eating by skipping the watching part of the equation. Do some stretching, or read a book instead.

3. **Get more sleep.** Not getting enough zzzz's can alter your glucose metabolism and negatively impact the appetite-regulating hormone leptin. If you get hungry after dinner, try heading off to bed instead of into the kitchen.

TIME YOUR MEALS ACTION PLAN: HOW TO EXTEND THE TIME YOU GO WITHOUT EATING

I'd never ask you to go run a marathon if you never trained. In much the same way, you can't go overnight from eating seventeen times a day to eating once a day; you need to gradually expand the number of hours between your meals. The following is a guideline for how to do just that. For the next three days, locate which step you are currently at, and take the corresponding next step that I've outlined here.

- *If you're currently eating at all hours of the day:* Stop eating three hours before bedtime.

- *If you've stopped eating three hours before bedtime but still rely on snacks to make it through the day:* Choose healthier snacks.

- *If you're already eating healthy snacks:* Wean yourself down to one snack at either midmorning or midafternoon.

- *If you're eating only one healthy snack a day:* Stop snacking altogether and eat only three meals a day.

- *If you don't require snacks, aren't eating anything within three hours of bedtime, and are already eating only three meals a day:* Delay your breakfast by an hour each day until you are going at least twelve hours without food. Say you normally eat dinner at 8 p.m. and eat breakfast at 7 a.m.; you want to push your breakfast back to 8 a.m. so that you're going twelve hours between your last meal of the day before and your first meal of the next day. This way, you are

INTERMITTENT FASTING

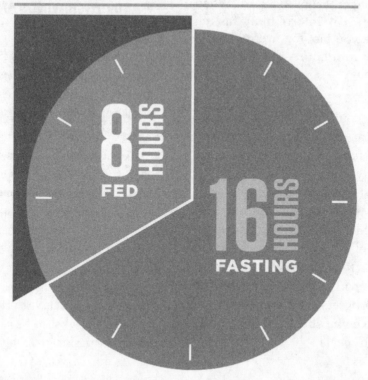

Over time, you want to get into a pattern of eating known as intermittent fasting, where you eat only during an eight-hour window most days.

asleep for seven to eight hours of your fasting time.

- *If you've already been going at least twelve hours between your last meal and the first meal of the next day:* Start working toward going sixteen hours without eating and having food only during an eight-hour window a day (what's known as a 16/8 eating pattern). So, if you typically have dinner at 7 p.m. and breakfast at 7 a.m., start pushing your breakfast back an hour (go at your own pace) to 8, then 9, then 10, then 11. To get there, continue pushing your first meal of the day back until you're eating only between 10 a.m. and 6 p.m., for example, or 11 a.m. and 7 p.m. Now you have arrived at intermittent fasting, where breakfast and lunch have merged and you're eating only two meals a day. Congratulations; your life is about to change!

- *If you're already able to go 16 hours without eating:* Now that you are here, let's take you one step further. See whether you can get that eating window down to six, five, or even four hours for the next three days. Once you fast for more than fifteen hours, autophagy (the body's process of getting rid of old, damaged cells) kicks in. When you hit the 20/4 intermittent fasting zone, where you fast for twenty hours, and feast for four hours, you are hitting max autophagy!

Remember, you don't want to eat less, you want to eat *less often*. You can still have as much food as if you were eating more frequently.

For the next three days, you just want to implement the right intermittent fasting strategy for you. As you continue through the Get Off Your Sugar program and make it a lifestyle (something we'll cover in Chapter 13), you can keep moving through this progression plan to acclimatize yourself to being able to go longer and longer between meals.

WHAT YOU CAN DRINK DURING YOUR HOURS SPENT FASTING

Just because you're "fasting," it doesn't mean that nothing can pass your lips. You can have as much as you like of the following:

Water

Hydration drink (⅛ tsp of Himalayan pink salt dissolved in 1 liter of water)

Green powder (with no sugar added)

Mineral powder (no sugar added)

Herbal teas

Organic coffee

HOW TO CHEAT YOUR FAST AND WARD OFF CRAVINGS AND HUNGER

Over the last twenty years, my good friend Jorge Cruise (jorgecruise.com) has written over thirty books, including *The Cruise Control Diet*, to help busy people shortcut fitness, and he says that intermittent fasting is *the most important tool* he's learned in his entire career.

The trick to make it a full sixteen hours without eating is to **use *healthy fats* to turn off your hunger without breaking your fast**—things like MCT oil, coconut oil, and on occasion, grass-fed butter (Jorge even loves beef tallow, which he says has helped him improve his immunity). You can use them to "cheat" your fast—take in calories without causing a rise in blood glucose—by adding them to a hot morning beverage, such as tea or coffee. Jorge starts his morning drinking a caffeine-free peppermint tea that he's added beef tallow to, or a cup of coffee with some of my Acid-Kicking Coffee Alkalizer. You can add up to 3 tablespoons of fat to your morning beverage of choice to help curb your appetite, and have up to three cups of fat-enhanced coffee or tea.

Jorge's other trick to stave off hunger is to drink 32 ounces of mineral water first thing in the morning—even before his coffee or tea—with ½ teaspoon of Redmond Real Salt or one scoop of Alkamind Daily Minerals. The minerals in the water and salt will help turn off your body's feeling of hunger, which is often simply dehydration and not true hunger.

Jorge's Flat-Belly Tea

Brew organic peppermint tea and add 1 to 3 tablespoons of your choice of healthy fat (MCT oil, coconut oil, or beef tallow) to curb appetite.

Jorge's Flat-Belly Water

Start your morning with 32 ounces of the highest-quality mineral water you can find—Jorge recommends the brand Mountain Valley. Then add half a teaspoon of Redmond's Real Salt. For flavor, add the juice of ½ lime and you're ready to rock and roll.

WHEN TO AVOID INTERMITTENT FASTING (WOMEN, YOU WILL WANT TO READ THIS)

It's important to tailor the Get Off Your Sugar program to your own body, and this is especially true if you are a premenopausal woman, because your body has different caloric needs at different times in your cycle. On Day 21 of your cycle (typically a week after ovulation and a week before your period starts), your progesterone levels spike. And your body needs glucose and insulin to be higher at that time because insulin is a master hormone regulator and plays an important role in the formation of progesterone and converting your hormones. That's why it's so common for premenstrual women to be craving carbs, such as chocolate, chips, sweets, and fries. Of course, I'm suggesting that you eat healthier fiber-rich, slow-burning carbs, such as sweet potatoes, quinoa, and squashes, instead of the sugary and/or processed stuff.

But that means you want to avoid fasting during this week before your period starts. Prioritize keeping your mineral and healthy fat intake up and eating more healthy complex carbs. You can still avoid eating three hours before bedtime, and do your best to have twelve to fourteen hours between your last meal of the day and your first meal of the next day, but I suggest not extending past that. Once your period starts, you can resume your fasting schedule.

You also want to avoid fasting if you are underweight, pregnant, breastfeeding, or have an eating disorder.

And finally, for *some* women, going sixteen hours or longer, or doing more frequent fasts (including daily intermittent fasting), especially when regularly doing intense exercise, can cause hormonal imbalances that can lead to fertility issues. In particular, it can affect the levels of luteinizing hormone, follicle-stimulating hormone, and progesterone. It may be that the women who experience this effect from intermittent fasting and intense exercise have more of a hormone called kisspeptin that makes them a little more sensitive to fasting. It should help to have healthy fats in the morning that won't break your fast, such as 1 tablespoon of chia seeds in 8 ounces of water, and to remember that you should still be getting plenty of calories during your eating window—it's not that you're eating fewer calories, it's that you're eating the same amount of calories in a smaller window of time. Lastly, instead of intermittent fasting every day, try every other day for a couple of weeks and see how you feel.

FIVE TO THRIVE

Wherever you are in your journey toward being able to go sixteen or more hours without eating, these five biohacks will help you crush cravings, boost energy, and become more fat-adapted.

The healthy fats and mineral salts will help you burn fat, give you energy, and help prevent any detox symptoms during your intermittent or partial fasting days (or what people call the "keto flu").

You don't have to do them all at once or even all of them in one day (although you absolutely can). Just listen to your body and give it what it is asking for. The whole purpose of this book is to help you succeed, and not fail; these will get you through any challenging times by helping you suppress hunger, crave less, and burn more fat for fuel.

Also, it's important to add—these won't break your fast!

1. ⅛ teaspoon of Himalayan pink salt or Redmond Real Salt in 1 liter of water

2. 1 tablespoon of raw almond, coconut, macadamia nut, or cacao butter

3. 1 tablespoon of omega-9 oil (avocado oil, extra-virgin olive oil, black seed oil, or macadamia nut oil)

4. 1 tablespoon of coconut oil or MCT oil (add a pinch of Himalayan pink salt), eaten right off the spoon

5. 1 tablespoon of chia seeds in 6 ounces of filtered water

TRACK YOUR JOURNEY

Record how the step is affecting your overall well-being by filling out the chart for Days 13 to 15 on page 209.

STEP 5: TIME YOUR MEALS ACTION PLAN

* Don't eat for three hours before going to sleep.

* Follow the Time Your Meals Action Plan on page 142 to extend the amount of time you go without eating (starting at the stage that makes sense for you).

* Do at least one of the daily steps in the "Five to Thrive" box on this page to reduce cravings and raise your energy.

* Continue eating your greens, healthy fats, moderate amounts of high-quality protein, and herbs and spices.

eleven

Step 6 (Days 16–18): Supplement Your Efforts

I BELIEVE WHOLEHEARTEDLY THAT FOOD IS OUR BEST MEDICINE. BUT THERE ARE some nutrients that foods just can't provide sufficient amounts of for us to be healthy in today's world. I wish it weren't the case, but it is. This step of the Get Off Your Sugar program is designed to get you up and running with the supplements that will deliver all the nutrients you need to heal from the damage sugar has caused and move toward optimal wellness. Once you have a smart supplement strategy in place (and at the end of these next three days, you will), you won't have to make any more decisions about which ones to take; you can just stick with your plan so that it becomes automatic.

As a bonus, supplements are like an umbrella insurance policy for your health—while you can't supplement your way out of a poor diet loaded with CRAP-py (completely refined and processed) carbs, they can support you through the inevitable times when you get off track.

What's the first thing you think of when you see a wilted plant—you think it needs water, right? Maybe some sunlight, some plant food?

You don't think, "That plant needs prescription drugs and surgery," right? Giving your body the right supplements is the equivalent of tending to a houseplant. It provides the components your body needs to flourish. From a nutritional standpoint, food can get you through three-quarters of a marathon; supplements carry you that last little way and get you over the finish line.

One note about supplements: before you start adding supplements to your daily routine, be sure to check with your health-care provider, as some supplements have contraindications with certain medications. As we all have different physiologies and health histories, we each require different nutrients in different amounts—it's really best to get an individualized recommendation.

WHY YOU NEED SUPPLEMENTS, NO MATTER HOW HEALTHY YOU EAT

Why can't we just eat a healthy diet and get everything we need to thrive? One major hurdle is that our soil has been depleted of nutrients as a result of modern farming practices, including consistently planting the same crops in the same fields (instead of using crop rotation, which replenishes any nutrients that the previous crops absorbed) and synthetic fertilizer and pesticide use. A 2004 study compared the mineral and vitamin content of forty-two plants in 1950 and in 1999—all of them saw significant declines in levels of calcium (16 percent), phosphorus (9 percent), iron (15 percent), riboflavin (38 percent),

and vitamin C (15 percent).[1] And that was more than twenty years ago.

Speaking of pesticides, we live in the most toxic time that's ever been. One hundred years ago, the soil was completely different than it is today. Now, even the minerals that *are* contained in our plants are negated by glyphosate, the herbicide in Roundup weed killer, which binds up half of the magnesium in the foods it's used on. Glyphosate is so ubiquitous that you can find traces of it in every single human being. It also destroys our gut bacteria, as do artificial sweeteners and antibiotics, which then further degrades our ability to assimilate the nutrients that are in our food.

Even people who have been eating very healthfully, with tons of organic vegetables, wonder why their hormones are out of balance or they're not feeling energized; it's because food doesn't have the good stuff in it that it used to.

On top of eating food that's been grown in depleted and toxic soil, we're also eating too much sugar, taking handfuls of medication every day, working too hard, drinking too much caffeine, and stressing too much, all of which drains our body of minerals and nutrients. For all these reasons, supplementing is a necessity for health. If you go to the supplement aisle of your drug store or grocery store, though, you'll probably get completely overwhelmed because there are so many available. That's why I'm introducing you to my personal top five supplements that I believe pretty much everyone should be taking.

THE TOP FIVE SUPPLEMENTS EVERYONE NEEDS TO GO FROM DEFICIENCY TO SUFFICIENCY

Supplement #1: Magnesium. You're probably thinking, "Yeah, we covered magnesium in Chapter 6"—that's true and you should check back there if you need a refresher, but it's worth repeating here: magnesium is the fourth-most-abundant mineral in your body, but it's the absolute most-important mineral in terms of function; researchers have detected more than 3,750 magnesium-binding sites on human proteins, and it is a cofactor for the activity of 700–800 enzymes. It's your number one most important neuroprotector, it helps keep your blood vessel walls nice and supple, it's essential for the absorption of calcium and vitamin D, it's necessary for insulin production, and it works in tandem with potassium to regulate blood sugar. It's important for energy production, as it activates six out of eight steps in the process (called the Krebs cycle) that your mitochondria use to manufacture adenosine triphosphate (ATP), the form of energy used by cells throughout your body. It's also the third-most-common mineral deficiency; if you have any health problems, it's likely that a magnesium deficiency might be a factor.

A note about testing your magnesium levels: If you get standard bloodwork at your annual physical, the magnesium levels it shows really aren't the full picture. The bloodwork measures only how much magnesium is in your blood, where only 1 percent of your magnesium is housed. Sixty percent of your magnesium is stored in your bones, 39 percent in the rest of your body—primarily the heart and the brain, which is why deficiency affects these two organs the most.

That 1 percent in the blood is there to neutralize acidity and inflammation—your body will always maintain that 1 percent. If your body is using up these stores (which happens with most people), it will steal it from the body, where it's not needed as urgently. So, you become deficient, even though your blood tests always show that 1 percent level is being maintained. And then, your doctor reads this test result and says you're fine, when you're not. If your standard blood test ever shows that your magnesium (that 1 percent) is *low*, you likely have a massive deficiency and you need to do a red blood cell magnesium test to look at your true numbers (see the Resources section for a source for this test if your doctor or health-care provider doesn't offer it).

You want to get magnesium from a variety of sources: foods (of course), green drinks (the center molecule of chlorophyll is magnesium), magnesium lotions and oils (as it can be absorbed through your skin; this is also a great way for kids to get it), by soaking in Epsom salts baths (Epsom salts are composed of magnesium sulfate), and from a magnesium supplement.

Dosage: There isn't one dosage that's right for everyone, although there is a guideline. Everyone needs between 500 and 600 mg of magnesium a day, and we can only really get about 200 mg from our food.

The way I counsel my patients to find their correct magnesium supplement dosage is to aim to get 3 to 4.5 mg per pound of body weight. So, if you weigh 100 pounds, that means you need between 300 and 450 mg a day in supplement form. The way to pinpoint from there is to start on the low end, and take 50 mg more per day until you get loose stools (because magnesium relaxes smooth muscle, including those in your GI tract, it is a great remedy for constipation, although there is such a thing as too much of a good thing), then back off on your dosage by 50 mg.

As for the form of magnesium to take, magnesium glycinate is the most bioavailable; magnesium threonate and magnesium citrate are also good.

Ideally, your magnesium supplement is in powder or liquid form. If it's a tablet, the most you can absorb is 30 percent, and if it's a capsule, your absorption will make out around 50 percent, making it very hard to assess how much you're actually getting. Remember, you are not what you eat, you are what you absorb and assimilate, which is why I prefer powders and liquids.

Supplement #2: Omega-3s. At their root, all chronic diseases are linked to inflammation, and the most critical driver of inflammation is your ratio of omega-3 fatty acids to omega-6 fatty acids.

Nearly everyone needs to supplement with omega-3 fatty acids to bring this crucial ratio into balance (I spend a lot of time in Chapter 7 on this important ratio, if you need a refresher).

The best source of omega-3s is fish oil that's been purified. Purified because there's not a milliliter of the ocean that's not contaminated with environmental pollutants, including heavy metals (e.g., mercury), PCBs, and plastic. And ideally, purified multiple times and tested by an FDA-registered facility. A bonus is for your fish oil to have been molecularly distilled, a process that concentrates the oil so that you have to take fewer softgels to get the dosage you need.

These extra steps do mean that quality fish oil supplements will probably be more money than you might like to spend on any one given supplement. *This is the one supplement you really don't want to cut costs on.* There are ninety-six thousand deaths per year related to an omega-3 deficiency—spending on good fish oil supplements can save you thousands in health care costs.

Ideally you want those omega-3s in a 2:1 ratio of EPA (which reduces inflammation) to DHA (which optimizes brain function); check the label, it should list the amounts of each of these essential fatty acids. The one exception to this ratio is children; because their brain is still developing, they need more DHA than EPA. (See the resources section for a specific omega-3 supplement recommendation.)

If you are vegetarian or vegan: I've got good news and bad news for you. The good news is that, as I mentioned in Chapter 7, there are vegetarian sources of omega-3s: flax, chia, and hemp seeds all contain alpha-linolenic acid (ALA), which is the plant-based form of omega-3s. The bad news is that your body has to convert ALA into EPA and DHA, and only about 1 percent of the ALA gets converted into a usable form. I respect vegetarians and vegans so much because they are often motivated by a love of animals. But really, the only way to ensure you get all the omega-3s you need is to take fish oil. If you just can't bring yourself to take fish oil, double up on your chia, flax, and hemp seeds and take an algae supplement (such as spirulina or chlorella), which provides small amounts of EPA and DHA (see Resources for a specific recommendation).

A note on krill oil: Some people recommend krill oil as an ideal source of omega-3s; krill are small, shrimplike creatures that live off of Antarctica, where the water is cleaner than most other parts of the world. Krill is high in the antioxidant astaxanthin, which gives it its pink color. But krill oil has low amounts of EPA and DHA, and they aren't in a good ratio to each other. Krill oil is also less absorbable than fish oil—you'd have to eat a whole handful of supplements to get the same amount of omega-3s in fish oil.

If you experience fish burps, either the oil has gone rancid, or you're not assimilating fat properly. If you know the fish oil is good, then you know it's a digestive issue—perhaps there's something off in your GI tract, or you have a gallbladder issue, or you don't have the necessary enzymes to digest it (I suggest everyone over the age of thirty-five take a digestive enzyme supplement—you'll read more about that shortly). Storing your fish oil supplements in the freezer will keep the oil fresher, longer. Also, be sure to take them before a meal so that it doesn't end up sitting on top of the food in your belly.

Dosage: 3,000 mg (or 3 grams) per day, with a 2:1 ratio of EPA to DHA. If you've never taken an omega-3 supplement before, start with taking one softgel a day, and gradually work your way up to the suggested dosage.

Supplement #3: Vitamin D. Vitamin D is actually a hormone, and it plays a critical role in so many systems of the body: it works in tandem with magnesium and vitamin K_2 and to absorb calcium and put it where the body truly needs it (i.e., the bones) and it's critical for immune system function and brain health. And it's estimated that one *billion* people around the world, and 90 percent of Americans, are deficient in it. There is even an increasing incidence in rickets, the bone-weakening disease caused by vitamin D deficiency that had been previously thought to be eradicated.

Your body will manufacture its own vitamin D from sun exposure—you need only about fifteen minutes of direct sunlight on a majority of your body to get all you need. But so few of us can do that, even in high summer. We're busy slathering on sunscreen and covering up (of course, you don't want to get burned, but we almost never get unfettered sun exposure that's not through a window or a layer of sunscreen). And if you live farther north than an imaginary line that runs from San Francisco to Philadelphia, the sun is not strong enough to cause the chemical reaction on your skin that creates vitamin D.

While I encourage everyone to get outside and let the sun hit as much of their skin as they are comfortable exposing for fifteen minutes a day, the vast majority of us need to supplement.

It's helpful to get a blood test to see where your vitamin D levels are so that you know how much supplementing you need to do. Also, what you *inspect* you'll *respect*.

The "normal" range on the blood test is 30 to 100 ng/ml, but you really don't want to be on the low end of that. You want to be in the 60 to 90 range; that's where you avoid the flu and degenerative disease. In fact, a 2016 study published in the journal *PloS One* found that a serum vitamin D level of at least 40 ng/ml is associated with a reduced risk of cancer by 67 percent compared to a level of 20 ng/ml or less.[2]

Dosage: A minimum of 5,000 international units (IUs) for adults. Make sure your supplement contains vitamin D_3, which is the natural form, and not D_2, which is the synthetic form. If I have a patient whose blood level is 40 ng/ml or lower, I'll have them take 10,000 IUs a day for a few months to get their levels up quickly.

Also, vitamin D is fat-soluble, which means it must be taken with a healthy fat. For this reason, I prefer a liquid vitamin that has coconut, extra-virgin olive, or MCT oil so that you can absorb it.

Supplement #4: Vitamin K_2. Vitamin K_2 works in tandem with magnesium and vitamin D to tell your body what to do with calcium. There are two primary forms of vitamin K: K_1 comes from vegetables, and then your body has to convert it to K_2, which is the usable form. If you don't have enough K_2, calcium will get deposited in your blood vessel walls (leading to atherosclerosis and cardiovascular disease), joints (contributing to arthritis), or the brain (increasing your odds of dementia) instead of to your bones.

There are also multiple forms of K_2. Based on what we know currently, you should look for a supplement with vitamin K_2 MK-7.

Dosage: 100 to 300 micrograms (mcg) per day of **vitamin K_2 MK-7** (the optimal form) for adults.

If you take a statin drug: Statins, which are prescribed for lowering cholesterol, block the conversion of K_1 to K_2. If you are taking statins, you need twice the amount. (Did your doctor tell you to take vitamin K_2 when they put you on a statin drug?)

If you have any blood-clotting disorders: Talk with your doctor before taking a K_2 supplement, as it can thin the blood.

If you have osteoporosis or osteopenia: Take 200 to 600 mcg per day to help ensure that your bones get all the calcium they need to stay strong.

Supplement #5: Probiotics. Probiotic supplements contain live bacteria that play a huge role in your health—they help heal leaky gut, reduce neuroinflammation, and improve mood (because 95 percent of your serotonin is in your gut). We're heavily deficient in these important creatures—we get one-millionth of the probiotics our ancient ancestors used to get.

Not only do we ingest fewer than we need, but there are many things we're exposed to—sometimes willingly and sometimes unknowingly—that harm the bacteria we do have. The word *probiotic* means "for life," and so many things we ingest are against life—sugar, artificial sweeteners, medicines, antibiotics, glyphosate, and pesticides all take a toll on our bacterial population.

One myth about probiotics is that you have good bacteria and bad bacteria residing in your body. You have bacteria, period. As living creatures, bacteria will adapt to terrain. If you have a gut that is acidic and inflamed, the bacteria that live in there will be transformed by the environment into harmful versions. So, while it's important to take a probiotic supplement, you also need to clean up the terrain (which is exactly what you're doing by following the Get Off Your Sugar program), *and* you need to eat the foods that nourish bacteria and keep them beneficial. These foods, called *prebiotics*, are at least as important, if not more so, than the probiotics, because without them, the bacteria you introduce via supplement won't live long.

Dosage: Aim to get 30 billion colony forming units (CFUs) per day; this will likely take two or three capsules that are best taken with your largest meal of the day. If the packaging of your supplement says it has 15 billion CFUs per capsule, there will be some degradation by the time you take it; assume you're getting only ten billion CFUs and take three capsules. Store your supplements in the fridge or freezer; the live bacteria will go dormant in the cold. It will also decrease moisture in the supplement, which will preserve the cultures for longer. Ideally, you'll switch up your probiotics every thirty to ninety days by buying a different brand. This will introduce different strains of bacteria into your gut.

You can, of course, also eat fermented foods, such as sauerkraut, kimchi, and miso, which are rich sources of bacteria. But if you have any level of leaky gut, the wild yeast that most fermented foods contain can leak into your bloodstream and wreak havoc. Let your gut heal first before making them a mainstay of your diet.

YOUR MOUTH NEEDS PREBIOTICS TOO

Your mouth is where your microbiome begins, and neglecting your oral health can actually be the cause of a number of gut issues. When I interviewed my good friend and top New York City biological dentist Dr. Gerry Curatola, with more than thirty years' experience (his practice is called Rejuvenation Dentistry), for the Get Off Your Sugar Summit, he shared that "Your mouth is a mirror for what's going on in your gut and your entire body."

The oral microbiome is extremely complex. It's as unique as your thumbprint and is made up of six to ten billion bacteria from about eight hundred different species. Yet what do we do with our chemical-laden toothpastes? Try to kill our oral bacteria!

The same bacteria that cause tooth decay and gum disease can be beneficial in a balanced environment. Improving your diet by following the Get Off Your Sugar program will improve the terrain for your oral microbiome as well as your gut microbiome.

But something else you should do to support your oral health is to stop using toothpastes that include the antibacterial chemical called triclosan, a chemical that has been shown to help prevent gingivitis *but* that has been linked to concerns about antibiotic resistance, endocrine disruption, and disruption of your oral (and gut) microbiome.[3] This ingredient is in your children's toothpaste as well—check your labels!

Dr. Curatola has created a prebiotic-rich toothpaste filled with essential oils, vitamins, enzymes, and minerals that's made for nurturing the microbiome, as opposed to every other chemical-filled toothpaste that is bacteria-destroying. See the Resources section for more information.

SUPPORTING PLAYERS

Some people need a bit more supplementation help to cover all their nutritional bases. The following are what I consider to be supporting players to the top five.

B Complex

Take if you are: vegetarian, vegan, and/or over age thirty-five.

The B vitamins, as I covered on page 29, are key to brain health. Taking a B complex ensures that you get the full suite of B vitamins, including: B_1, B_2, B_3, B_5, B_6, B_7, B_9, and B_{12}.

B vitamins enhance brain performance and increased alertness. Research shows that a vitamin B deficiency can cause neurological problems. People who suffer from depression or anxiety can often trace their problems to a lack of vitamin B in their diet. Specifically, a vitamin B_6 deficiency can cause depression and swelling of the tongue, whereas a vitamin B_{12} deficiency can produce a type of anemia, fatigue, and memory and cognitive impairment. In addition to optimizing brain function, they play important roles in energy production; the synthesis and repair of DNA and RNA; and carbohydrate, protein, and fat metabolism.

B vitamins are found in dark green leafy vegetables, animal proteins, and whole grains.

Unfortunately, many of us don't get enough B vitamins on a daily basis. Industrial farming, depleted soils, highly processed foods, and food allergies and intolerances all lead to vitamin B deficiencies, specifically B_6, B_{12}, and B_9 (folate). Industrial farming robs the soil of magnesium and trace minerals that are essential for the plants to create B vitamins. Both humans and animals are consuming food that is deficient in B vitamins.

Dosage: B-complex supplements vary widely in composition and dosage. For this reason, it's best to follow the dosage recommendations on the label, as different companies use different concentrations, and dosage may vary between brands. Look for a B-complex formula that contains only the active forms. "Active" means that the Bs are in a form that the body can utilize immediately. Some examples of active or methylated forms are:

- **Benfotiamine** for thiamine or B_1
- **Methylcobalamin** for B_{12}
- **L-5-MTHF** for folic acid

Finally, and most important, look for a formulation that provides a slow release. Why is this so important? B vitamins are water-soluble; they flush through us. That means that whatever the cells cannot absorb in approximately sixty minutes is eliminated via the kidneys into urine. So, even the best B complexes will only be bioavailable for a very short period of time. A slow-release formula allows the active Bs to be in circulation four or five times longer, increasing the window of opportunity that each cell has to absorb these key nutrients. This is a huge advantage over regular B formulations, significantly benefitting those individuals experiencing stress, chronic fatigue conditions, and cognitive impairment.

The next time you are shopping for a B complex use this checklist to help choose the right one:

- Look for bioactive forms where possible.

- Look for higher dosages; because B vitamins are water-soluble, any excess will be excreted through your urine (you will notice that they turn your urine bright yellow).

- Look for brands that don't use any artificial dyes or coloring.

- Try to find products with no fillers or extra ingredients (if you can't pronounce it, you probably can't digest it!).

- If you have specific allergens make sure your B complex is free of those allergens.

- The better brands will add labels indicating that they are hypoallergenic, gluten-free, and vegetarian/vegan.

Do You Need Extra B$_{12}$?

There are also instances where taking additional individual B vitamins may be appropriate. For example, vitamin B$_{12}$ may be useful for those who use stomach acid–controlling drugs, including H2 blockers and proton-pump inhibitors, or who take Metformin to treat type 2 diabetes. But I really don't want you throwing darts at a dartboard. Before you decide to take any additional individual B vitamin supplements, verify any deficiencies with a blood test.

Digestive Enzymes

Take if you are: over age thirty-five.

Starting around age thirty-five, you produce less stomach acid. This may *sound* like a good thing (particularly if you read my first book, *Get Off Your Acid*, about the dangers of eating too many acidic foods that can upset your body's delicate pH balance), but it actually makes it harder for your body to break down the food you eat and assimilate the nutrients contained in your food. This is particularly true of fat, because your body can kind of forget how to burn fat if you've spent years and years primarily eating and burning sugar. Stress also takes a toll on digestive enzymes because the body shuts down digestion—including the release of digestive enzymes—when it perceives a threat. And we are all stressed to varying degrees every day, no matter our age. Taking digestive enzymes before meals can help fire up your fat-burning engines as well as break down—

and thus, assimilate—the nutrients in the food you eat.

Classic signs of insufficient digestive enzymes include frequent burping while eating, gas and bloating, heartburn, and a sensation of food feeling "stuck" somewhere in your GI tract, because it actually *is* stuck in transit.

Dosage: Aim for a high-potency digestive enzyme that minimally contains the enzymes protease, lipase, and amylase, to assist in the optimal digestion of proteins, fats, and carbohydrates in your diet. Take one capsule right before your meal, or after the first or second bite.

Extra Omega-3s

Take if you are: pregnant or postnatal.

I recommend pregnant women take extra omega-3s, especially in the first trimester, as the baby's brain is forming at that time and DHA is a crucial ingredient for healthy brain development.

When Chelsea was pregnant with our two kids, she would take three grams of an adult omega-3 supplement daily, and then take an additional baby omega-3 supplement, with 750 milligrams of omega-3s in the baby-appropriate DHA:EPA ratio (since babies need more DHA than adults do).

Also, the baby will take all the nutrients it needs from the mom, and that can mean a pregnant mom can get deficient in omega-3s and vitamin D. And low levels of these two things are a big factor in postpartum depression. So, make sure you are getting ample amounts of these two top five, both through food and through supplements.

Iodine

Take if you are: tired and sick all the time, and/or female, and/or over age thirty-five, or pregnant, or have thyroid problems, such as hypothyroidism or Hashimoto's.

Iodine is a mineral that's used in your bones and to manufacture thyroid hormone. The thyroid rules your metabolism; if your thyroid hormones are off, even a little bit, it can feel as if someone either took their foot off the gas pedal of your body, or have stepped on the gas and are revving your engines way too high. Common symptoms of insufficient thyroid hormone include gaining weight that you can't seem to lose, hair loss, sensitivity to cold, heavy or irregular menstrual cycles, or chronic fatigue.

As with vitamin B_{12}, your body cannot make iodine. You have to get it through food—sea vegetables, such as kelp or dulse; wild-caught fish; shellfish; egg yolks (from pastured organic chickens); and lima beans are all good food sources of iodine—or supplements. Himalayan pink salt has trace amounts.

Iodine deficiency is the number one cause of thyroid issues, such as Hashimoto's and hypothyroidism. If you are iodine deficient and pregnant, it can impair the baby's brain development, particularly in the third trimester, so it's very important for pregnant and breastfeeding women to make sure they're getting enough.

Dosage: Adults need 150 mcg a day; if you're pregnant, that number goes up to 220 mcg; and if you're breastfeeding, it's 290 mcg. To make up for a likely deficiency,

I recommend taking 500 to 1,000 mcg per day.

If you have thyroid concerns but are not on thyroid medication, begin by adding different kinds of fresh and dried seaweeds into your diet. Fresh is always best, but if seaweeds are scarce, alternate between kelp powder (brown algae) and dulse flakes (sea lettuce), which are both highly alkaline sea vegetables. Start with ⅛ teaspoon daily for one month and see how you feel, and then go up steadily from there.

If you are on medications, speak with your health-care practitioner before implementing any changes.

Antioxidants

Take if you are: alive (i.e., anyone).

Pick one or two of the following to have daily:

Black seed oil. I'm putting this one at the top of the list because it is three times more anti-inflammatory than turmeric and one thousand times more active than vitamin E, echinacea, and elderberry as an antioxidant. When Covid-19 hit, this powerful antioxidant was something I gave to my family, clients, and patients because it has been extensively researched for its antiviral activity and ability to help your immune system defend against invaders. It also helps regulate blood sugar and lessens risk of many cancers, including colon, pancreatic, liver, lung, breast, and cervical cancer. Because of its potency, this is the antioxidant I recommend, but you can also choose from the list below.

Dosage: 500 mg daily (see Resources section for a specific recommendation)

N-acetyl cysteine (NAC). This amino acid is essential for making glutathione, a powerful antioxidant that lessens free radical damage and helps the body detox heavy metals. NAC is also great for your liver, and can help protect against hangover.

Dosage: 240 mg daily for adults

Vitamin C. This essential vitamin (meaning it can't be produced by the body) can increase your levels of circulating antioxidants by 30 percent. It also boosts the production and function of white blood cells, an important component of your immune system. Because now we understand that we need to prepared for the next pandemic—whether it's Covid-19 or something we don't even know about yet—vitamin C is a crucial piece of having an immune system that is tuned up and at the ready, but not overstimulated. There's a saying: the best time to prepare for an emergency was two years ago; the second-best time is today. Let's be ready.

Dosage: 1,000 mg daily (ideally in liposomal or buffered form)

Molecular hydrogen (H2). Technically a gas, hydrogen targets the most harmful free radicals and neutralizes them. Your gut bacteria produce hydrogen when they digest fiber, so molecular hydrogen is completely safe to take.

Dosage: Take it in the form of a water filtration unit, or tablets or drops that you add to a glass of water. (See the Resources section for a recommendation.)

TOP THREE SUPPLEMENTS FOR BRAIN HEALTH

Remember, your body is electrical, and the health of your nervous system is crucial for its operation. You're not pronounced dead when your heart stops, it's when your brain stops, so you must do whatever you can to support your nervous system function. The top three most powerful supplements to protect your brain and nervous system health are **magnesium**, **omega-3 fish oil**, and **B complex**.

If you've been experiencing brain fog or forgetfulness, you need to take all three. And if you don't have those symptoms, guess what—you still need to take all three! Don't wait for a toothache to start brushing your teeth, know what I mean?!

TRACK YOUR JOURNEY

Assess how this step is impacting you by filling out the chart for Days 16–18 on page 209.

STEP 6: SUPPLEMENT YOUR EFFORTS ACTION PLAN

* Buy the top five supplements.
* Identify what supporting players make sense for you.
* Take your supplements every day—I take mine either at lunch or dinner, about fifteen minutes after I've started eating, so that my digestion is humming, and they're more easily broken down and thus more easily assimilated.
* Continue doing each of the previous steps.

twelve

Step 7 (Days 19–21): Amp Up Your Workout

By now, you've incorporated all the major components of the Get Off Your Sugar eating plan: You've upped your intake of minerals, healthy fats, plant-based protein, herbs and spices, and slow-burning, fiber-rich carbs. You've moderated your protein intake. You've gone a long way toward nudging your body into the fat-burning zone. Now it's time for the final piece—the cherry on top of your Avocado Chocolate Mousse. And that is to amp up your exercise habits.

When you pair exercising with a healthy diet, the game changes.

Don't worry; that doesn't mean you have to start running ultra marathons (although you might be surprised how burning fat can help you do physical feats of endurance you never thought possible!). While, of course, some forms of exercise are more beneficial than others, you simply need to move your body more. When you do, you'll boost energy, improve circulation, detoxify through your lymphatic system, and manage stress better.

MOVE MORE, STRESS LESS, STAY OFF SUGAR

You likely know that going for a walk or a run can clear your head. That's because exercise triggers the production of numerous chemicals that help your body respond better to stressors. Those chemicals include endorphins—which improve mood and lower pain—and neurotransmitters, such as serotonin and dopamine, which literally make you happier. It also lowers your levels of stress hormones, including adrenaline and cortisol. Or, as I like to say, *motion* is *emotion*. Moving makes you feel good. When you feel better, you make healthier choices. You will *want* to eat a salad or have a green drink. On the other hand, when you're sedentary and you don't have a healthy means of bringing your stress levels down, you'll reach for CRAP-py (completely refined and processed) carbs to soothe yourself.

When you know *why* something is good for you, you're much more likely to *comply*, so here are all the things exercise does for you:

- Helps insulin sensitivity or resistance to heal. Exercise causes your blood glucose levels to go down; that means you have to release less insulin, which gives your insulin sensitivity or resistance a chance to heal. Exercise-improved insulin/leptin receptor sensitivity is perhaps the most important factor for optimizing your overall health and preventing chronic disease.

- Increases circulation all the way down to your capillaries, which deliver oxygen and other nutrients deep into your tissues. This process, known as microcirculation, is responsible for 75 percent of all circulation in the body.

- Spurs the development of new blood vessels (a process known as angiogenesis), increasing microcirculation.

- Lowers blood pressure; because exercise (particularly aerobic exercise, which I'll cover in just a moment) strengthens your heart, it helps your heart pump more blood, more efficiently, which brings your systolic blood pressure (the first number in your blood pressure reading) down.

- Encourages your brain to work at optimum capacity by causing your nerve cells to multiply, strengthening their interconnections and protecting them from damage.

- Boosts the function of the lymphatic system, meaning your detoxing abilities are enhanced.

- Strengthens your joints and bones, as they respond to the forces placed upon them, and exercise can expose them to forces that are as much as six times more than your body weight.

- Reduces risk of breast cancer by as much as 40 percent in women who exercise regularly.

- Decreases pain levels, thanks in large part to the pain-relieving chemicals known as endorphins of which exercise triggers the release.

- Helps you dislodge and release the toxins that have been stored in your fat.

I'm not talking about really going for the burn here. You don't have to push yourself to the limit in a spinning or hot yoga class for exercise to count. You can absolutely do the exercise that you actually enjoy. Just make it your goal to get up and move your body at an appropriate level. As we did with food, start by adding more good. If you're fairly sedentary, start with a fifteen-minute walk. Just do it with the mindset of "this is my exercise," so it's not an aimless ramble down the street. Put on your real workout clothes; get off your phone and into a healthy healing environment.

I love going out and playing soccer with my son or scootering with my daughter, and both completely count as movement. When you enjoy your exercise, you'll do it on a regular basis. Better yet, you'll improve your quality of life, because you'll be having more fun. And that's how I'd like you to approach these next three days—with an attitude of fun and experimentation.

SUGAR-BURNING VS. FAT-BURNING EXERCISE

Just as with diet, a major ingredient of exercise success is variety. You don't want to do the same workout every day. (There is a routine I'll share with you in just a minute that you could do every day if it feels good to you, but it takes only eight minutes! You should still do other forms of exercise, and those need to be varied.)

That said, there are two different basic types of exercise that you should be aware of, so that you can make sure that you're doing both of them. They are aerobic and anaerobic:

Aerobic

What it is: Most exercise that we would call "cardio"—running, walking, cross-country skiing, hiking. It is fueled by oxygen. (Unless you do it so intensely that you start gasping for air—running up a hill, for example; then it becomes anaerobic.)

Stimulates: Parasympathetic nervous system activity (the rest-and-digest functions of the body) and heart rate variability (HRV; the prime predictor of cardiovascular health). Most of us get stuck in the sympathetic nervous system realm (which rules the fight-or-flight response) thanks to our constant exposure to low levels of stress, whether it's physical, chemical, or emotional stress. A healthy HRV means you can easily switch between a sympathetic and parasympathetic state—and that's what aerobic exercise helps you build.

Burns: Primarily fat. Aerobic metabolism is your fat-burning friend, as it takes the fat out of the connective tissues and cells and burns it to produce energy for the muscle. It also burns up the available and stored sugars (glycogen) in your liver and muscles, which allows your body to begin to access and burn off its stored fat.

Good for: Burning fat, lowering inflammation[1], building endurance, and improving cardiovascular health and longevity (by preserving the length of telomeres—the genetic material that seals the ends of your DNA).[2]

Examples: Walking (and speed walking), yoga, tai chi, Pilates, jogging, swimming, easy running, biking, spinning, playing sports, dancing, and boxing (as long as you can still pass the talk test and carry on a conversation without huffing/puffing).

Anaerobic

What it is: Brief, intense bursts of energy that require more oxygen than you have access to, so the body breaks down the stored glucose (called glycogen) in your muscles and liver, followed by your stored fat, to meet your energy demands.

Stimulates: Sympathetic nervous system (fight or flight).

Burns: Primarily sugar. Anaerobic metabolism primarily uses glucose and glycogen; however, when done the right way, at the right time (i.e., before breaking your fast), with the right diet, you can use this type of workout to fuel your fat-burning engine.

Good for: Building lean muscle, strengthening bones, increasing stamina, losing weight.

Examples: Heavy weightlifting, general strength training, sprinting, high-intensity interval training (HIIT—more on this on pages 170–172).

Neither aerobic nor anaerobic exercise is better; they are both important for your health and longevity, and both types of exercise can burn fat. Although it's long been thought that low-intensity cardio is optimal for fat loss, that thinking is starting to evolve. Whereas aerobic exercise does use a higher percentage of fat for energy as opposed to anaerobic exercise, which relies primarily on muscle glycogen, the total amount of energy burned during aerobic exercise is *lower* than during anaerobic exercise for a given period of time.

This means that, for most people, extended periods of aerobic exercise are needed to achieve significant fat loss, whereas anaerobic exercise can get you to your weight loss goals with less time spent working out.

With that said, the key to getting the best results is either to have a workout that incorporates both forms of exercise, or regularly doing exercise from each category, so that your body can continuously adapt.

WORKOUT FAQS AND STRATEGIES

When Is the Best Time to Work Out?

There isn't a *wrong* time to work out or train, but there is an *optimal* time; and that's when your blood sugar levels are at their lowest, which means before you have your first meal of the day, whether that's at a traditional breakfast time or later in the day because you're intermittent fasting. Why? Because it will force your body to burn fat for energy as you won't have a lot of glucose just lying around. So, booking that early-morning spin class or going for a jog before work works well if you're fasting.

As I talked about in Chapter 10, when your blood sugar levels are low, your insulin is also low. And when your insulin levels are low, your body doesn't have any sugar lying around to burn off for fuel, so instead, it goes to its *preferred* source of energy, which is fat. Here's the best part: when you tap into this fat-burning state, not only will you see your belly become flatter, you will have endless energy throughout your workout and your day.

If that wasn't enough motivation, when you exercise before breaking your fast, the beta receptors on the fat cells in the belly area are activated. That makes them much more likely to be burned (remember, the *b* in *beta* also stands for burn). So, forget about fueling up before your workout—fasting in advance will increase your results.

That being said, the best workout is the one you actually *do*. So, if the only time you have to exercise is after work, that's totally fine. You may have heard that working out in the evening can throw your bodily rhythm out of whack and lead to difficulty sleeping, but evening workouts have their benefits. Evenings are typically when we have our biggest stretch of time when we're not at work; fitting in a workout at night can be a lot easier than squeezing it in before work. One study (although, admittedly, it was small) also found that anaerobic capacity increases in the evening, leading to more productive workouts.[3] First, just develop the habit of exercising regularly, doing it whenever works for you and your schedule. You can always optimize the timing later.

What Should I Eat Before, During, and After My Workout to Burn Fat?

Before. As I just covered, the ideal time to work out is before you've had your first meal of the day, so ideally, you don't have to think much about what to eat *before* you work out. When you're in ketosis, your body is in prime fat-burning mode. This means your body can use the calories stored in its own fat to fuel your workout. Research has shown that people on a ketogenic diet burn over twice as much fat when they exercise than those who are eating a high-carb diet.[4]

If you choose to work out in a fasted state, you can have a cup of green tea—or better, matcha (which has 120 times the antioxidants of regular green tea; see Resources for my favorite brand)—before your workout to increase the levels of the fat-burning enzyme lipase to burn through your adipose tissue faster. I recommend this biohack only when you don't have any preworkout snacks.

I understand that everyone's goal may not be fat loss, or that you may be transitioning to this lifestyle and may still need some fuel or energy before you exercise.

If you need a preworkout snack, have a vegetable puree, as it is high in minerals and easy to digest, so it won't tax your digestive system or divert energy that you need for your workout. You can also have a chia shot (one of my favorite biohacks from "Five to Thrive" on page 146): Fifteen to thirty minutes before your workout, drink a 6-ounce glass of water with 1 to 2 tablespoons of chia seeds plus the juice from a slice of fresh organic lemon. Chia seeds are the perfect superfood to fuel your workout, as they are 50 percent omega-3 fatty acids to boost energy, 20 percent protein to give your muscles the amino acids they need to perform and repair themselves during exercise, and magnesium and other alkaline minerals to neutralize the acidity from whatever exercise you decide to do.

You never want to do cardio on a full stomach, as the sudden demand for blood flow from the muscles will steal vital blood flow needed by the digestive system for digestion and assimilation of nutrients.

A lot of protein right before a workout can cause cramping, since protein is acidic and requires more fluids to be metabolized than carbs and fat do. Cramping occurs when the body is less hydrated and when it has to use its mineral reserves to neutralize any acidic foods or toxins entering it. Protein is for building muscles, not for fueling them.

BIOHACK YOUR EXERCISE WITH PREWORKOUT GLUCOSE

If you're able to burn fat for fuel, here's a good biohack that I learned from Drew Manning (the celebrity trainer and bestselling author of *Fit2Fat2Fit*) that will give you instant fuel and energy to boost your performance during your workout:

Eat a boiled potato with Himalayan pink salt twenty to thirty minutes before you exercise.

Your body sees the glucose from the potato as damaging to your cells, and it wants to burn it off immediately, which in turn ignites your energy to give you that extra push you may need to go the extra distance.

You want to wait until you have become fat adapted before trying this trick, because once your body gains more metabolic flexibility, it knows how to use the glucose you strategically throw at it. So, by adding 10 to 20 grams of carbs before your workout, which the boiled potato provides, you give your body instant energy without compromising your ability to build lean muscle mass or to burn fat.

During. This really depends on how long your workout is. For a short (less than 60 minutes), low-intensity workout, you really don't need anything. If you're doing HIIT or doing a high-energy gym class for more than thirty minutes, you may want to sip on some water in which you've dissolved a pinch of Himalayan pink salt to replenish some of the trace minerals you're sweating out; whenever I take an intense class or have a workout longer than thirty minutes, I dissolve a scoop of my Alkamind Acid-Kicking Minerals into my water bottle to neutralize the lactic acid that exercise produces in my muscles to promote faster recovery.

If you are an endurance athlete, you can exercise for about ninety minutes without eating anything, as long as you stay well hydrated and supplement your water with trace minerals or Himalayan pink salt.

When I would run marathons or ultramarathons that required me to exercise for more than ninety minutes, I would use this biohack: I took a sprouted Ezekiel tortilla (sprouting denatures nearly all of the gluten), spread some raw sprouted almond butter on it, and topped it with a drizzle of manuka honey, some cinnamon, sea salt, and chia seeds. I would roll the wrap and then slice it into little bite-size pieces. Then, I wrapped those pieces in some cellophane wrap and put them in my pocket. It gave me an easily digestible source of fats and carbs that my body could burn right away.

You can also make your own energy gel (since most of the ones that are available in stores are loaded with sugar) by soaking 2 to 3 tablespoons of chia seeds in 4 to 6 ounces of water until it forms a gel. Then, put it into a snack-size resealable plastic bag and eat it as needed.

After. Once your workout is complete, you have a very small window of opportunity—about fifteen minutes—to neutralize all the lactic acid from your workout. If you didn't take minerals during your workout by adding $1/8$ teaspoon of Himalayan pink salt or a scoop of Alkamind Acid-Kicking Minerals to your water bottle, have some now, ideally dissolved in 4 to 6 ounces of water.

What you put into your body *after* your workout is one of the most important meals of the day. My number one rule for this meal is that it be low-carb. If you were to put sugar, carbs, or grains in your system at this time, your body would preferentially use these dirty fuels first, as sugar in all forms is inflammatory and your body

wants to burn it off. This would immediately pull you out of your fat-burning state, and possibly trigger the storage of fat.

Ideally, I recommend some form of a nutrient-dense drinkable meal that has a healthy balance of minerals, plant-based protein, and healthy fats for fast recovery, nutrient replenishment, and to maintain a fat-burning state. If you are in a hurry, you can simply go for a plant-based protein shake blended with some unsweetened almond or coconut milk, or even some full-fat coconut milk.

Otherwise, I suggest making your own superfood smoothie with a base of unsweetened almond or coconut milk, or full-fat coconut milk. Add two or three additional healthy fats, such as chia seeds, coconut oil, MCT oil, unsweetened coconut flakes, and/or some hemp seeds, which are also high in protein. Top it off with some cacao powder, cacao nibs, Himalayan pink salt, and a scoop of dehydrated greens for more minerals and alkalinity. Again, be sure to avoid carbs and fructose, even in the form of moderate-sugar fruits, such as blueberries or bananas. You can consume this superfood smoothie as soon after your workout as you like, or within a two-hour window.

Also keep in mind that if you are working out on a regular basis, you need to increase your protein intake. Research shows that consuming only 20 percent of your calories from protein when you exercise regularly can lead to muscle loss.[5] This tells us that your body requires more protein if you are exercising, likely closer to 30 percent of your total daily calories. To set a target for yourself, take the calculation you made of how much protein you need in a day (on page 115), and double it.

How Hard Do I Need to Work Out to Burn Fat?

When you're doing what's considered "cardio" exercise—such as walking or running—you want your exertion level to be between a 5 and a 7 (if 1 is ambling and 10 is sprinting up a big hill). You'll know you're in the sweet spot because you can still carry on a conversation without gasping for air. That means you're in an aerobic zone and are running on oxygen, not sugar (which is what happens when you exercise anaerobically). When you can do that, you're burning fat.

Another key thing to keep in mind, which a lot of people don't know, is that you don't want to zoom right up to level 7 intensity. When you walk out your door and immediately start running, your body goes into fight or flight—it doesn't know you're trying to do something beneficial. For all it knows, you could be running from a saber-toothed tiger. So, it will release cortisol, and you'll start burning sugar immediately. And when that happens, you can't tap into your fat stores, meaning you'll run out of energy quickly *and* you won't be able to burn fat. Start off walking slowly for seven to ten minutes or, if you're at the gym, ride the bike at a low speed. Have a slow and gentle warm-up so that your body knows you're not in danger, and you'll be much more likely to burn fat.

It may take a few workouts to get familiar with what your 5–7 exertion zone feels like. Whenever I exercise, I always do a self-check-in and ask myself, what is my exertion level? This allows me to always know which state my body is in—sugar burning or fat burning. If it's sugar burning, I know I need more minerals.

Are There Any Tricks to Maximize My Fat-Burning After My Workout Is Through?

Aside from making the next meal you eat after working out low-carb, the best way to keep your fat-burning engine stoked is to immerse yourself in cold water—either in the shower or jumping into a cold pool or bath—for two to five minutes.

Your body burns more calories when it's cold in an attempt to generate body heat and maintain a healthy core temperature. As your body temperature dips slightly, you enter a phase called "nonshivering thermogenesis," during which you increase your calorie and fat-burning capabilities.

A study published in *Cellular Metabolism* in 2014 revealed that the cold chill activates stores of good fat in your body called brown adipose fat (BAT; the T is for *tissue*), which helps turn up your metabolism and burn more fat and calories.[6] The heat is generated by mitochondria, little energy factories in a cell that turn glucose, fat, and other nutrients into a form of energy the cell can use.

When you cool off, your metabolism heats up! It's as if your mitochondria keep working out for you, even after your exertion is through.

How Do I Find the Motivation to Work Out Regularly?

Here's a tip to get the most from whatever exercise you do: do it with others. Not only will you be more likely to show up, but also your exercise will seem to be easier and take less time. It's not your imagination: taking an exercise class or having an exercise partner increases endorphins and tolerance to pain better than exercising alone.[7]

With two kids, work, and everything else, it's harder and harder for Chelsea and me to do date night. So, we work out together every Tuesday at 12:30 p.m. at a class taught by my good friend and celebrity trainer Anna Kaiser. Anna, who trains Kelly Ripa, Shakira, and Alicia Keys (among others), designed her classes to move the body functionally in all planes of motion, challenging every muscle, with the right ratio of cardio to strength training. Literally, it is the perfect workout for total body health and peak performance. When Chelsea and I go on these fitness "dates," we are doing something good for us, it makes us feel great, and because we are together, it motivates us more. It helps us feel more connected, and we can be more present when we're with the kids. Working out can absolutely be together time.

THE MISSING INGREDIENT FROM MOST WORKOUT PLANS

As I've said, one of the key components of a long-term healthy diet is variation. Your body is designed to be adaptable, and when you eat the same thing over and over, year-round, you are not giving it anything to adapt to. The same is true of exercise. You've got to switch it up to make it effective. That means you have full permission to do a bunch of different things for exercise. You can still have your favorites, but don't do them to the exclusion of other things. You can also choose a class or other workout that changes things up for you. That's another reason I love Anna Kaiser's class, because she changes it every three weeks. Just when I'm starting to get the hang of the routine, boom, she switches it up on us!

Varying your exercise keeps your body on its toes. It also encourages neuroplasticity, which is the capacity of neurons and neural networks in the brain to change in response to new stimulation, because your brain has to orchestrate the different things you're doing with your body, and if it can't anticipate what's coming next, it has to adapt. People who do the same exercise every day, whether that's hot yoga, spinning, or running, lose adaptability. When it comes to fitness, you've got to mix it up.

Your ideal workout program should include cardiovascular exercise, strength training, and a HIIT workout. Do some spinning, some gentle cardio, some HIIT, some yoga or tai chi, some strength training, swimming, running—mix it up and do what feels right for your body. Here is a sample workout week that incorporates both aerobic and anaerobic workouts, designed to accelerate your fat-burning state:

- **Day 1:** Strength/resistance training and 8-Minute Acid-Kicking Workout (see page 173)
- **Day 2:** Cardio (30–60 minutes) and 8-Minute Acid-Kicking Workout
- **Day 3:** HIIT (plus optional 8-Minute Acid-Kicking Workout)
- **Day 4:** Yoga, Pilates, or tai chi (take an optional day off from the 8-Minute Acid-Kicking Workout if you feel you need a rest—otherwise do it too)
- **Day 5:** Strength/resistance training and 8-Minute Acid-Kicking Workout
- **Day 6:** HIIT (plus optional 8-Minute Acid-Kicking Workout)
- **Day 7:** 8-Minute Acid-Kicking Workout

With this workout schedule, you give your body a chance to burn fat fast with strength and resistance training and HIIT intervals, but you also get to utilize easier days to burn fat with some moderate-intensity cardio, without quite as much strain on the body as when you do the same workout day in and day out.

Here are some great cardio options:

Walking

Jogging

Dancing

Rollerblading

Strength training

Functional exercise (body weight movements, such as squats and push-ups)

Cycling

Rowing

Gardening

Dancing

Zumba

Tennis

Basketball

Swimming

Cross-country skiing

Hiking

YET ANOTHER REASON TO EXERCISE: MOVING LYMPHATIC FLUID

The lymphatic system is an unsung hero of the human body. Basically, it's our garbage disposal, responsible for filtering our system and eliminating toxins.

Your lymph system parallels your circulatory system. But unlike your circulatory system, which has blood that is moved by the contractions of your heart, you don't have a pump for your lymphatic fluid. It is circulated by gravity and the contractions of your muscles—in other words, your lymphatic system is moved by movement.

Without movement, the toxins, poisons, and heavy metals that we ingest from our food, water, and environment will stagnate in our body and tissues. Not flushing your lymphatic system is like filling your wastebasket with trash and letting it pile up for weeks on end. That is not a pretty sight! But this is what is happening inside your body if you are not consciously moving it every day. Instead of being flushed from the body, toxins get trapped in small fat pockets. Since toxicity plays a huge roll in weight gain, premature aging, inflammation, and chronic disease, this system *must* be addressed when we are seeking optimal health.

Although all exercise will help circulate your lymph, my favorite way to move this important fluid is to bounce on a rebounder, otherwise known as a mini trampoline. (I jump on a rebounder most mornings for eight to ten minutes.) You can also encourage lymphatic drainage with lymphatic massage, dry skin brushing, or using a whole-body vibration plate.

NASA SAYS THIS WORKOUT IS MORE EFFECTIVE THAN RUNNING

Many adults haven't jumped on a trampoline since they were very young, but bouncing on a rebounder comes with some serious health benefits—even though it doesn't necessarily look like real exercise.

Rebounding jumpstarts the metabolism, stimulates the lymphatic system (an important component of the immune system that collects toxins and waste from the cells), and improves cardiovascular health. It also helps people lose weight, even if they have physical limitations that keep them from participating in higher-impact exercise. It is the only exercise that strengthens, cleanses, and tones every cell in the body.

Think for a minute about what you felt the last time you bounced on a trampoline. At the very top of your bounce, that split second when you were in the air before you came back down, you experienced weightlessness. At the bottom of your bounce, you felt much heavier than normal as the g-force intensified. You fluctuated between zero gravity and three times the normal amount. The fluctuation in gravity is what makes rebounding one of the best ways to stimulate your lymphatic system.

If you are sedentary and not moving enough, your body won't have enough energy to propel these toxins out of your system. Instead, your body stores these toxins bound to fat in your connective tissue, or what I call the acid magnets or catchers of the body. It "parks" them here for safekeeping so that these toxins can't harm your more important organs and systems in the body.

In the short run, the fat you gain is protective. In the long run, you'll gain more weight, and these inflammatory toxins and acids that your fat is buffering will damage your body, your energy, and your health.

When you rebound, you help dislodge the toxins stored in your fat cells and then eliminate them from the body. The fat that stores the toxins is swept away too. The result? Weight loss (particularly in the form of fat).

In the 1980s, NASA commissioned a study to find a form of exercise that could allow astronauts to stay fit in a weightless environment. They found rebounding is even more effective than running. Athletes who jumped on a trampoline experienced less stress on their ankles and legs than those who ran. At the same level of exertion, athletes who rebounded gained 68 percent more oxygen uptake than those who were running, which is great for energy, immunity, and weight loss.[8] (And it's better for your back, spine, and knees than running too!)

You can use the rebounder as gently as you like—I even have clients who have difficulty walking who bounce just their legs, sitting in a chair. Kids can do it (just teach them how to stay in the middle and keep an eye on them), and it's great for burning off some of their energy too.

My favorite rebounder is a Bellicon—it is top-of-the-line and has foldable legs so you can store it under a bed and uses bungee cords instead of springs, so it doesn't ever squeak (and it will also last longer). With that said, you don't need one with all the bells and whistles; you can also find a rebounder for as little as $50. It's a small investment of time and money that will pay big dividends in improved immunity and decreased toxins.

HOW TO REBOUND

* **Warm up.** Step on the trampoline and gently shift your weight between one foot and the other. Gradually add a little bounce. Loosen your hips and lower back, and start to swing your arms as you bounce. The balls of your feet stay on the rebounder at all times, while your heels elevate with each movement.

* **Bunny hops.** Use your toes, calf muscles, and legs to propel yourself in a series of small hops. Keep your knees soft as you land. Feel the work in your thighs and buttocks.

* **Jumping jacks.** Elevate your heart rate by doing the same exercise you did in high school gym class, only with a bounce.

* **Hop squats.** This moves the legs the same way as a jumping jack. When you land with your legs shoulder width apart, drop your weight by bending your knees to a 90-degree angle, as if you're sitting in a chair.

* **Oblique twists.** Do a twist while you jump, to define your waist. As you jump, turn your hips one way and your shoulders the other.

THE MOST EFFICIENT EXERCISE (I PROMISE, YOU HAVE TIME FOR THIS)

You probably know it's a good *idea* to be active—yet if you're like most people, it probably feels like you don't have the time to exercise.[9] If you can relate, I've got such good news for you. There is a form of exercise that is highly effective and *highly* time efficient. In fact, it can take only eight minutes—at home, using nothing more than your body for equipment—to give yourself more benefits than a typical forty-five- to ninety-minute exercise class. This too good to be true–sounding workout is high-intensity interval training (HIIT)—a fitness approach characterized by bursts of effort followed by short periods of rest. True to its name, HIIT is fairly *intense*. But it's that intensity (interspersed with periods of rest, don't forget!) that offers maximal health benefits in minimal time, including the following:

Torching calories in a short period of time

HIIT allows you to burn about the *same* amount of calories, but spend *less* time exercising than other workouts: one study had participants either do thirty minutes of HIIT, weight training, running, or biking. The HIIT group burned 25 to 30 percent more calories than the other groups did. Keep in mind that in this study, the HIIT folks did circuits of twenty seconds of maximal effort, followed by forty seconds of rest—meaning they were actually exercising only for one-third of the time that the running and biking groups were.[10]

Summary: HIIT helps burn more calories than other forms of exercise in less time.

Boosting your metabolism for hours after your workout is through

It's about more than just the calories you burn *during* the workout, though. Several studies show that HIIT can boost your metabolic rate for hours after your workout is through, meaning you keep burning additional calories even after you're done exercising. HIIT provides this long tail of metabolic benefit even more than jogging and weight training—all while nudging

your body more toward using fat than carbs for energy.[11] It does it by raising levels of catecholamines (the family of neurotransmitters that includes epinephrine, adrenaline, and norepinephrine and that drive the breakdown of fats) and human growth hormone.

Another study showed that just **two minutes of HIIT—in the form of sprints—increased metabolism over 24 hours as much as 30 minutes of running.**[12] **Two minutes!**

Summary: HIIT helps you give yourself hours of a boosted metabolism after just a short duration of effort.

Helping you shed fat— including belly fat

One review that looked at thirteen studies that included a total of 424 people found that HIIT reduces both body fat and waist circumference, which means less visceral fat—the dangerous fat that accumulates around your organs.[13]

Another study found twelve weeks of doing twenty-minute HIIT sessions three times a week resulted in an average of 4.4 pounds of body fat lost—and this was without any dietary changes! It also meant a 17 percent reduction in visceral fat.[14]

Summary: HIIT blasts body fat in general, and belly fat in particular.

Reducing blood sugar and lessening insulin resistance

Studies have shown that doing HIIT for twelve weeks or less can bring down blood sugar levels,[15] including in those with type 2 diabetes.[16] Even more important, a review of fifty different studies found that HIIT also does a better job at reducing insulin resistance than more traditional workouts.[17]

Summary: HIIT helps resolve insulin resistance more efficiently than do diet changes alone, which in turn helps you become more fat-adapted (since when you're insulin resistant, your body's primary source of fuel is sugar, impeding its ability to burn fat).

IN ADDITION TO all these benefits that help you get off your sugar, HIIT has also been shown to be especially useful for people over age fifty:

- Preserves muscle mass as you age (which typically declines as much as seven pounds every ten years), meaning that you lose fat and not muscle.
- Reduces inflammation. HIIT can help upregulate the genes that promote mitochondrial function so that you have more energy and experience less oxidative stress that leads to . . . inflammation.
- Promotes cognitive function and wards off age-related cognitive decline[18] through its contribution to the formation of new mitochondria in the brain.

That's not even the best part! I asked Anna Kaiser to take something that usually takes thirty or sixty minutes and create an effective HIIT workout that you can complete in just eight minutes. Even better, the workout Anna created is high intensity but *low impact* (known as HILIIT, for high-intensity, low-impact interval training), meaning it won't take a toll on your joints the way higher-impact workouts can.

YOU NEED EXTRA HYDRATION WHEN DOING HIIT WORKOUTS

Like the name says, HIIT is *intense*. That intensity means it dehydrates the body more. If you're not drinking enough water, the toxins that you liberate from your fat cells won't get filtered by your kidneys and excreted through your urine; instead, your body will send those toxins out through your sweat, and you may start to break out. If they don't get pushed out into your sweat, the body will simply redistribute them, meaning you'll hold on to fat as well as toxins—not what we're after! Although I normally suggest drinking 3 to 4 liters of water daily, you want to add an extra liter to the days you do HIIT. When you drink more water, you'll excrete more toxins and lose more fat. Always go with my motto: **the solution to pollution is dilution**.

YOUR 8-MINUTE ACID-KICKING W
BY ANNA KAISER

Anna masterminded this highly efficient aerob
help you burn more fat for a longer period of
treadmill for thirty minutes. In only eight
build cardiovascular endurance, and be
those toxins are acidic, and getting rid of them

Best of all, you can do it at home, which is alw
nience sake, but also, as the coronavirus pandemic s
have options beyond going to gyms and workout classe
healthy.

The workout consists of two circuits of four exercises each. Yo
first circuit for four minutes, then switch to the second for four minu
Then you're done! No time to get bored, and at only eight minutes of total
work, no excuses that you don't have the time.

Here's how the timing works:

CIRCUIT 1

Round 1: Do each exercise (exercises 1–4) continuously for 30 seconds (2 minutes total to complete all four exercises)

Optional rest: 30 seconds before starting round 2

Round 2: Do each exercise continuously for 15 seconds (1 minute total)

Optional rest: 30 seconds before starting round 3

Round 3: Do each exercise continuously for 15 seconds (1 minute total)

Total time for circuit 1: 4 minutes (not including optional rest)

CIRCUIT 2

Optional rest: 1 minute before starting circuit 2

Round 1: Do each exercise (exercises 5–8) continuously for 30 seconds (2 minutes total to complete all four exercises)

continues

al rest: 30 seconds before starting round 2

nd 2: Do each exercise continuously for 15 seconds (1 minute total)

tional rest: 30 seconds before starting round 3

Round 3: Do each exercise continuously for 15 seconds (1 minute total)

Total time for circuit 2: 4 minutes (not including optional rest)

Total time to complete both circuits: 8 minutes (not including optional rest)

As you move through each round, try to increase the intensity by either moving faster, increasing your range of motion, or adding weights.

Exercises

CIRCUIT 1

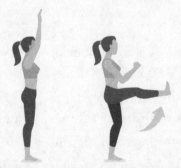

Karate Kicks

This move warms up and engages every muscle in your body, including a dynamic stretch for your hamstrings.

Directions:
- Kick forward on alternate sides, stepping foot to foot.

Advanced:
- Alternate sides by jumping foot to foot.

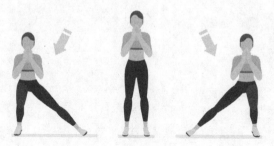

Alternating Lateral Lunges

Side lunges work your glutes, quads, and adductors, helping to shape and tone your legs and your core.

Directions:

- Stand with your feet hip-width apart. Keeping your feet parallel and your core engaged, step your right foot wide to the right.

- Keeping your left leg straight, your chest up, and your back flat, bend your right knee, sit your hips back, and lower your body until your right thigh is parallel to the floor.

- Return to the starting position and repeat on the left side.

Advanced:

- Perform the same exact motion, holding a pair of light weights in your hands. When stepping out to the right side, the dumbbells should frame your right leg at the bottom of the move. Same for opposite side.

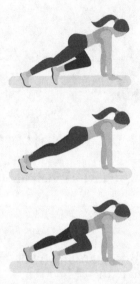

Cross-Body Dynamic Plank

This full-body exercise strengthens and targets every muscle of your core in a very powerful way. You won't need to do many of these to get results!

Directions:

- Resting your hands on the edge of a table or a chair with your feet on the floor, arms and legs straight, and core fully engaged (basically, you're in an inclined push-up position), pull one knee at a time toward the opposite elbow, alternating sides (make sure chair or table is stable).

Advanced:

- Perform the plank on the floor, bringing one knee to the opposite elbow, alternating sides. If you have a wrist problem or experience wrist pain, perform the plank on your forearms instead.

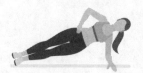

Side Plank

The side plank improves balance, spinal stability, and upper-body and core strength, with an emphasis on the obliques and deep core stabilizers.

Directions:

- Lie on your side with your forearm flat on the floor (do the plank on a chair, couch, or coffee table to decrease intensity), bottom elbow lined up directly under your shoulder. Your feet can be either staggered for more stability, or stacked for more of a challenge.

- Engage your core and lift your hips off the floor, forming a straight line from your head to your feet. Your top hand can be on your hip (easier) or reaching up to the ceiling (harder).

- Round 1: hold for 15 seconds, then switch sides. Round 2: hold for 15 seconds on the right side only. Round 3: hold for 15 seconds on the left side only.

Advanced:

- Keep switching sides in continuous dynamic movement, for all three rounds.

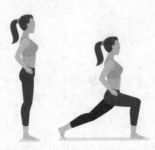

Switching Lunges

Lunges are a quintessential exercise; you can do them anywhere, and the effects can be seen in no time, in the form of shapely, toned legs and backside.

Directions:

- Step forward into a lunge position, leading with your heel, keeping your front knee behind your toe and your chest up, trying to hit a 90-degree angle every time. Step back to neutral.

- Switch legs to bring the opposite foot forward into a lunge. Continue alternating.

Advanced:

- Option 1: Jump into a lunge position, keeping your front knee behind your toe and your chest up.

- Jump to switch legs (holding hands in prayer position during jump). Continue alternating.

- Option 2: Perform step *or* jump lunges with light weights in hand—this will be your true leg burner!

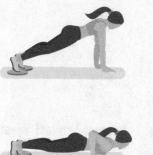

Push-up

Push-ups are basic strength-building total body exercises that strengthen the upper body and improve core strength.

Directions:

- Use the floor, or for less intensity, a coffee table, chair, wall, or desk.

- Place your hands flat on the ground, directly under your shoulders with your feet slightly wider than hip-width apart. Bend your elbows to 45 degrees and **aim to graze your chest on the floor or table** to engage every muscle in your upper body.

- Push your body away from the ground to straighten your arms and come back to the starting position. For *modified push-up*, bring your knees down to floor.

- **Most important is the range of motion**, with the goal of getting your chest to tap whichever surface you are using (chair, couch, or floor). Keep your core engaged—no sagging or slumping.

Advanced:

- Volume is king! Perform more on the floor, faster, with full range of motion, without compromising form.

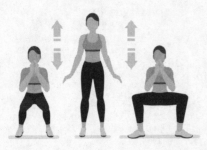

Internal-External Squat & Stand

Love them or loathe them, squats are one of the most effective exercises you can do. Squats are also highly versatile: you can do them anywhere—even while brushing your teeth. Multitask by adding bicep curls and other moves to make them harder.

Directions:

- Place your feet shoulder-width apart or slightly wider, while extending your hands straight out in front of you (or in prayer position) to help keep your balance.

- Sit back and down like you're sitting into an imaginary chair, keeping your head facing forward as your upper body bends forward a bit (thighs parallel to floor with knees over ankles).

- Do four squats straight up and down, then *externally rotate your hips* (feet point outward at 45 degrees), and do another four squats in that position. Repeat until the time is up.

Advanced:

- Perform an internal squat, then jump to an external squat, back to internal, and so on.

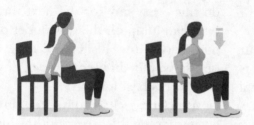

Triceps Dip

This is a great total-body exercise that works the muscles in your shoulders, upper back, and triceps. In addition to targeting the upper body, the movement also strengthens the glutes and quadriceps muscles that work to support your body weight during the movement.

Directions:

- Sit on the edge of a stable chair (or bench, ottoman, couch, or sturdy coffee table, which helps with sensitive wrists or carpal tunnel) with your arms mostly straight (just a little bend in your elbows to keep tension on your triceps and off your elbow joints) and your palms resting on the chair seat with your fingers facing forward, your hands shoulder-width apart.

- Slide your butt off the front of the chair with your knees bent, feet on the floor, and core engaged.

- Slowly bend your elbows straight back to lower your body toward the floor until your upper arms come parallel to the floor. Keep your back close to the chair and your shoulders down as you lower and raise your body.

- Once you reach the bottom of the movement, press down into the chair to straighten your elbows and return to the starting position. This completes one rep.

- Repeat until your 30 seconds (round 1) or 15 seconds (rounds 2 and 3) are up.

- If you need a modification to make it less intense, walk your feet in closer to the chair.

Advanced:

- Have your legs straight.

When and How Often to Do This Workout

Because this is such a great boost for your metabolism, this eight-minute workout is best to do before you have your first meal of the day, to help you burn more fat. It's also a great way to perk you back up during that late afternoon slump (around four o'clock) and get your digestion humming for dinner. But don't get too hung up on timing—the most important thing is that you do it!

As for frequency, if you're new to exercise, do it just once during these next three days to give yourself the experience of pushing yourself and to reap the benefits that HIIT provides. If you're already work-ing out at least somewhat regularly, aim to do this every day for the next three days (you can jump on the rebounder on these days, too—either just before your workout or at a wholly different time of day, what-ever works best for you).

After these three days are through, I suggest doing this workout three days in a row and then taking one day off to rebuild. Your long-term goal is to do it daily—it's only eight minutes, after all! If you are do-ing another workout, you can still do it that same day. If you're not doing any other workouts, you can even do this *twice* daily, as it's a great functional workout that is highly beneficial for whole-body detoxification, metabolism, and the health of your cardiovascular system.

STEP 7: AMP UP YOUR WORKOUT ACTION PLAN

* Pick a workout.

* If you haven't been moving much, commit to doing something active ev-ery day, even if it's only for five minutes.

* Consider getting a rebounder and making it part of your morning and/or evening routine to help keep your lymphatic system humming.

* If you're already exercising at least somewhat regularly, do the 8-Minute Acid-Kicking Workout by Anna Kaiser each of the three days.

* Consider getting a workout partner so you have someone to hold you accountable and help you get some good social time too.

TRACK YOUR JOURNEY

Assess how adding exercise (if you weren't moving much before) or HILIIT (if you're up for the challenge) over the next three days affects how you feel, and then record your insights in the chart on page 210.

PHASE 3: FEED

90 DAYS

thirteen

Your Life After Sugar

By now, you've weaned yourself off snacks, retrained your taste buds to appreciate new flavors, and jump-started your fat-burning engines. You've done great work to transition from *stress eating* to *strength eating*. Now, it's time to lock in those new habits and make them a lifestyle—a process that takes about ninety days.

This chapter includes a recap of everything we've covered and the bird's-eye view of how all the changes you've made add up to a daily strategy that can keep you in the fat-burning zone, optimize your hormones, and help you prevent all the chronic diseases associated with eating too much sugar. By the end of the next three months, by following these principles, all your new habits will become second nature and you'll get the same results with only 25 percent of the effort, all because of the stacking effect that happens when you follow the "add, don't take away" approach that the Get Off Your Sugar program follows. You'll notice that your cravings have completely transformed in that you'll crave for the healthy stuff because you feel so *good* when you eat them— it won't feel like a sacrifice at all to live this way. Especially when I tell you what I'm about to tell you.

And that piece of good news is: **you don't have to eat perfectly to completely transform your health**. Going forward, your goal is to simply make 80 percent of your diet follow the "Get Off Your Sugar Food Pyramid" (see page 188); 20 percent of what you eat can be outside these guidelines. Even a 70/30 ratio of on-the-program food versus off-the-program food will keep you moving forward without losing any of the good ground that you've gained. I know if you're an over-achiever, you'll probably aim for 90/10, but the sweet spot of sustainability and effectiveness is 80/20.

You can break this 80/20 down in a few ways:

- **Per meal.** Make 80 percent of the foods on your plate Get Off Your Sugar approved; the other 20 percent can be something else.

- **Per day.** If you know you're going to a party where you'll have some wine or sweets or if you're going out to a steak dinner, eat as well as you possibly can during the day and save the whole 20 percent for when you're at the event.

- **Per week**. If you're having three meals a day, or twenty-one meals total, make

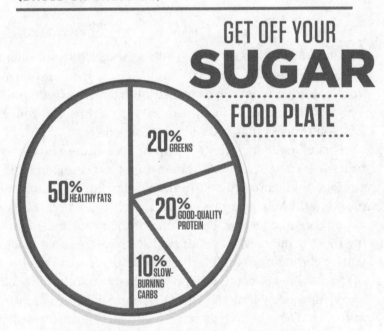

(BASED ON CALORIES)

GET OFF YOUR
SUGAR
FOOD PLATE

20% GREENS

20% GOOD-QUALITY PROTEIN

50% HEALTHY FATS

10% SLOW-BURNING CARBS

Get Off Your Sugar Food Plate—Caloric Breakdown

seventeen of those meals chock-full of good foods, and give yourself a little more leeway for four meals out of your week. If you're eating two meals a day, that's eleven meals "on" and three meals "off."

Remember, Get Off Your Sugar isn't about deprivation, it's about moderation. I want you to enjoy your life—I'm not asking you to give up absolutely every guilty pleasure. If you want to have a glass of wine, have a glass of wine. If you want a piece of chocolate, have a piece of chocolate. Just make your indulgences the best

you can make them—if you're going to have chocolate, make it 100 percent dark chocolate with no added sugar, or 100 percent raw cacao, instead of milk chocolate. If you're going to have wine, make it red wine (due to its higher levels of antioxidants) and make it organic and low-sulfite. When I interviewed my good friend Bobbi Brown, the makeup and beauty guru, she said something I thought was really profound, and I'll share it with you here: when you focus on making every food you eat the *best* possible version of that food, you can become the *best* version of yourself.

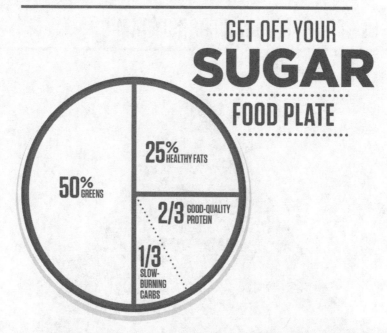

Get Off Your Sugar Food Plate—Visual Breakdown

It's important at least for the next ninety days that you pay close attention to making your food intake align with the food plate—both the caloric breakdown and the visual representation shown on these pages. But I also want you to know that you will start to be able to sense exactly what your body needs to stay off sugar and feel good, and that this will naturally change a little bit day to day, as life is a little different every day and so are you. After about three months, you'll have your dietary needs dialed in, and you will need only to refer back to this page during those rare times when you notice you've gotten sidetracked by life and need a little visual reminder to help you get back on track right away.

On a *per-meal* basis, your servings will look like this:

- 2 to 3 cups of nonstarchy, mineral-rich vegetables (leafy greens and cruciferous vegetables)

- 2 to 3 tablespoons of high-quality plant-based fats/oils (see table on page 108 for serving sizes)

- 2 to 4 ounces of high-quality, wild-caught or pasture-raised animal protein, if eating meat. Ideally, add more plant-based proteins.

- No more than ½ cup of fiber-rich, slow-burning carbs (starchy vegetables) and/or fruit per meal, not to exceed 1 cup per day

GET OFF YOUR SUGAR FOOD PYRAMID

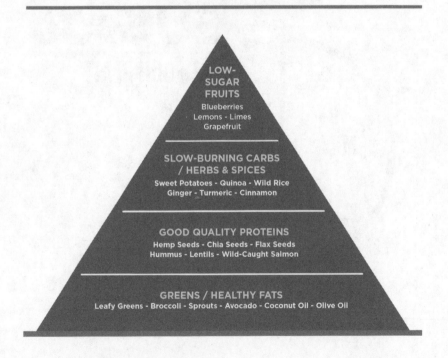

LOW-SUGAR FRUITS
Blueberries
Lemons - Limes
Grapefruit

SLOW-BURNING CARBS / HERBS & SPICES
Sweet Potatoes - Quinoa - Wild Rice
Ginger - Turmeric - Cinnamon

GOOD QUALITY PROTEINS
Hemp Seeds - Chia Seeds - Flax Seeds
Hummus - Lentils - Wild-Caught Salmon

GREENS / HEALTHY FATS
Leafy Greens - Broccoli - Sprouts - Avocado - Coconut Oil - Olive Oil

On a *per-day* basis, you are aiming for:

- 7 to 10 servings of nonstarchy, mineral-rich vegetables
- 7 to 10 servings healthy fats
- 1 to 2 servings of high-quality protein
- 1 to 2 servings of fiber-rich, slow-burning carbs
- 3 to 4 liters of water—or 1 ounce of water for every 2 pounds of body weight—with an extra liter on the days when you do high-intensity exercise and 1½ ounces of extra water for every ounce of alcohol or caffeinated beverage you drink

STRATEGIES FOR FAT-BURNING

* Demand organic when you can.

* Eat 7 to 10 servings of low-carb green vegetables throughout the day.

* Eat 2 to 3 tablespoons of fat with every meal.

* Be mindful of the *quantity* and the *quality* of your protein.

* Add herbs and spices into every meal.

* When cravings strike, or even if you anticipate cravings, use one or all of the "Five to Thrive" (see box on page 146).

* Move your body (at least) a little bit every day.

* Don't eat three hours before bed.

* Don't eat less; eat less often.

* Aim for two meals a day, eaten within an eight-hour window.

* Get at least 3 liters of filtered water a day, supercharged with minerals, Himalayan pink salt, dehydrated greens powder, or molecular hydrogen.

GOING FORWARD: THE OPTIMAL DIET VARIATION STRATEGY

Once you become comfortable following the guidelines I just listed, you want to adopt an eating plan that ensures you get ample fast time as well as ample feast time.

The formula that I recommend is called 5:1:1. That refers to **5 days of intermittent fasting**, with all your eating done within an eight-hour-or-less window, and ideally, 50 grams of net carbs or fewer; **1 day of partial fasting**, with only one meal of 500 to 1,000 calories (and also 50 grams or fewer of net carbs, and no more than 20 grams of protein on the partial fast day); and **1 day of feasting**, when you can have up to 150 grams of net carbs from slow-burning carbs, such as squash, quinoa, and sweet potatoes. That way, you let your body know that it is not starving, and therefore not in danger. Varying your diet by going through periods of fasting and feasting is designed to help you keep burning fat for fuel over the long term, while making sure that you still take in all the nutrients you need to keep your body replenished and renewed for the long haul.

I recommend splitting up your five days of intermitting fasting throughout the week, like so:

Sunday, Monday, Tuesday: Intermittent Fasting— Fast and Feast Days

(*Note:* You can do this any days of the week, but I find this schedule works best, especially having the partial fast day on a workday and the feast day on a weekend when you're with family or friends.)

Ideally, keep your net carbs to 50 grams or less; your basic calorie breakdown to 50 percent from healthy fats, 20 percent from mineral-rich vegetables, 20 percent from protein (favoring plant-based), and 10 percent from starchy, slow-burning, fiber-rich carbs; your fasting window to sixteen hours; and your feasting window to eight hours. Depending on where you're at, you can further stretch that window to 18/6, or even 20/4, where maximum autophagy happens.

Wednesday: Partial Fasting— OMAD (One Meal a Day)

Have one meal, either at three p.m. or six p.m. (or somewhere in between). Keep your total intake to somewhere between 500 and 1,000 calories; limit protein to 20 grams and net carbs to 50 grams or less. Eat primarily greens and healthy fats.

I find it really helpful to do my partial fast on a busy day. If I am cranking at work, I don't think twice about it. Remember, you can also have the beverages listed on page 144. And if you are hungry, use the "Cheat the Fast" biohacks on page 144, or my "Five to Thrive" from the box on page 146.

Thursday and Friday: Intermittent Fasting—Fast and Feast Days

Again, keep your net carbs to 50 grams or less and your fasting window to sixteen hours, and your eating window to eight hours (unless you want to compress that to 18/6 or 20/4), and keep following the protein guidelines outlined in Chapter 8.

Saturday: Feast Day

Increase net carbs to 100 to 150 grams, making sure they come from healthy fiber-rich, slow-burning carbs (such as squashes, sweet potatoes, and quinoa—no processed carbs or refined sugars), and continue eating the appropriate amount of protein for you (that you calculated in Chapter 8). The purpose of this day is to let your body know that it is not in starvation mode. Believe it or not, having a feast day will help your body burn more fat, because it knows it is *not* in danger, it is *not* starving, it is *not* in fight or flight.

On each of these days, when you eat, eat until you are full, no more, no less.

IIIIIIIIIIIIIIIIIIIIIIIIIIIIIIIIIIIIIIIIIIIIIIIIIIIIIIIIIIIIIIIIIIIIIIIIIIIIIIIIIIIIII

SAMPLE REGIMENS FOR EACH OF THE DIFFERENT 5:1:1 DAYS

Feast *and* Fast Days (intermittent fasting— five days per week)

6:00 a.m. wake-up call: Mineral powder, or Alkamind Acid-Kicking Greens powder mixed with water, or one of the healing tonics from the recipe section that starts on page 219.

6:45 a.m. lymphatic jump-start: 10 minutes on rebounder or 2 minutes dry brushing your skin.

7:00 a.m. cheat your fast: 1 tablespoon of coconut oil with ⅛ teaspoon of Himalayan pink salt for energy, either eaten straight off the spoon or mixed into organic coffee (or turn your next cup of coffee into a cup of acid-kicking coffee, with Dr. Daryl's Acid-Kicking Coffee Alkalizer, see Resources for more information—just know that you need 1½ ounces of water for every ounce of coffee you drink to offset that beloved morning beverage's diuretic effects); or add 2 tablespoons of chia seeds in 6 ounces of water, allow to sit for 10 minutes until it forms a gel and brighten up with a squeeze of lemon juice.

11:45 a.m. workout: The 8-Minute Acid-Kicking Workout on page 173 (you can even do it in your office).

11:55 a.m. prelunch hydration and postworkout recovery: A glass of water with Himalayan pink salt or a scoop of Mineral Powder or Alkamind Acid-Kicking Minerals in water; digestive enzyme.

12 noon lunch: Spinach salad with broccoli, cucumber, red bell pepper, red onion, sliced avocado, walnuts, extra-virgin olive oil, lemon juice, and a 3-ounce piece of wild-caught salmon; or a smoothie from the recipe section that starts on page 215. Add a tablespoon of coconut oil or raw nut butter, if needed.

6:00 p.m. dinner: Raw Zucchini Pesto Pasta (page 237); dessert (optional): Avocado Chocolate Mousse (page 263).

6:15 p.m. middinner supplements (could also be taken at lunch if you prefer): Once your digestion is in full swing and your enzymes are kicked in, take your fish oil, probiotic, vitamin D_3, vitamin K_2, and your choice of antioxidant.

9:30 p.m., 30 minutes before bed: Mineral powder, Alkamind Acid-Kicking Minerals, or water with a pinch of Himalayan pink salt.

Fast Day (Partial fast—one day per week, I find it works best to do it on a busy midweek day, such as Wednesday)

6:00 a.m. wake-up call: Mineral powder, or Alkamind Acid-Kicking Greens powder mixed with water, or one of the healing tonics from the recipe section that starts on page 219.

6:45 a.m. lymphatic jump-start: Ten minutes on rebounder or two minutes dry skin brushing.

7:00 a.m. cheat your fast: 1 tablespoon coconut oil with ⅛ teaspoon of Himalayan salt pink for energy, either eaten straight off the spoon or mixed into organic coffee (or turn your next cup of coffee into a cup of acid-kicking coffee, with Dr. Daryl's Acid-Kicking Coffee Alkalizer, see Resources for more information—just remember to drink an extra 1½ ounces of water for every ounce of coffee you drink to offset its diuretic effects); or add 2 tablespoons of chia seeds in 6 ounces of water, allow to sit for 10 minutes until it forms a gel and brighten up with a squeeze of lemon juice.

10:00 a.m. energizer: Chia seed drink—mix 2 tablespoons of chia seeds with 6 ounces or water and a squeeze of lemon juice, let it sit for ten minutes until a gel forms, then drink.

11:00 a.m. de-stress: Five minutes of 3:6:5 Power Breath (see page 74) or 4:8 Extended Exhale breath (see page 195); skip a formal workout this day so you can expend your energy on healing instead.

Anytime between 3:00 and 6:00 p.m. meal: Aim for 500 to 1,000 calories from lots of greens, lots of fats, and 20 grams, max, of high-quality proteins, such as a rainbow salad with avocado, a green soup, and a tablespoon of raw nut butter.

15 minutes into your meal: Once your digestion is in full swing and your enzymes are kicked in, take your fish oil, probiotic, vitamin D_3, vitamin K_2, and your choice of antioxidant.

9:00 p.m. evening detox: Detox Bath (see page 92).

30 minutes before bed: Mineral powder or Alkamind Acid-Kicking Minerals or water with a pinch of Himalayan pink salt.

Feast Day (one day per week—Saturday is often a good day since you're with family and friends)

6:00 a.m. wake-up call: Mineral powder or Alkamind Acid-Kicking Greens powder mixed with water, or one of the healing tonics from the recipe section that starts on page 219.

6:45 a.m. lymphatic jump-start: Ten minutes on rebounder or two minutes of dry skin brushing.

7:00 a.m. breakfast (optional): Choose from 30-Minute Apple Cinnamon Chia Pudding (page 264); ½ avocado with extra-virgin olive oil, Himalayan pink salt, black pepper, cumin, and chia seeds; or plant-based protein powder in 8 ounces of coconut milk with 1 tablespoon each of chia seeds and raw almond butter and a pinch of Himalayan pink salt. If you're having coffee, make it organic and include a tablespoon of coconut or MCT oil (or turn your next cup of coffee into a cup of acid-kicking coffee, with Dr. Daryl's Acid-Kicking Coffee Alkalizer, see Resources for more information) and be sure to drink 1½ ounces of water for every ounce of coffee you drink to offset its diuretic effects.

11:45 a.m. workout: The 8-Minute Acid-Kicking Workout on page 173.

11:55 a.m. prelunch hydration: A glass of water with ⅛ teaspoon of Himalayan pink salt or a scoop of Alkamind Acid-Kicking Minerals in water.

12 noon lunch: Spinach salad with broccoli, cucumber, red bell pepper, red onion, sliced avocado, walnuts, extra-virgin olive oil, lemon juice, and a 3-ounce piece of wild-caught salmon, plus 1 tablespoon of coconut oil or raw nut butter, if needed.

6:00 p.m. dinner: Cauliflower Rice–Stuffed Peppers (page 235); dessert (optional): Chocolate Chia Pudding (page 260).

6:15 p.m. middinner supplements: Once your digestion is in full swing and your enzymes are kicked in, take your fish oil, probiotic, vitamin D_3, vitamin K_2, and your choice of antioxidant.

9:30 p.m., 30 minutes before bed: Mineral powder or Alkamind Acid-Kicking Minerals or water with a pinch of Himalayan pink salt.

OUTSMART POTENTIAL DERAILMENTS

The truth is, everyone's going to experience things that will make it more challenging to stick to your Get Off Your Sugar goals, and your nice 80/20 ratio of "good" foods to "bad" may shift to more like 20/80. It's not a question of if, it's a matter of when. Take some time to think through the two most common challenges—travel (whether for work or for pleasure) and periods of intense stress or busy-ness—now, so that they don't catch you by surprise. **If you're failing to plan, you're planning to fail.**

That being said, everyone will derail from time to time; the key is to catch it as soon as you can so that you only have to make minor adjustments to get back on track and don't have to start again from scratch.

Travel. When you're on the road, it's so important that you bring at least a little bit of good food with you; if you don't you can almost guarantee that you'll derail. It's too easy to find CRAP-py (completely refined and processed) carbs when you're out and about—they're in every vending machine and corner store—but you're a lot less likely to find an avocado or raw nuts. Your best bet is to keep a couple of things in your carry-on bag or your glove compartment so that if you get held up, you can refuel without getting back on the stress-eating sugar yo-yo.

When you're eating out while on the road, and you're having a feast day, you can even order a dessert to end your meal—share it with someone and stick to only three bites. And if it's one of those foods that in the past you couldn't stop eating what you started, skip it altogether.

FOODS TO BRING ALONG WHEN TRAVELING

* (At least) two avocados: a ripe one for the trip, and a semiripe one for the next day
* Grain-Free Granola (recipe on page 222)
* Raw nuts, such as almonds, walnuts, macadamia nuts, or Brazil nuts
* Hemp seeds, chia seeds, flaxseeds
* High-fat, low-sugar bars (Yes, bars are one of my favorites, particularly the black sesame sea salt flavor)
* Kale chips
* Roasted seaweed
* Plant-based protein powder; you can always add it to your water bottle on the go
* Raw almond/coconut/cacao butter packets (such as those by Artisana Organics)
* Coconut oil packets
* A 2-ounce Redmond Real Salt shaker

Superbusy. Everyone will have times where it feels like there's no time—or bandwidth—to eat healthfully. The good news is that once you get to a fat-adapted state, you can go longer periods without eating. I've been flying to California a lot for work, and I notice that if the flight attendants are not handing out the snacks quickly enough, people start freaking out. It's sad that people can't go one five-hour flight without the CRAP-py snacks. When you are burning fat, it's not a big deal to go this long without eating. That means when you're superbusy, you don't have to spend as much time thinking about food, preparing food, and eating food. You can just keep it supersimple and get the fat, fiber, and protein you need without a lot of fuss, yet still get a ton of flavor (see "Supereasy and/or Quick Meals for Busy Times," on the next page).

These busy times are also when the "Five to Thrive" on page 146 become so important—they will help make sure you get the fats and minerals to stay strong and energized.

SUPEREASY AND/OR QUICK MEALS FOR BUSY TIMES

There are certain ingredients that you should keep on hand because they can help you stay on the Get Off Your Sugar program with only about five minutes of prep. With these around, a lack of time won't derail you.

Roasted sweet potatoes. Stick a sweet potato in a 350°F oven when you get home from work and let it cook for forty-five minutes (or less, depending on how big your sweet potato is) while you transition from work to home. Then, load it up with coconut oil, cinnamon, and a pinch of Himalayan pink salt, and make a salad out of whatever veggies you have in the fridge and boom, you've got dinner.

Adzuki Butter Tacos. For those nights when you don't have time to really cook, try this go-to healthy taco recipe: Put a couple of tablespoons of canned adzuki beans (Eden Organics preferred, drained and rinsed) plus a couple of slices of avocado in a piece of butter lettuce for a healthy taco. Sprinkle it with Himalayan pink salt, a little ground cumin, some hemp seeds, red onion, and a little salsa or hot sauce if you like things spicy (see page 246 for an alkaline hot sauce recipe), and then eat with your hands. This is a tasty, easy way to get fiber, protein, and fats in minimal time.

Chocolate Chia Pudding (page 260). This is so easy to make, and it keeps great in the fridge, so make some on Sunday night and have it to eat all week long. This creamy pudding works for breakfast, lunch, dinner, or dessert. The only hitch is it takes five hours to thicken; if you need it faster than that, throw it in the freezer for fifteen minutes. (This is a tip from my good friend Shayna Taylor.) And if you want to vary the flavor, add ¼ cup of raw cacao powder, ½ cup pure pumpkin puree, or some fresh blueberries—it's as easy as that.

Dr. Daryl's Favorite Salad Dressing. This dressing, which appeared in my book *Get Off Your Acid*, was everybody's favorite. So, even though I've already shared it, I had to add it in this book for anyone who doesn't already have it. Every Sunday, we make this dressing and cut up a bunch of vegetables, such as fennel, sugar snap peas, broccoli, celery, cucumber, and red bell pepper, so that there's always something grab-able (and delicious) in the fridge. It is the most delicious salad dressing you will *ever* make. (We make it so often, in fact, that I had to name it after myself!) The vegetables give a great crunch and the dressing (see page 234 for recipe) provides a flavor blast that's supersatisfying. It's great to pull these veggie sticks and dressing out a few minutes before dinner when your kids (and you) are hungry.

IF YOU'RE NOT HANDLING YOUR STRESS, YOUR STRESS IS HANDLING YOU

Going forward, the key to being able to maintain your new taste buds and your fat-burning state is to manage your stress levels. That's because most of the time, the common root of all derailments is stress, whether it's work stress, physical stress, or emotional stress. Thanks to the fact that the body needs glucose to fuel it when it's in fight or flight, stress creates cravings for sugar. When you eat something high-carb or a sugary meal in this stressed-out, fight-or-flight state, in response, your blood sugar takes up to six times longer to go back to normal. And we are all subject to varying levels of stressors all the time. **I've said it before, but I'll say it again: we are marinating in cortisol.**

It sounds overly simple, but your best tool for counteracting stress is breathing. There's actually a third stress response in addition to fight or flight, and that's to freeze—think of a deer caught in headlights. When you're frozen, you stop breathing deeply. That makes stress worse, because it cuts down on oxygenation that's so vital for health and mood. Breathing has been proven to shift your body out of sympathetic nervous system activation and bring your parasympathetic nervous system, which rules the rest and digest functions of the body, online. Just like you need balance between omega-3s and omega-6s, and calcium and magnesium, you also need balance between the sympathetic nervous system and the parasympathetic nervous system. And breathing can help you achieve just that.

Your breath impacts your circulatory, lymphatic, and digestive systems too. In fact, I learned by reading *The Tao of Natural Breathing* by Dennis Lewis that up to **70 percent of our body's waste products are eliminated via our lungs**. The rest are excreted through urination, defe-cation, and perspiration (pee them out, poop them out, sweat them out). If you're not breathing enough, your cells aren't getting sufficient amounts of oxygen. Without enough oxygen, your blood and lymphatic flow slows down, which lessens the removal of toxins, waste products, and the delivery of immune cells. It also slows down your digestive process.

Did you know that the average breath rate is 14 breaths per minute, when it should be 5 to 6? Did you also know that the average breath rate of someone fighting cancer is over 25 times per minute? Why is that? Because cancer is induced by toxicity, and when you become more toxic, your body innately works harder, breathing more rapidly yet with more shallowness, all in effort to get these toxins *out*!

When you breathe more slowly and more deeply, you assist the body's ability to detoxify. Doing a simple breathing exercise every morning takes only a few minutes, and here's the best part—it's free. You don't need to buy anything in order to be able to do it.

Proper breathing is critical to getting off your sugar. It will help shift you from sympathetic (fight or flight) to parasympathetic (rest and digest), which will ultimately help you move from burning sugar to burning more fat.

We've already covered the 3:6:5 Power Breath; taking ten of those can reset your mental state and your stress levels. Another breathing technique that can literally help you blow off stress is the 4:8 Extended Exhale Breath—breathing in for a count of 4 and exhaling for a count of 8.

Squeezing that much air out forces you to engage your diaphragm, which can get locked up when you've been taking shallow stress breaths. Getting your diaphragm to move with each breath again sends the "all clear" signal to your nervous system. Also, expelling all that stale air out invites big, oxygen-rich breaths back in, and that oxygen makes your whole being feel better.

In addition to breathing, journaling is a proven stress reliever; you can use it to write down your feelings (so that they don't swirl around in your head and contribute to your stress) and your goals.

Another fantastic way to make sure your stress doesn't derail you is to get yourself an accountability partner and make a plan to check in with them a minimum of once a week to talk through any challenges you're facing and share strategies for meeting your goals. **When you share your goals with someone, you're significantly more likely to achieve them . . . so the takeaway is to write and share!**

WHEN STRESS STRIKES: NO-SUGAR SURVIVAL STRATEGIES

Here are simple things you can do *instead* of reaching for something sweet to take the edge of your stress.

1. Take a hot bath with Epsom salts, baking soda, and essential oils.

2. Do a few yoga poses.

3. Meditate, or listen to the BrainTap app (see Resources section for more info on BrainTap).

4. Take ten 3:6:5 Power Breaths.

5. Try twenty 4:8 Extended Exhale Breaths.

6. Do the 8-Minute Acid-Kicking Workout.

7. Drink a green juice.

8. Take a walk.

9. Write in your journal—what are you grateful for *today*?

10. Put on a power song to instantly change your mental state.

11. Read something empowering.

12. Go back and reread your *why* (that you wrote on page 203).

GETTING MORE SLEEP HELPS YOU STAY OFF SUGAR

When you're tired, it's so tempting to eat something sugary because you know it will perk you right up, temporarily at least, until you crash and feel even more tired than you were before. But the link between sugar and sleep goes deeper than an energy fix.

Research has shown that after four nights of poor sleep (4.5 hours per night), insulin sensitivity takes a hit—particularly the insulin sensitivity of your fat cells.[1] That means losing sleep contributes to insulin resistance. Turns out, even your fat cells need sleep to be their best!

A 2010 study found that sleeping only four hours for two consecutive nights also reduced the hunger-regulating hormone, leptin.[2] (This helps explain why eating the sugary thing when you're tired feels like such a good idea—your body can't calibrate leptin correctly, your hunger and satiation signals get blunted, and you stay hungry and never full.)

You've probably noticed that losing sleep affects your mood and maybe your ability to recall words and names, but sleep affects more than your brain—it also impacts your bones! A 2019 study found that **women who slept five hours or less per night had 0.012 to 0.018 grams per square centimeter (g/cm²) lower bone mineral density than women who slept seven hours or more a night**. That may not sound like much, but it's equivalent to about one year of aging. They were also 22 percent more likely to have osteoporosis of the hip, and 28 percent more likely to have osteoporosis of the spine than the seven-plus-hours-per-night group.[3]

You've really got to prioritize your sleep for all kinds of reasons.

||||||||||||||||||||||||||||||||||||||||||||||||||||||||||||||||||||||||||||||

TOP SIX HACKS TO GET MORE SLEEP

1. **Snuff out any light sources**. Light, especially the light from LEDs (which now includes street lamps) and electronic devices, is stimulating to your brain and disruptive to your sleep cycles. For deep sleep, use blackout shades, keep the light from any electronics to a bare minimum (including digital clocks and nightlights), and use a sleep mask.

2. **Keep it cool.** Your body temperature drops to its lowest levels when you're sleeping, so if it's too warm in your bedroom, it can keep you from entering deep sleep. Keep your room somewhere between 60° and 68°F.

3. **Stick to morning (not afternoon) caffeine.** Caffeine has a half-life of five hours. This means the amount of caffeine in your bloodstream is reduced by 50 percent every five hours. This means if you consume 200 mg of caffeine at midday, you would still have 100 mg in you at around 5:45 p.m. If you're going to drink coffee, have it only in the morning (and make it organic!), and drink 1½ ounces of water for every ounce of coffee you drink, to offset its diuretic effects.

4. **Stop screen-ing yourself to sleep.** I know so many people who like to watch TV—or videos on their phones, tablets, or laptops—in bed, but the light from these devices is stimulating blue light, which leads to lower levels of the sleep-regulating melatonin.[4] The result? Less sleep. Try reading instead, or listening to something soothing—I love the sleep program on the BrainTap app.

5. **Shut down the Wi-Fi and wean from the screen.** A 2008 study found a link between exposure to radiation from cell phones in the three hours before bed and difficulty either falling asleep and/or staying asleep.[5] I know it's hard to do, but you've got to wean from the screen before bedtime—and make sure that your kids do too. A good way to stop the

late-night streaming is to turn the Wi-Fi off at a certain time each night—an automatic timer makes this effortless.

6. **Don't eat three hours before bedtime.** Theoretically, you're already doing this (right??), but if you need more of a reason to stop eating at night, know that when you eat too close to bedtime your body won't have the bandwidth to repair itself because it will be distracted by digestion, and you'll be likely to wake up less refreshed because of it.

DON'T WAIT TO MAKE CHANGE

Now you have the knowledge about *why* you need to get off your sugar as well as *how* to do it. And yet, contrary to popular belief, knowledge isn't power. It's the *potential* for power. Action is what takes that potential and turns it into actual power. So, the question before you now is . . . what will you do with your new knowledge? Will you get into action? Or will you wait?

So many people choose the latter and wait for bad news from their doctor before they decide to make a change. Or they don't think twice about their health until someone they know has a health crisis. They keep saying they'll make a change tomorrow, or Monday, or January 1, or after "things calm down." But procrastination is the killer of dreams. Your current and future health, as well as the current and future health of your children if you're a parent, depends on you. I beg you to stop telling yourself the same stories you've been telling yourself your whole life—such as that it doesn't really matter what you eat or that you can't make changes. Stop waiting for conditions to be perfect before you start doing things differently. I did that for so many years, and I can tell you this: it's never going to be perfect.

I outlined the step-by-step process that has helped me and thousands of my patients get off their sugar and given you a timeline so that you don't have to ever wonder what you should do next; you can just follow the trail of hemp seeds (I can't bring myself to say bread crumbs!). I sincerely believe that following it will make your path as painless and as effective as possible.

All that being said, I know that not everyone is truly ready to turn their health around in twenty-one days. Some people naturally move at a slower pace, and that is perfectly fine. You *can* take it one step at a time. Even if you start by making just one small change—such as not eating three hours before bedtime, or having a green juice before you have a Diet Coke—do it. That one little thing will help you have more energy and feel more confident in your ability to change, which will inspire you to add in the next small change. Keep adding and you will build up momentum like a snowball rolling down a hill.

Whenever you feel like you've stalled out or gotten off track, go back and review your why. Remind yourself of who you want to become and what changes you need to make to become that person.

Also, resist the urge to do this all by yourself. It's so important to your success that you enroll people to do this program with you. Share this book with the people you love, and tell them that you want to create better health for you and for them. Ask them to make this journey with you. And if they aren't on board—do it anyway. Sometimes the most powerful thing you can do to help someone else change is to change yourself. And please, come connect with me on Facebook and Instagram (I'm @drdarylgioffre in both places), where you can get support and answers from the source (me!) and everyone else who is dedicated to getting off their sugar so that they can feel more energized, strong in their body, and clear in their mind than they have in years—maybe ever.

Health is the most valuable asset we have; it's too important to leave to chance, or to be haphazard about. Sugar is depriving us of our most precious gift and creating millions of new cases of cancer, diabetes, Alzheimer's, or dementia every year. It's making us vulnerable to viruses—those we've known about forever, such as influenza and the cold, as well as those that are new, such as Covid-19. As I write this, America is number one in the developing world in health-care spending, but only number thirty-seven on the list of healthiest countries. On top of that, we in the United States were blindsided by the coronavirus pandemic. Too many of us had the comorbidities that made us vulnerable to the worst outcomes. And to make matters worse, when the virus hit and the quarantine was slapped on us, most of us went into *stress eating*, and many gained weight, known as the *quarantine 15*. The majority of my clients, however, thrived despite the virus and the stress it brought with it, because they were *strength eating* the right foods, finding a way to stay fit, and finding ways to manage stress better.

I did receive a call from one client who got the virus. She was scared. She wanted guidance on what she could do in that moment to help her fight off the infection. But she also said, "I wish I had listened to you about getting off my sugar earlier." (I'm so happy and thankful to report that we got her through it.)

They say that the best time to prepare for an emergency was two years ago, and the second-best time is *today*. What got you to this point where you picked up this book isn't what's important. What matters is what you do now that you have this information. We got surprised by Covid-19, but now we know to expect the next pandemic. It's up to us to be prepared. Self-care is no longer optional. It's a necessity. We've got to start taking care of ourselves, and we've got to *keep doing it*. We may not know the road ahead, but we can be ready.

Now you have everything you need— your *why* and your MAP (massive action plan)—to free yourself from the sugar addiction that is impacting too many of the people you know and love, to turn your stress into strength, and to spend your time, energy, and resources on wellness instead of illness.

Having suffered my entire life from acid reflux and heartburn, chronic migraines, and fibromyalgia, I just assumed that I would never experience a day without discomfort. Every time I saw a doctor it kicked off a cycle of pain, medication, repeat. Then I found Dr. Daryl. In as little as one week my fibromyalgia pain was unbelievably improved. I had the energy to run errands, that I hadn't had in years. Walking up and down the stairs didn't feel like a marathon. I lost 20 pounds without even trying. My chronic migraines reduced in frequency. I felt like a different person!

Having been told my whole life that the only route to relief was a never-ending cocktail of prescriptions, I couldn't believe how a simple change of no sugar and a common sense nutritional regimen could make such a drastic improvement. The ailments of my past no longer define me. This is a lifestyle change that truly works. Dr. Daryl has transformed my life for the better. —KATHY H. F.

Your Full Get Off Your Sugar MAP (Massive Action Plan)

PREPARE TO GET OFF YOUR SUGAR

❑ Take the How Sugar-Addicted Are You? Quiz on page 8.

❑ Use the chart on the following page to write down everything you ate in the previous forty-eight hours. Be sure to include beverages, too, and anything you added to those beverages (e.g., sugar, creamer, or milk).

	DAY 1	DAY 2
Breakfast		
Midmorning snacks		
Lunch		
Afternoon snacks		
Dinner		
Nighttime snacks		

- ❏ Assess your candida levels with the at-home test on page 24.
- ❏ Follow the candida protocol on page 25 if you determine you do have candida overgrowth.
- ❏ Go through the "Seven Ways to Neuroprotect Your Brain" checklist on page 29 and make sure you're regularly doing these activities.
- ❏ Determine how you'll track your transition to fat burning and purchase any supplies you need (such as a ketone meter or urine strips).
- ❏ See how many of the actions of a fat burner you're taking with the self-assessment on page 43.
- ❏ Follow the three-step snack strategy on page 55 anytime a craving strikes and make a list of the craving-crushing snacks (see page 50) that you'll have on hand. Remember the old adage—if you fail to prepare, you prepare to fail.

PHASE 1: WEED
7-DAY MIND/PANTRY/BODY DETOX

Day 1: Calculate your wellness quotient (see page 69).

Day 2: Get clear on your desired outcome and write out your why (see page 71).

My desired outcome is: _____

_____

My *why* for getting off sugar is: _____

_____

Day 3: Commit to your journey (see page 72), decide which digital detox strategies you'll implement going forward, and teach yourself the 3:6:5 Power Breath.

Day 4: Detox your pantry.

Day 5–7: Capture your before, then detox your body with a 3-Day Alkaline Cleanse.

Phase 1: 3-Day Alkaline Cleanse

	DAY 1	DAY 2	DAY 3
7–8 a.m.	Hydration (Detox Tea, page 220, or lemon water) and five minutes of the 3:6:5 Power Breath	Hydration (Detox Tea, page 220, or lemon water) and five minutes of the 3:6:5 Power Breath	Hydration (Detox Tea, page 220, or lemon water) and five minutes of the 3:6:5 Power Breath

continues

continued

	DAY 1	**DAY 2**	**DAY 3**
8–9 a.m.	Green Juice (choose 1): A high-quality greens powder mixed with water Shot of wheatgrass juice Organic celery juice Fresh green juice (with no fruit other than ½ green apple) made at home or from a juice bar (or the beverage case)	Green Juice (choose 1): A high-quality greens powder mixed with water Shot of wheatgrass juice Organic celery juice Fresh green juice (with no fruit other than ½ green apple) made at home or from a juice bar (or the beverage case)	Green Juice (choose 1): A high-quality greens powder mixed with water Shot of wheatgrass juice Organic celery juice Fresh green juice (with no fruit other than ½ green apple) made at home or from a juice bar (or the beverage case)
9–10 a.m.	Dr. Green Detox Smoothie, page 215	Skinny Mint Green Smoothie, page 217	Coco-Berry Smoothie, page 217
10–11 a.m.	Hydration (lemon water)	Hydration (lemon water)	Hydration (lemon water)
11 a.m.–1 p.m.	Chilled Green Detox Soup, page 225	Creamy Spinach Basil Soup, page 226	Chilled Cucumber Avocado Soup, page 227
1–2 p.m.	Hydration (lemon water)	Hydration (lemon water)	Hydration (lemon water)
2–3 p.m.	Afternoon smoothie or snack; choose from: Dr. Green Detox Smoothie (leftover from the morning) 5-Minute Hummus, page 255 Easy Choose-Your-Own-Flavor Kale Chips, page 255	Afternoon smoothie or snack; choose from: Skinny Mint Green Smoothie (leftover from the morning) Clean Keto Garlic Dip, page 251 Crispy Chickpeas, page 252	Afternoon smoothie or snack; choose from: Coco-Berry Smoothie, (leftover from the morning) Superpower Alkaline Treats, page 252 Cacao Almond Fat Bombs, page 256
3–4 p.m.	Hydration (lemon water)	Hydration (lemon water)	Hydration (lemon water)
5–7 p.m.	Avocado, Kale, and Pepita Salad, page 232	Salad with Spicy Salsa Verde, page 230	Perfect Salad in a Jar, page 234

	DAY 1	DAY 2	DAY 3
7–8 p.m.	Hydration (lemon water)	Hydration (lemon water)	Hydration (lemon water)
30 minutes before bed	Alkamind Acid-Kicking Minerals in 4 ounces of water or ⅛ teaspoon Himalayan pink salt dissolved in 6–8 ounces of water	Alkamind Acid-Kicking Minerals in 4 ounces of water or ⅛ teaspoon Himalayan pink salt dissolved in 6–8 ounces of water	Alkamind Acid-Kicking Minerals in 4 ounces of water or ⅛ teaspoon Himalayan pink salt dissolved in 6–8 ounces of water

Phase 1: Tracking Your Journey

So that you can see how your efforts are paying off, each day I want you to give yourself a score of 1 to 10 in the following categories, with 1 being absolutely terrible and 10 being off-the-charts amazing. It will be motivating to see how these change over time, as well as to see which steps make the biggest difference for you. Be sure to start it the day *before* you start making any changes, to give yourself a baseline.

DAY	MY ENERGY LEVEL IS . . .	I SLEPT . . .	MY MOOD IS . . .	MY MENTAL CLARITY IS . . .	MY BODY FEELS . . .
DAY 0 *Before You Start*					
DAY 1 *Find Your Wellness Quotient*					
DAY 2 *Name Your Why*					
DAY 3 *Commit to Your Journey*					

continues

continued

DAY	MY ENERGY LEVEL IS . . .	I SLEPT . . .	MY MOOD IS . . .	MY MENTAL CLARITY IS . . .	MY BODY FEELS . . .
DAY 4 Detox Your Pantry					
DAY 5 Alkaline Cleanse					
DAY 6 Alkaline Cleanse					
DAY 7 Alkaline Cleanse					

PHASE 2: SEED
21 DAYS TO GET OFF YOUR SUGAR

Days 1–3: Start eating at least three green foods a day (choose from juices, smoothies, salads, and soup), but ideally aim for seven to ten servings of greens per day, spread out over three meals, to increase your mineral intake.

Days 4–6: Begin eating two to three servings of healthy fats with each meal (omitting between-meal snacks if you feel ready).

Days 7–9: Calculate how much protein you should be eating and adjust how much protein you're eating each day; switch to more plant-based proteins and improve the quality of the animal-based proteins you eat.

Days 10–12: Begin incorporating at least one herb or spice into everything you eat.

Days 13–15: Stop eating three hours before bedtime. If you are currently snacking between meals, swap any carbohydrate or sugar-filled snacks with healthier snacks. If you are already eating healthy snacks, transition to eating only one healthy snack and three meals a day. If you're already only having one snack a day, omit snacks altogether and stick to three meals a day. If you're eating three meals a day, push your breakfast back by an hour until you're having only two meals a day within an eight-hour window (otherwise known as intermittent fasting); if you're already regularly eating only two meals a day, start having only one meal a day (a partial fast) one day a week.

Days 16–18: Start taking your top five supplements and determine any supporting players you need.

Days 19–21: Do the 8-Minute Acid-Kicking Workout by Anna Kaiser (see pages 173–181) every day during these three days; if you have a rebounder, add a five- to ten-minute bounce in the morning and/or the evening to stimulate your lymphatic system (if you don't, do two minutes of dry skin brushing to get that lymph moving).

Phase 2: Tracking Your Journey

STEP/DAY	MY ENERGY LEVEL IS . . .	I SLEPT . . .	MY MOOD IS . . .	MY MENTAL CLARITY IS . . .	MY BODY FEELS . . .
Step 1 DAY 1 *Re-Mineralize*					
Step 1 DAY 2 *Re-Mineralize*					
Step 1 DAY 3 *Re-Mineralize*					
Step 2 DAY 4 *Add More Healthy Fats*					
Step 2 DAY 5 *Add More Healthy Fats*					

continues

continued

STEP/DAY	MY ENERGY LEVEL IS . . .	I SLEPT . . .	MY MOOD IS . . .	MY MENTAL CLARITY IS . . .	MY BODY FEELS . . .
Step 2 DAY 6 *Add More Healthy Fats*					
Step 3 DAY 7 *Get Protein Smart*					
Step 3 DAY 8 *Get Protein Smart*					
Step 3 DAY 9 *Get Protein Smart*					
Step 4 DAY 10 *Spice Things Up*					
Step 4 DAY 11 *Spice Things Up*					
Step 4 DAY 12 *Spice Things Up*					

STEP/DAY	MY ENERGY LEVEL IS . . .	I SLEPT . . .	MY MOOD IS . . .	MY MENTAL CLARITY IS . . .	MY BODY FEELS . . .
Step 5 DAY 13 *Time Your Meals*					
Step 5 DAY 14 *Time Your Meals*					
Step 5 DAY 15 *Time Your Meals*					
Step 6 DAY 16 *Supplement Your Efforts*					
Step 6 DAY 17 *Supplement Your Efforts*					
Step 6 DAY 18 *Supplement Your Efforts*					

continues

STEP/DAY	MY ENERGY LEVEL IS . . .	I SLEPT . . .	MY MOOD IS . . .	MY MENTAL CLARITY IS . . .	MY BODY FEELS . . .
Step 7 DAY 19 *Amp Up Your Workout*					
Step 7 DAY 20 *Amp Up Your Workout*					
Step 7 DAY 21 *Amp Up Your Workout*					

PHASE 3: FEED
90 DAYS TO MAKE GET OFF
YOUR SUGAR A NEW LIFESTYLE

❏ Make 80 percent of the food you eat in line with the "Get Off Your Sugar Food Pyramid" (page 188) and stick to the macros on "Get Off Your Sugar Food Plate (Based on Visual Appearance)" (page 187).

❏ Stick to the "Strategies for Fat-Burning" (page 189).

❏ Incorporate the "Five to Thrive" (on page 146).

❏ Work your way up to following the 5:1:1 eating plan (five days of intermittent fasting, one day of partial fasting, and one feast day per week).

❏ Make a list of three strategies for improve sleep and/or manage stress better.

Get Off Your Sugar Recipes

LIGHT MEALS

SNACKS/ FOOD TO GO

FAT BOMBS (AND OTHER HEALTHY KETO SNACKS)

DESSERTS

SMOOTHIES

CHOCOLATE ALMOND SMOOTHIE

SERVES 1

You'll feel like you're cheating on your healthy lifestyle when you start your day off with this delicious smoothie. Despite its rich, chocolaty taste, you're actually getting greens, protein, healthy fats, and a lot of vitamins and minerals to power through your day.

- 2 handfuls of fresh spinach
- 1 cup unsweetened almond or coconut milk from a carton
- 1 frozen banana
- ½ Hass avocado, peeled and pitted
- 2 tablespoons raw cacao powder
- 2 tablespoons raw almond butter
- ¼ teaspoon ground cinnamon

In a blender, blend together the spinach and almond milk until smooth. Then, add the banana, avocado, cacao powder, almond butter, and cinnamon and blend until smooth.

NUTRIENT TOTALS (BASED ON ALMOND MILK)

Calories: 515	Dietary Fiber: 21 g	Net Carbs: 26 g
Protein: 12 g	Total Fat: 35 g	
Carbohydrate: 47 g	Saturated Fat: 5 g	

DR. GREEN DETOX SMOOTHIE

SERVES 1

The powerhouse blend will put a pep in your step and a zing on your tongue as it also escorts toxins out of your body (cilantro is a powerful purifier). As a bonus, the greens in this smoothie will help retrain your taste buds. If the ginger kick is too strong for your taste, use a smaller piece.

continues

continued

1 handful of spinach

½ lemon, peeled

1 (1-inch) piece fresh ginger, peeled and grated

½ cucumber, peeled

1 small handful of fresh cilantro

1 small handful of fresh parsley

1 cup coconut water or filtered water

Liquid organic stevia (optional)

Handful of ice (optional)

Combine all the ingredients in a blender and puree for 45 to 60 seconds.

NUTRIENT TOTALS

Calories: 153

Protein: 5 g

Carbohydrate: 14 g (using water; 31 g using coconut water)

Dietary Fiber: 6 g

Total Sugars: 3 g (using water; 15 g using coconut water)

Total Fat: 1 g

Saturated Fat: 0.5 g

Net Carbs: 8 g (using water; 16 g using coconut water)

MACA POWER BREAKFAST SHAKE

SERVES 1

This energizing morning blast utilizes maca powder. Maca is a nutrient-dense vegetable root that is rich in immunity-boosting vitamin C as well as minerals, such as iron and amino acids. Not only can maca contribute to overall well-being, but it can also balance hormone levels, boost energy, suppress hot flashes, and support a healthy libido. Its nutty, earthy flavor adds to this smoothie's chocolate almond taste for a treat you'll love.

½ cup unsweetened almond or coconut milk from a carton

1 tablespoon raw almond or macadamia nut butter

½ Hass avocado, peeled and pitted

¼ cup raw cacao powder

2 teaspoons maca powder

2 or 3 drops organic liquid stevia

½ cup ice

Combine all the ingredients in a blender, and puree for 45 to 60 seconds.

NUTRIENT TOTALS (BASED ON ALMOND MILK)

Calories: 390

Protein: 6 g

Carbohydrate: 27 g

Dietary Fiber: 16 g

Total Sugars: 5 g

Total Fat: 29 g

Saturated Fat: 6.5 g

Net Carbs: 11 g

SKINNY MINT GREEN SMOOTHIE

SERVES 1

Drinking your greens has never been this delicious! The mint in this smoothie will refresh you; the lime and ginger will help give you all the energy you need to face your day.

1 cucumber, peeled
6 or 8 leaves romaine lettuce, or
1 large bunch spinach
1 cup coconut water or filtered
water

Juice of 1 lime
1 (1-inch) piece fresh ginger,
peeled
1 bunch fresh mint, leaves only

1 date, or organic stevia to taste
(optional)
Handful of ice (optional)

Combine all the ingredients in a blender and puree for 45 to 60 seconds.

NUTRIENT TOTALS (USING FILTERED WATER)

Calories: 88
Protein: 3 g
Carbohydrate: 21 g

Dietary Fiber: 5 g
Total Sugars: 6 g
Total Fat: 1 g

Saturated Fat: 0 g
Net Carbs: 16 g

NUTRIENT TOTALS (USING COCONUT WATER)

Calories: 178
Protein: 5 g
Carbohydrate: 39 g

Dietary Fiber: 8 g
Total Sugars: 24 g
Total Fat: 1 g

Saturated Fat: 0 g
Net Carbs: 31 g

COCO-BERRY SMOOTHIE

SERVES 1

This raspberry and coconut smoothie is a delicious way to get plenty of healthy fats first thing in the morning. Feel free to substitute blueberries or blackberries for the raspberries, or use a mix of all three.

2 cups fresh spinach
2 cups unsweetened almond or
coconut milk from a carton
1 cup fresh or frozen raspberries

¼ cup unsweetened coconut
flakes
2 tablespoons coconut oil
1 teaspoon pure vanilla extract

2 drops organic liquid stevia
(optional)

continues

continued

Combine all the ingredients in a blender and puree for 45 to 60 seconds.

NUTRIENT TOTALS (BASED ON ALMOND MILK)

Calories: 604
Protein: 6 g
Carbohydrate: 40 g

Dietary Fiber: 20 g
Total Sugars: 13 g
Total Fat: 50 g

Saturated Fat: 42 g
Net Carbs: 11 g

JUICES

If you own a juicer (or if you've been thinking about getting one, perhaps these will inspire you to take the plunge), here are two options that will get you plenty of minerals and taste great without a lot of sugar.

THE CRIMSON KICKER

SERVES 1

Although there's plenty of sweet, earthy flavor in this tasty juice, it's low in sugar and high in nutrients.

2 red beets, peeled
½ lemon, peeled

1 cup fresh spinach
½ green apple, cored

1 tablespoon chia seeds

Juice together all the ingredients, except the chia seeds. Top with the chia seeds and serve.

NUTRIENT TOTALS

Calories: 79
Protein: 2 g
Carbohydrate: 18 g

Dietary Fiber: 2 g
Total Sugars: 15 g
Total Fat: 0.5 g

Saturated Fat: 0 g
Net Carbs: 16 g

GREEN DETOX JUICE

SERVES 1

The ginger, lemon juice, greens, and chia seeds in this juice are all detox superfoods that taste great.

1 cup kale or spinach
1 small green apple, cored
½ cucumber

1 tablespoon freshly squeezed
  lemon juice

1 (1-inch) piece fresh ginger,
  peeled
1 tablespoon chia seeds

Juice together all the ingredients, except the chia seeds. Top with the chia seeds and serve.

NUTRIENT TOTALS

Calories: 226
Protein: 8 g
Carbohydrate: 34 g

Dietary Fiber: 13 g
Total Sugars: 19 g
Total Fat: 6 g

Saturated Fat: 0.5 g
Net Carbs: 21 g

OTHER HEALING TONICS

MORNING FAT BURNER TONIC

SERVES 1

This hot tea is a great way to start your morning, but you can also enjoy it at night. It delivers alkalizing, hydrating ingredients that boost your immune system and metabolism, helping you burn fat throughout your day or even while you sleep!

continues

continued

8 ounces hot filtered water

2 tablespoons freshly squeezed lemon juice

2 tablespoons apple cider vinegar

1 (1-inch) piece fresh ginger, peeled and grated

1 drop organic liquid stevia

Pinch of ground cinnamon

Pinch of cayenne pepper (optional)

In a mug, pour the hot water over the lemon juice, apple cider vinegar, and ginger. Then, add the stevia, cinnamon, and cayenne (if using). Stir to combine and drink while it's warm, or pour over ice if you prefer it chilled.

NUTRIENT TOTALS

Calories: 17	Dietary Fiber: 1 g	Saturated Fat: 0 g
Protein: 0 g	Total Sugars: 1 g	Net Carbs: 3 g
Carbohydrate: 4 g	Total Fat: 0 g	

DETOX TEA

SERVES 4

Lemon, ginger, and turmeric are a trifecta of anti-inflammatory superstars. In addition this tea helps cleanse your lymph system, which boosts immunity. This tea is easy to make and a great start to your day.

16 to 20 ounces filtered water

1 (1-inch) piece fresh organic turmeric, peeled and minced

1 (1-inch) piece fresh ginger, peeled and minced

Pinch of freshly ground black pepper

Pinch of cayenne pepper (optional)

1 lemon slice

1 scoop dehydrated green juice powder (optional)

Pour the water into a pot and bring to a boil. Once the water begins to boil, remove from the heat, then add the turmeric, ginger, black pepper, and cayenne (if using) to the pot, and let steep for 10 minutes. The longer you steep it, the more potent and concentrated your Detox Tea will be. Pour the tea into a cup and squeeze the lemon juice into it. Store any leftovers in the fridge in an airtight container for a healthy Detox Iced Tea, and feel free to add a scoop of dehydrated green juice powder to give it even more power.

NUTRIENT TOTALS

Calories: 2	Dietary Fiber: 0 g	Saturated Fat: 0 g
Protein: 0 g	Total Sugars: 0 g	Net Carbs: 0
Carbohydrate: 0 g	Total Fat: 0 g	

MORE BREAKFAST OPTIONS

ALMOND BUTTER & BANANA GREEN SMOOTHIE BOWL

SERVES 2

Who says you need to drink your smoothie? This is thicker than a typical smoothie but has many of the same clean, green ingredients that make an alkaline breakfast, served in a bowl and topped with more delicious goodness!

2 handfuls of kale

¼ cup coconut milk, full-fat canned if you prefer thicker (Native Forest is great), unsweetened carton if you prefer thinner

1 frozen banana

1 tablespoon chia seeds

3 tablespoons almond butter

2 tablespoons sliced raw almonds

1 tablespoon unsweetened coconut flakes

1 tablespoon shelled raw pepitas (pumpkin seeds)

A few fresh banana slices and/or a handful of berries, for garnish

In a blender, blend together the kale and coconut milk until smooth. Add the banana, chia seeds, and almond butter and blend, adding more liquid if needed. The consistency should be thicker than a smoothie. Pour into a bowl and top with the almonds, coconut flakes, pumpkin seeds, and a few banana slices and/or berries. Serve immediately.

NUTRIENT TOTALS (BASED ON CANNED FULL-FAT COCONUT MILK)

Calories: 429
Protein: 14 g
Carbohydrate: 28 g

Dietary Fiber: 13 g
Total Sugars: 9.5 g
Total Fat: 32 g

Saturated Fat: 9 g
Sodium: 26 mg
Net Carbs: 15 g

GRAIN-FREE GRANOLA

SERVES 6 SERVINGS OF ½ CUP EACH

Make a batch of this grain-free granola for quick access to a healthy crunch all week long! This golden granola is delicious and addictive, and it's better than anything you can buy at the store. It's a very versatile recipe to have on' hand for breakfast or a nutritious snack. Use it to top your favorite breakfast smoothies or chia seed puddings, or eat it as a traditional granola with nut milk poured over it.

¾ cup raw almonds

½ cup raw pistachio nuts

½ cup macadamia nuts

1 tablespoon coconut oil, melted

½ teaspoon sea salt (Celtic Grey, Himalayan pink, or Redmond Real Salt)

½ teaspoon ground coriander

½ teaspoon ground ginger

⅛ teaspoon ground cinnamon

⅛ teaspoon cayenne pepper (optional; add more or less to heat preference)

⅓ cup unsweetened coconut flakes

¼ cup shelled raw pepitas (pumpkin seeds)

Unsweetened almond or coconut milk, for serving (optional)

Preheat the oven to 350°F. Place the almonds, pistachio nuts, and macadamia nuts in a baking pan and add the coconut oil. In a small bowl, stir together the sea salt, coriander, ginger, cinnamon, and cayenne (if using). Sprinkle the seasoning mixture over the nuts and stir well to fully coat the nuts with the oil and seasonings. Bake for 10 minutes more, stirring at the 5-minute mark.

Next, add the coconut flakes and pepitas to the pan. Bake for 3 minutes, or until the mixture is toasted. Remove from the oven and let cool, then store in an airtight container. Serve, if desired, in a bowl with almond or coconut milk.

NUTRIENT TOTALS

Calories: 205

Protein: 9 g

Carbohydrate: 8 g

Dietary Fiber: 4 g

Total Sugars: 2 g

Total Fat: 18 g

Saturated Fat: 3 g

Net Carbs: 4 g

CHICKPEA VEGGIE FRITTATA

SERVES 4

If you've ever wondered how you might live without eggs, wait until you try this plant-based frittata. It's so tasty and so easy.

2 tablespoons extra-virgin olive oil

1 cup chopped onion
1 cup chopped cauliflower

2 cups packed fresh spinach
½ teaspoon sea salt

BATTER

1½ cups chickpea flour

½ teaspoon freshly ground black pepper

1½ cups filtered water

Preheat the oven to 375°F and use 1 tablespoon of the olive oil to oil a 10-inch Pyrex (or any type) baking dish. Set aside. Meanwhile, heat the remaining tablespoon of oil in a large sauté pan over medium heat. Add the onion and cauliflower and cook until the vegetables are tender, about 4 minutes. Then, remove from heat and fold in the spinach and salt until spinach is wilted.

Prepare the batter: In a medium-size bowl, mix the chickpea flour with the pepper and water. Mix in the cooked vegetables. Pour the mixture into the prepared baking dish. Spread to smooth the top.

Bake for 30 minutes, or until the top is cracked and feels firm and set in the middle. Remove from the oven and let cool for 5 minutes before slicing. Leftovers can be stored, tightly covered, in the refrigerator for up to four days.

Notes: If using a smaller baking dish (for example, a 9-inch pan), bake for 40 to 45 minutes. Also, you may use any vegetable combination of your liking. For example, instead of using spinach and cauliflower, you can use broccoli (chopped) and red bell peppers (thinly sliced), or scallions and asparagus, etc.

NUTRIENT TOTALS

Calories: 202
Protein: 7 g
Carbohydrate: 25 g

Dietary Fiber: 10 g
Total Sugars: 2 g
Total Fat: 8.5 g

Saturated Fat: 2.5 g
Net Carbs: 15 g

KELLY'S PANCAKES WITH RHUBARB COMPOTE

SERVES 2 TO 4

Kelly Ripa made this grain-free, low-sugar recipe on her show, *Live with Kelly and Ryan*. This is a perfect way to convince anyone who is skeptical about getting off sugar just how delicious it can be. Top the pancakes with the barely sweet rhubarb compote and enjoy.

3 bananas

2 large pasture-raised, grass-fed eggs

½ cup almond butter

2 teaspoons ground cinnamon

1 teaspoon pure vanilla extract

Pinch of sea salt (Celtic Grey, Himalayan pink, or Redmond Real Salt)

1 tablespoon coconut oil

Combine all the ingredients, except the coconut oil, in a blender, and blend until smooth. Heat the coconut oil in a medium-size skillet over medium heat. Pour ¼ cup of the batter on the skillet and cook over medium heat until golden brown, about 1 minute, flip over, and cook until the other side is golden brown. Repeat until all the batter is cooked.

RHUBARB COMPOTE

2 rhubarb stalks, chopped

1 pint strawberries, hulled and chopped

Zest and juice of 1 lemon

Combine all the ingredients in a medium-size saucepan and cook over medium-low heat until fruit is soft and jamlike, about 15 minutes. Add a little water, if necessary. Top the pancakes with the compote and serve.

NUTRIENT TOTALS FOR PANCAKES (BASED ON 3 SERVINGS)

Calories: 352.6

Protein: 9 g

Carbohydrate: 25 g

Dietary Fiber: 6 g

Total Sugars: 9 g

Total Fat: 25 g

Saturated Fat: 5 g

Net Carbs: 19 g

NUTRIENT TOTALS FOR COMPOTE (BASED ON 3 SERVINGS)

Calories: 31

Protein: 1 g

Carbohydrate: 7 g

Dietary Fiber: 3 g

Total Sugars: 4 g

Total Fat: 0 g

Saturated Fat: 0 g

Net Carbs: 4 g

RAW GREEN SOUPS

CHILLED GREEN DETOX SOUP

SERVES 4

This savory soup is a mega-dose of greens and minerals—all it takes is a quick whiz in the blender and you're ready to power up!

2 cups filtered water

2 medium-size cucumbers, chopped

½ bunch of your favorite greens (kale, spinach, arugula, Swiss chard), chopped

2 celery stalks, chopped

¼ cup freshly squeezed lemon juice

½ cup extra-virgin olive oil

1 garlic clove, minced

1 teaspoon sea salt (Celtic Grey, Himalayan pink, or Redmond Real Salt)

Small handful of fresh parsley and/or cilantro (optional)

Fresh basil, paprika, or cayenne pepper, for garnish

Place all the ingredients, including the parsley or cilantro, if desired, but omitting the garnish, in a blender. Blend at high speed to your desired consistency and enjoy immediately, or serve chilled. Garnish with basil, paprika, or cayenne.

NUTRIENT TOTALS

Calories: 156

Protein: 2 g

Carbohydrate: 7 g

Dietary Fiber: 2 g

Total Sugars: 2 g

Total Fat: 14 g

Saturated Fat: 2 g

Net Carbs: 5 g

SPICY MOROCCAN TOMATO-GINGER SOUP

SERVES 4

This flavor-packed soup is naturally raw, vegetarian, vegan, and gluten-free. Even better, it takes only five minutes in a blender to make. This will make plenty extra, so feel free to have it as a snack later in the day, or let all of those spices and flavors meld overnight.

continues

continued

3 tomatoes
¼ cup sun-dried tomatoes
4 ounces fresh ginger, minced
½ cup tahini
1 teaspoon ground cardamom
1 teaspoon ground cumin

½ teaspoon caraway seeds
2 garlic cloves
¼ cup chopped fresh basil
¼ chopped fresh parsley
¼ cup extra-virgin olive oil

1 teaspoon salt (Celtic Grey, Himalayan pink, or Redmond Real Salt)
Fresh basil, paprika, or cayenne pepper, for garnish

Place all the ingredients, omitting the garnish, in a blender, blend at high speed to your desired consistency, and enjoy immediately or serve chilled. Garnish with basil, paprika, or cayenne.

NUTRIENT TOTALS

Calories: 345
Protein: 8 g
Carbohydrate: 16 g

Dietary Fiber: 5 g
Total Sugars: 4 g
Total Fat: 30 g

Saturated Fat: 4 g
Net Carbs: 11 g

CREAMY SPINACH BASIL SOUP

SERVES 4

This quick soup gets a huge taste boost, thanks to the basil; it's the flavors of pesto in soup form.

4 cups filtered water
1 bunch spinach, chopped
½ bunch basil (about 2 cups, loosely packed)
¼ small red onion, chopped

1 medium-size cucumber, chopped
1 medium-size tomato, chopped
2 celery stalks
½ cup pine nuts
½ cup extra-virgin olive oil

1 garlic clove, chopped
1 teaspoon sea salt (Celtic Grey, Himalayan pink, or Redmond Real Salt)
Pinch of cayenne pepper (optional)

Place all the ingredients in a blender, blend at high speed to your desired consistency, and enjoy immediately, or serve chilled.

NUTRIENT TOTALS

Calories: 204
Protein: 3 g
Carbohydrate: 7 g

Dietary Fiber: 2 g
Total Sugars: 3 g
Total Fat: 20 g

Saturated Fat: 2 g
Net Carbs: 5 g

CHILLED CUCUMBER AVOCADO SOUP

SERVES 2

This easy soup is refreshing and flavorful. The avocado makes it creamy and filling, even though it's vegan, clean keto, and completely alkaline.

2 Hass avocados, peeled, pitted, and sliced

2 medium-size cucumbers, roughly chopped

¼ cup fresh cilantro

Juice of 1 lime

½ teaspoon sea salt (Celtic Grey, Himalayan pink, or Redmond Real Salt)

Freshly ground black pepper

¼ teaspoon cayenne pepper (optional)

½ cup filtered water (optional)

Reserve half of one of the avocados for garnish. Place the other ingredients, except the water, in a blender and blend until smooth. Add filtered water to thin to your desired consistency. Taste for seasoning and adjust as needed. Serve garnished with the reserved avocado slices.

NUTRIENT TOTALS (INCLUDES ½ AVOCADO PER SERVING)

Calories: 248
Protein: 4 g
Carbohydrate: 18 g
Dietary Fiber: 7 g

Total Sugars: 4 g
Total Fat: 20 g
Saturated Fat: 3 g
Net Carbs: 11 g

HOT SOUPS

VEGAN PROTEIN BONELESS BROTH

SERVES 6

This rich, superfood boneless broth can serve as a base for so many different soups, and each one of them will help you detox. It's very easy to pull together—just chop everything and throw it in a slow cooker or Instant Pot. Yes, you could substitute organic, yeast-free vegetable broth, but this tastes so much better!

continues

continued

10 cups filtered water

1 tablespoon coconut oil

2 small garlic cloves, peeled and finely chopped

1 (1-inch) piece fresh ginger, peeled and finely chopped

1 onion, chopped

1 leek, finely chopped

2 celery stalks, chopped

2 carrots, chopped

1 cup kale or collard greens

1 tablespoon freshly squeezed lemon juice

2 (4-inch) pieces kombu (sea vegetables found in the Asian section of the supermarket)

2 teaspoons ground turmeric

½ cup fresh parsley leaves

2 teaspoons sea salt (Celtic Grey, Himalayan pink, or Redmond Real Salt)

½ teaspoon freshly ground black pepper

Place all the ingredients in a slow cooker and cook on LOW for 4 hours *or* use an Instant Pot on the SOUP setting. If you're cooking on the stovetop, put all ingredients into a big pot and bring to a boil over high heat, and then lower the heat and let simmer, covered, for 2 hours.

After cooking, let cool, and then pour through a wire mesh strainer. Store in the fridge for use over the next few days. If you are making it ahead of time, freeze in 1- to 1½-cup portions.

NUTRIENT TOTALS

Calories: 36	Dietary Fiber: 0.5 g	Saturated Fat: 1 g
Protein: 1 g	Total Sugars: 2.5 g	Net carbs: 2 g
Carbohydrate: 2.5 g	Total Fat: 1.5 g	

FARMER'S LENTIL SOUP

SERVES 4

Once you have the basics for this hearty, warm-your-soul soup, you can substitute veggies depending on what's in season and what you like.

2 tablespoons coconut oil

1 small yellow onion, diced

4 large carrots, thinly sliced

4 celery stalks, thinly sliced

2 medium-size or 1 large garlic clove, peeled and minced

Pinch of sea salt (Celtic Grey, Himalayan pink, or Redmond Real Salt)

Pinch of freshly ground black pepper

4 cups Vegan Protein Boneless Broth (for homemade, see page 227) or organic vegetable broth

1 cup dried green lentils, rinsed and drained (or any color lentil you choose)

2 cups chopped kale or spinach

2 teaspoons fresh thyme leaves

In a large pot or Dutch oven, heat the coconut oil on medium heat. Once melted, add the onion, carrots, celery, and garlic. Season with a pinch of salt and pepper, then sauté, stirring occasionally, for 4 minutes. Add the broth and increase the heat to bring to a boil. Add the lentils, then lower the heat, cover, and simmer for 15 minutes, or until the lentils are tender. Add the kale and thyme and cook long enough for the kale to wilt (a few minutes at most) and taste for seasoning. Serve in a bowl.

NUTRIENT TOTALS

Calories: 298	Dietary Fiber: 19 g	Saturated Fat: 6 g
Protein: 14.5 g	Total Sugars: 7.5 g	Sodium: 516 mg
Carbohydrate: 42 g	Total Fat: 8 g	Net Carbs: 23 g

ZUCCHINI, APPLE, AND BASIL-FENNEL SOUP

SERVES 6

The recipe for this flavorful soup comes from the COMO Parrot Cay resort in Turks and Caicos, where my wife and I enjoyed a wonderful family trip—the restaurant's many delicious vegan recipes made the experience even better. This soup, with its unique taste combinations, was our favorite choice from their Shambhala menu.

¼ cup extra-virgin olive oil

1 yellow onion, diced

4 garlic cloves

3 fennel bulbs, trimmed, cored, and shaved (e.g., with a mandoline)

Sea salt (Celtic Grey, Himalayan pink, or Redmond Real Salt)

3 zucchini, seeded and diced

5 cups vegetable broth (for homemade, see page 227)

2 Granny Smith apples, peeled, cored, and sliced

1 cup fresh basil leaves, or zucchini ribbons, red pepper flakes, and a drizzle of extra-virgin olive oil, for garnish (optional)

Heat the olive oil in a large saucepan over medium heat. Then, add the onion, garlic, and fennel, season to taste with sea salt, and cook for 15 minutes, or until the vegetables appear soft and translucent. Next, add the zucchini and cook for 5 more minutes. Add the vegetable stock, bring to a boil, then lower the heat to a simmer and cover.

Cook for 30 minutes, then add the apples and simmer for another 15 minutes. Remove from the heat, transfer to a blender, and puree until a smooth creamy consistency is reached (this may need to be done in two batches; use caution when blending hot liquids). Serve in a soup bowl, garnished with basil leaves or zucchini ribbons, red pepper flakes, with a drizzle of olive oil.

NUTRIENT TOTALS

Calories: 173	Dietary Fiber: 6 g	Saturated Fat: 1.5 g
Protein: 4 g	Total Sugars: 8 g	Net Carbs: 16 g
Carbohydrate: 22 g	Total Fat: 9.5 g	

SALADS AND DRESSINGS

SALAD WITH SPICY SALSA VERDE

SERVES 2

The spicy, Mexican-inspired salsa verde that serves as the dressing on this salad makes it crave-worthy compared to your standard salad. And with two healthy sources of fat—the avocado and extra-virgin olive oil—you'll stay full for hours while you enjoy a big energy boost from the greens.

SALSA VERDE

2 tablespoons extra-virgin olive oil

2 garlic cloves, peeled

Handful of fresh cilantro

½ teaspoon sea salt (Celtic Grey, Himalayan pink, or Redmond Real Salt)

Freshly ground black pepper

½ to 1 jalapeño pepper, seeds removed (optional)

SALAD

2 big handfuls arugula or baby romaine lettuce

1 cup cherry or grape tomatoes, sliced lengthwise

1 Hass avocado, diced

Prepare the salsa verde: In a blender, blend together the salsa verde ingredients until smooth.

Combine the salad ingredients in a big bowl, toss with salsa verde, and serve.

NUTRIENT TOTALS

Calories: 258

Protein: 3 g

Carbohydrate: 11 g

Dietary Fiber: 6 g

Total Sugars: 3 g

Total Fat: 24 g

Saturated Fat: 3.5 g

Sodium: 297 mg

Net Carbs: 5 g

ADZUKI BEAN AND ASPARAGUS SALAD

SERVES 2

This salad is *so* satisfying. It makes a great dinner on its own or travels to work easily for lunch. The great thing about this recipe from a nutritional standpoint is that the only fruit in the salad (fresh lemon juice) is a low-sugar fruit that helps alkalize your body.

1 bunch thin asparagus, rough ends trimmed off
¼ cup extra-virgin olive oil
Zest and juice of 1 lemon

½ bunch parsley, chopped
1 (15-ounce) can adzuki beans, drained and rinsed (Eden Organics is great)

2 cups baby arugula
Sea salt (Celtic Grey, Himalayan pink, or Redmond Real Salt)
Freshly ground black pepper

Bring a pot of water to a boil. Blanch the asparagus for 5 to 8 minutes, until tender. Remove from the water and pat dry with paper towels. Chop into 1-inch pieces. In a small bowl, whisk together the olive oil, lemon zest and juice, and parsley.

In a medium-size bowl, combine the beans, asparagus, and arugula. Toss with the dressing and season to taste with salt and pepper.

NUTRIENT TOTALS

Calories: 269	Dietary Fiber: 9 g	Saturated Fat: 2 g
Protein: 9 g	Total Sugars: 1.5 g	Net Carbs: 18 g
Carbohydrate: 27 g	Total Fat: 14 g	

POMEGRANATE AND WHITE BEAN SALAD WITH TARRAGON DRESSING

SERVES 2

This salad is a delicious mix of flavors and textures. If you're tired of eating the same old salads, give this a try. Because of the white beans and avocado, you'll get a good dose of protein and fat that will keep you full for hours.

SALAD

4 cups baby spinach
Seeds from 1 pomegranate, or ⅓ cup seeds
2 baby leeks, thinly sliced
1 Hass avocado, peeled, pitted, and diced

½ cup canned white beans, drained and rinsed (Eden Organics is great)
¼ cup pine nuts or sliced raw almonds

continues

continued

DRESSING

3 tablespoons apple cider vinegar

½ cup extra-virgin olive oil

2 garlic cloves, peeled and minced

1 tablespoon whole-grain mustard

2 tablespoons chopped fresh tarragon

Sea salt (Celtic Grey, Himalayan pink, or Redmond Real Salt)

Freshly ground black pepper

Prepare the salad: Mix together all the salad ingredients in a bowl.

Prepare the dressing: In a small bowl, combine all the dressing ingredients, including salt and pepper to taste. Toss with the salad.

NUTRIENT TOTALS

Calories: 266
Protein: 6 g
Carbohydrate: 18 g

Dietary Fiber: 6 g
Total Sugars: 3.5 g
Total Fat: 21 g

Saturated Fat: 2.5 g
Net Carbs: 12 g

AVOCADO, KALE, AND PEPITA SALAD

SERVES 4

This salad is such a great source of healthy fats. Between one whole avocado per person (yum!), the coconut oil, and the pepitas, it's a healthy fat-filled power lunch!

2 tablespoons coconut oil

2 large bunches kale, stemmed and chopped

1 tablespoon coconut aminos or gluten-free tamari

4 Hass avocados, peeled, pitted, and chopped

¼ cup shelled raw pepitas (pumpkin seeds)

Melt the coconut oil in a large skillet over medium-high heat. Add the kale and stir-fry for 5 minutes. The kale should be tender and bright green. Remove from the heat and toss with the coconut aminos. Serve with the avocado and pepitas on top.

NUTRIENT TOTALS

Calories: 399
Protein: 11 g
Carbohydrate: 22 g

Dietary Fiber: 13 g
Total Sugars: 0.5 g
Total Fat: 33 g

Saturated Fat: 9.5 g
Net Carbs: 9 g

MEDITERRANEAN CHOPPED SALAD

SERVES 2

This simple salad is a taste explosion in your mouth. And here's a time-saving tip for you: double the ingredients for the dressing and keep it (in the fridge) right in the jar you mix it up in. It will give you a head start on making this salad again (it's so good, you'll definitely be thinking about it tomorrow).

SALAD

1 medium-size cucumber, chopped

½ cup canned chickpeas, drained and rinsed (Eden Organics is great)

½ cup black olives

¼ red onion, diced

½ cup cherry tomatoes

DRESSING

¼ cup extra-virgin olive oil

1 tablespoon apple cider vinegar

2 tablespoons freshly squeezed lemon juice

1 teaspoon chopped garlic

1 teaspoon dried basil

½ teaspoon dried oregano

Pinch of sea salt (Celtic Grey, Himalayan pink, or Redmond Real Salt)

Freshly ground black pepper

Prepare the salad: Place the cucumber, chickpeas, black olives, red onion, and cherry tomatoes together in a bowl.

Prepare the dressing: Combine the dressing ingredients, including salt and pepper to taste, in a jar with a tight-fitting lid and shake well. Add the dressing to the salad, gently toss, and serve.

NUTRIENT TOTALS

Calories: 299

Protein: 3 g

Carbohydrate: 10 g

Dietary Fiber: 3 g

Total Sugars: 1 g

Total Fat: 29 g

Saturated Fat: 4 g

Net Carbs: 7 g

PERFECT SALAD IN A JAR

Why is this salad "perfect"? First, it's got the Asian flair and crunch of a Chinese chicken salad (without all the sneaky sugar in the dressing). Next, it delivers a huge helping of mineral- and fiber-rich greens; and the nuts, seeds, and almond butter bring along a nice amount of healthy fats. But what really puts it over the top is that it's so easily portable, making it an ideal grab-and-go lunch for those busy days when you don't have time to make or even go out and pick up a healthy meal.

3 tablespoons raw almond butter

1 tablespoon freshly squeezed lemon juice or apple cider vinegar

1 tablespoon pure maple syrup (I use low-carb ChocZero maple syrup, which has 1 gram net carbs)

2 teaspoons sesame oil

½ Granny Smith apple, cored and diced

4 or 5 cherry tomatoes

4 radishes, sliced

2 celery stalks, diced

¼ cup of your favorite raw nuts and seeds (slivered almonds, walnuts, pumpkin seeds, hemp seeds, etc.)

4 to 6 cups of your favorite greens (spinach, kale, mixed greens, etc.)

Combine the almond butter, lemon juice, maple syrup, and sesame oil in a small bowl and whisk until smooth. Next, add the apple to the dressing (so it's covered and won't brown), and divide between two 16-ounce mason jars.

Layer the tomatoes, radishes, celery, nuts and seeds, and greens on top and seal. When ready to eat, shake up the jar, open and enjoy immediately, or pour it into a large bowl to mix more thoroughly.

NUTRIENT TOTALS

Calories: 332
Protein: 10 g
Carbohydrate: 27 g

Dietary Fiber: 15 g
Total Sugars: 8 g
Total Fat: 25 g

Saturated Fat: 2 g
Net Carbs: 12 g

DR. DARYL'S FAVORITE SALAD DRESSING

There's a reason this one is named my favorite dressing—we make it a few times per week, and it never lasts long. It makes the perfect salad dressing, and a healthy dipping sauce for raw vegetables. The chipotle and optional cayenne gives this dressing a kick that will leave you coming back for more. Consider doubling the recipe—it's that good.

- ½ cup extra virgin olive oil
- 2 tablespoons freshly squeezed lime juice
- 2 tablespoons Bragg Liquid Aminos
- 2 tablespoons minced red onion
- 1 garlic clove
- ½ teaspoon chipotle powder
- 1½ pitted dates
- ¼ teaspoon sea salt (Celtic Grey, Himalaya pink, or Redmond Real Salt)
- Pinch of cayenne pepper (optional)

Place all the ingredients in a blender or small food processor and blend to your desired consistency. Serve as a salad dressing with your favorite leafy greens, or with your favorite vegetable sticks (peppers, carrots, broccoli, etc.).

NUTRIENT TOTALS

Calories: 179
Protein: 1 g
Carbohydrate: 5 g

Dietary Fiber: 0.5 g
Total Sugars: 4 g
Total Fat: 18 g

Saturated Fat: 2.5 g
Net Carbs: 4.5 g

ENTRÉES

MAIN DISHES (PLANT-BASED KETO, STIR-FRIES, WILD OMEGA-3 FISH)

CAULIFLOWER RICE–STUFFED PEPPERS

SERVES 4

These stuffed peppers are better than any pepper stuffed with acidic ingredients you've ever had, I guarantee. They take a little more time in the oven than my recipes typically do, but it's worth the wait. And you'll have leftovers for lunches or another dinner.

continues

continued

2 tablespoons coconut oil

4 red bell peppers, cut in half lengthwise and seeded

Sea salt (Celtic Grey, Himalayan pink, or Redmond Real Salt)

1 head cauliflower, riced or finely chopped, or 1 (12-ounce) package frozen cauliflower rice

2 garlic cloves, minced

1 red onion, diced

2 teaspoons ground cumin

2 teaspoons chili powder

Juice of 1 lime

⅔ cup healthy salsa (use Salsa Verde from page 230)

1 (15-ounce) can adzuki beans, drained and rinsed (Eden Organics is great)

Freshly ground black pepper

OPTIONAL TOPPINGS

Chopped fresh cilantro

1 Hass avocado, peeled, pitted, and sliced

Freshly squeezed lime juice

Jalapeño peppers

Salsa

Preheat the oven to 400°F. Brush a large baking dish (glass works well) with a little of the coconut oil. Then, place the bell peppers, cut side up, in the dish and coat the outsides and insides with the coconut oil. Sprinkle with sea salt. Heat a skillet over medium-low heat and add the rest of the coconut oil. Add the cauliflower rice, garlic, red onion, spices, lime juice, and salsa. Sauté for 2 to 3 minutes as you incorporate the ingredients. Add the adzuki beans and remove from the heat.

Stuff the pepper halves with the mixture, taste, and add salt, pepper, and lime to taste. Place the pepper halves, stuffing side up, in a lidded cast-iron pot and bake for 40 minutes. If you don't have a cast-iron pot, you can use a Dutch oven, or you can use a glass baking dish that you cover loosely with foil and bake for 25 minutes, then remove the foil and bake for another 15 minutes. Top with your choice of cilantro, avocado, lime juice, or jalapeños, and serve with salsa.

NUTRIENT TOTALS (2 PEPPER HALVES PER SERVING, WITHOUT TOPPINGS)

Calories: 258	Dietary Fiber: 14 g	Saturated Fat: 6 g
Protein: 11 g	Total Sugars: 10 g	Sodium: 725 mg
Carbohydrate: 36 g	Total Fat: 8 g	Net Carbs: 22 g

CITRUS-HERB ROASTED SALMON WITH ASPARAGUS

SERVES 4

This is an elevated but easy keto meal that comes together quickly. It's perfect for having company over for dinner or just enjoying with your family. It delivers a ton of healthy omega-3 fats in addition to vitamins and minerals.

1 tablespoon coconut oil

4 (6-ounce) Pacific wild-caught salmon fillets

1 bunch asparagus, ends trimmed

Sea salt (Celtic Grey, Himalayan pink, or Redmond Real Salt)

Freshly ground black pepper

1 tablespoon chopped fresh parsley or thyme

Juice of ½ lemon

Preheat the oven to 450°F. Coat a roasting pan with some of the coconut oil and place the salmon, skin side down, in the pan. Use the remaining coconut oil to coat the asparagus and spread out on the roasting pan. Sprinkle the whole pan with the seasonings, transfer to the oven, and roast for 8 to 12 minutes, depending on desired doneness. Remove from the oven, sprinkle the salmon with parsley or thyme leaves and a squeeze of lemon, and serve on a plate.

NUTRIENT TOTALS

Calories: 282

Protein: 35 g

Carbohydrate: 2 g

Dietary Fiber: 1 g

Total Sugars: 1 g

Total Fat: 14 g

Saturated Fat: 4.5 g

Net Carbs: 1 g

RAW ZUCCHINI PESTO PASTA

SERVES 4

Zucchini noodles, or "zoodles," are a gluten-free, low-calorie substitute for traditional pasta in this easy and fresh vegan dinner. And the sauce is dairy-free and completely plant-based, combining walnuts and basil in a flavorful pesto. When eating vegan, anti-inflammatory food tastes this good, why would you eat any other way?

ZOODLES

3 medium-size zucchini, peeled

continues

continued

WALNUT BASIL PESTO

2 cups packed fresh basil leaves, plus more for garnish

⅔ cup raw walnuts, ideally soaked in water overnight and drained

2 small garlic cloves, peeled

2 teaspoons freshly squeezed lemon juice

Sea salt (Celtic Grey, Himalayan pink, or Redmond Real Salt)

Freshly ground black pepper

2 tablespoons extra-virgin olive oil

Prepare the zoodles: Spiralize the zucchini into curly or straight zoodles and place in a bowl. If you don't have a spiralizer, you can use a vegetable peeler to give you wide, fettuccine-like slices.

Prepare the pesto: Combine the basil, walnuts, garlic, lemon juice, and salt and pepper to taste in a food processor or blender, drizzling olive oil in as the mixture pulses, until it reaches a pesto consistency. Taste for salt and pepper. Mix the pesto with the zoodles, garnish with basil leaves, and serve.

NUTRIENT TOTALS

Calories: 198
Protein: 5 g
Carbohydrate: 8 g

Dietary Fiber: 3 g
Total Sugars: 3 g
Total Fat: 18 g

Saturated Fat: 2 g
Net Carbs: 5 g

GREEN CURRY WITH SUMMER VEGGIES

SERVES 4

If you normally avoid curries because they're too spicy, you'll love this mild, tasty version, which utilizes a ton of fresh, organic produce. If this exact combo is not in season or in your kitchen, you can use whatever veggies you've picked up at the farmers' market or grocery store.

2 tablespoons coconut oil

1 onion, peeled and diced

3 garlic cloves, peeled and minced

1 tablespoon green curry paste

1 medium-size summer squash, diced

1 zucchini, diced

2 baby bok choy, chopped

½ cup sugar snap peas

1 (15-ounce) can chickpeas, drained and rinsed (Eden Organics is great)

1 (15-ounce) can full-fat coconut milk (I recommend Native Forest brand)

1 cup vegetable broth (for homemade, see page 227)

2 bunches kale, collards, or other greens, washed and cut

Sea salt (Celtic Grey, Himalayan pink, or Redmond Real Salt)

Freshly ground black pepper

Cooked quinoa, for serving (optional)

Fresh basil and/or cilantro, for garnish

In a large pot, heat the coconut oil and sauté the onion until soft, 6 to 8 minutes. Add the garlic and green curry paste and sauté for 2 to 3 more minutes. Add the vegetables, chickpeas, and coconut milk. Bring to a simmer and add the vegetable broth. Simmer until the veggies are tender, 10 minutes at most. Add the greens to wilt, then season with salt and pepper to taste.

Serve in a bowl, and for some added protein and fiber, serve over cooked quinoa. Garnish with basil and/or cilantro.

NUTRIENT TOTALS

Calories: 383	Dietary Fiber: 9 g	Saturated Fat: 22 g
Protein: 9.5 g	Total Sugars: 4 g	Net Carbs: 21 g
Carbohydrate: 30 g	Total Fat: 27 g	

CHINESE TAKEOUT BROCCOLI WITH "FRIED RICE"

SERVES 2

Yes, you *can* turn your favorite takeout foods into anti-inflammatory, alkaline dishes you make at home in just minutes. You won't miss the meat with this tasty broccoli main dish.

1 (12-ounce) package frozen cauliflower rice; 1 head cauliflower, riced or finely chopped; or 1 cup cooked quinoa or wild rice

1½ teaspoons arrowroot starch

1½ tablespoons coconut aminos

1½ teaspoons Bragg liquid aminos or gluten-free tamari

1 (1-inch) piece fresh ginger, peeled and minced or grated

2 teaspoons water

1 tablespoon coconut oil

3 cups chopped broccoli florets

1 garlic clove, minced

Cook the cauliflower rice, if using, according to the package directions and set aside. Combine the arrowroot starch, coconut aminos, liquid aminos, and ginger in a blender and blend, adding water slowly to reach your desired consistency.

Heat a large saucepan over medium heat and add the coconut oil. Add the broccoli and garlic and cook until the broccoli is bright green, 4 to 5 minutes. Add the sauce mixture to the saucepan and cook for 2 minutes more.

Divide the cauliflower rice between two plates, top with the broccoli and sauce, and serve.

NUTRIENT TOTALS

Calories: 167	Dietary Fiber: 8 g	Saturated Fat: 6 g
Protein: 9 g	Total Sugars: 6 g	Net Carbs: 12 g
Carbohydrate: 21 g	Total Fat: 7.5 g	

"RANCH" ROASTED CAULIFLOWER

This zesty blend of herbs and spices give you the flavor of ranch dressing with none of the acid. Added to cauliflower, it makes a delicious and flavorful "steak" that won't leave you missing meat.

1 garlic clove, peeled
¼ yellow onion
1 tablespoon fresh dill
1 tablespoon fresh parsley
1 teaspoon fresh chives

1 teaspoon sea salt (Celtic Grey, Himalayan pink, or Redmond Real Salt)
Freshly ground black pepper

1 teaspoon freshly squeezed lemon juice
2 tablespoons coconut oil, melted
1 head cauliflower, cut lengthwise into ¾- to 1-inch-thick steaks

Preheat the oven to 400°F. In a blender or food processor, combine the garlic, onion, all of the herbs, salt and pepper to taste, the lemon juice, and 1 tablespoon of the coconut oil. Pulse to incorporate.

Brush the remaining tablespoon of coconut oil over the cauliflower and then brush the mixture over both sides of each steak. Roast the steaks on a baking sheet for 30 minutes, or until they turn golden. Remove from the oven and serve.

NUTRIENT TOTALS

Calories: 103	Dietary Fiber: 4 g	Saturated Fat: 6 g
Protein: 3 g	Total Sugars: 4.5 g	Net Carbs: 6 g
Carbohydrate: 10 g	Total Fat: 7 g	

BOWLS

ROASTED BEET AND LENTIL BOWL WITH AVOCADO CILANTRO SAUCE

This zesty bowl combines asparagus and beets on a bed of lentils and tops them with a creamy avocado lime dressing that you won't be able to get enough of. Consider yourself warned—you might want to double the recipe. All of this can be made in advance and stored in the fridge for a few days.

- 1 cup dried lentils, rinsed
- 2 cups water, vegetable broth, or Vegan Protein Boneless Broth (page 227)
- 4 medium-size beets
- 1 bunch asparagus, chopped into bite-size pieces
- 2 teaspoons extra-virgin olive oil
- 1 large Hass avocado, peeled and pitted
- ½ cup fresh cilantro leaves
- 1 garlic clove, peeled
- 2 teaspoons freshly squeezed lime juice
- Sea salt (Celtic Grey, Himalayan pink, or Redmond Real Salt)
- Freshly ground black pepper
- 2 tablespoons water or unsweetened coconut water

Preheat the oven to 400°F.

Combine the lentils and water or broth in a pot over medium-high heat and cook until the water is absorbed and the lentils are tender, about 15 minutes.

Wash and peel the beets. Place in a Dutch oven, or other lidded, oven-safe pot, and roast in the oven for 35 minutes, or until almost tender. Brush the asparagus with the olive oil and add to the baking sheet with the beets for the last 10 minutes of cook time. Once cooled, chop the beets into bite-size cubes.

In a blender, combine the avocado, cilantro, garlic, lime juice, and salt and pepper to taste and blend. Add the water slowly until you have a sauce consistency.

Divide the lentils between two bowls, top with chopped asparagus and beets, and drizzle with the avocado sauce.

NUTRIENT TOTALS

Calories: 296	Dietary Fiber: 21 g	Saturated Fat: 1 g
Protein: 15.5 g	Total Sugars: 8 g	Net Carbs: 21 g
Carbohydrate: 42 g	Total Fat: 8 g	

THAI SPRING ROLL VEGGIE BOWL

SERVES 2

If you love fried veggie spring rolls, this recipe will give you the crunch you crave without the inflammation. The Thai sauce is sweetened with ChocZero low-carb maple syrup, which has only 1 gram of net carbs and no artificial ingredients. If you can't find that (it's available online or at health food stores), you can substitute liquid stevia.

continues

continued

THAI SAUCE

½ cup unsweetened almond butter

1 tablespoon ChocZero sugar-free maple syrup, or 2 drops organic liquid stevia

½ cup water

1 teaspoon red pepper flakes

2 tablespoons coconut aminos

1 garlic clove, peeled

1 teaspoon peeled and minced fresh ginger

Pinch of sea salt (Celtic Grey, Himalayan pink, or Redmond Real Salt)

Pinch of freshly ground black pepper

SPRING ROLL BOWL

½ head purple cabbage, thinly chopped

2 cups snow peas, sliced

5 medium-size carrots, shredded

1 Hass avocado, peeled, pitted, and cubed

4 green onions, sliced thinly

2 tablespoons chopped fresh cilantro

1 tablespoon black sesame seeds

1 lime, cut into wedges

OPTIONAL WRAPS

Romaine or butter lettuce

Turmeric coconut wraps

Ezekiel brand tortillas

Put all the Thai sauce ingredients into a blender and blend until smooth.

Toss the spring roll ingredients together and portion out into bowls, and save any remaining ingredients for leftovers. Drizzle the sauce over the veggies bowl, reserving any extra sauce for the leftovers in a separate container.

You can eat the Thai veggies in a bowl, or roll them into a wrap using romaine or butter lettuce, turmeric coconut wraps, or an Ezekiel tortilla.

NUTRIENT TOTALS

Calories: 512
Protein: 17.5 g
Carbohydrate: 49 g

Dietary Fiber: 21 g
Total Sugars: 21.5 g
Total Fat: 31 g

Saturated Fat: 3 g
Net Carbs: 28 g

VEGAN, GRAIN-FREE TEX-MEX BOWL

SERVES 4

Who needs taco Tuesday when you can eat these delicious Tex-Mex bowls any day of the week? Start with cauliflower rice, add the flavors of your favorite tacos, and then finish up with a rainbow of ingredients that creates a satisfying dinner that's ready in just a few minutes.

- 2 tablespoons coconut oil
- 1 head cauliflower, riced, or 1 (12-ounce) package frozen cauliflower rice
- 1 garlic clove, peeled and minced
- ¼ teaspoon sea salt (Celtic Grey, Himalayan pink, or Redmond Real Salt), plus more to taste
- ½ teaspoon ground cumin
- ¼ teaspoon cayenne pepper (optional)
- Juice of 1 lime, plus more for garnish
- 1 romaine lettuce heart, chopped
- 1 (15-ounce) can adzuki beans, drained and rinsed
- 1 Hass avocado, sliced
- ½ cup cherry tomatoes, halved
- ¼ cup red onion, minced
- ¼ cup fresh cilantro, chopped
- Fresh cilantro and guacamole, for garnish

Heat the coconut oil in a large pan over medium heat. Add the cauliflower rice, then the garlic, sea salt, cumin, and cayenne. Sauté for 3 to 4 minutes, or until soft and evenly seasoned.

Remove the cauliflower from the heat and squeeze in the lime juice. Portion the lettuce into four bowls, add the cauliflower rice, and top with the beans, avocado, cherry tomatoes, and red onion. Garnish with cilantro, more lime juice, and guacamole as desired. (*Note:* You can substitute 2 cups cooked quinoa for cauliflower if you prefer.)

NUTRIENT TOTALS

Calories: 286
Protein: 12 g
Carbohydrate: 35 g

Dietary Fiber: 18 g
Total Sugars: 6.5 g
Total Fat: 13 g

Saturated Fat: 6.5 g
Net Carbs: 17 g

MEXICAN SPICE IMMUNE-BOOSTING GREEN BOWL

SERVES 2

You could put avocado, tomato, and cilantro on just about anything and it would taste great. This lentil bowl is no exception. Plus, it's full of anti-inflammatory, detoxifying ingredients so you'll feel great after you eat it too.

- 1 tablespoon coconut oil
- 1 small red onion, diced
- 1 tablespoon chili powder, or less, if desired
- About ½ teaspoon sea salt (Celtic Grey, Himalayan pink, or Redmond Real Salt), or to taste
- 2 cups cooked lentils
- 1 medium-size red bell pepper, seeded and diced
- 1 Hass avocado, peeled, pitted, and sliced
- 1 cup cherry tomatoes, halved
- 2 tablespoons finely chopped fresh cilantro
- A few slices of jalapeño pepper, seeds removed (optional)
- Freshly ground black pepper

continues

continued

Heat the coconut oil in a large sauté pan over medium heat. Add the red onion and cook for 7 to 8 minutes, or until translucent. Add the chili powder, salt, and lentils and stir well. Cook for a further 5 minutes, or until fragrant. To serve, spoon the lentils into two bowls and top with the avocado, cherry tomatoes, red pepper, cilantro, and jalapeño (if using). Sprinkle with black pepper as desired.

NUTRIENT TOTALS

Calories: 454
Protein: 21 g
Carbohydrate: 51 g

Dietary Fiber: 27 g
Total Sugars: 10 g
Total Fat: 18.5 g

Saturated Fat: 7.5
Net Carbs: 24 g

TURMERIC QUINOA POWER BOWL

SERVES 2

Quinoa is already a nutrition superstar on its own, but when you add anti-inflammatory powerhouse turmeric and the delicious fiber delivery system of broccoli to it, you're basically eating health in a bowl.

2 cups filtered water
¾ cup uncooked quinoa, rinsed
2 tablespoons coconut oil
1 medium-size onion, diced
1½ teaspoons ground turmeric

1 red, yellow, or orange bell pepper, seeded and chopped
Pinch of sea salt (Celtic Grey, Himalayan pink, or Redmond Real Salt)

Pinch of freshly ground black pepper
2 cups chopped broccoli

Place the filtered water in a medium-size saucepan and bring to a boil. Lower the heat, add the quinoa, and simmer until the water is fully absorbed, 10 to 15 minutes.

Next, melt the coconut oil in a medium-size skillet over medium-high heat. Add the onion, turmeric, bell pepper, sea salt, and black pepper and sauté for a few minutes. Add the broccoli and sauté for 5 to 6 minutes, or until it becomes softened. Remove from the heat, add the cooked quinoa, and stir everything together. Transfer to a bowl and serve.

NUTRIENT TOTALS

Calories: 428
Protein: 13 g
Carbohydrate: 49 g

Dietary Fiber: 12 g
Total Sugars: 6 g
Total Fat: 18 g

Saturated Fat: 12 g
Net Carbs: 37 g

LIGHT MEALS

LEMONY ROASTED CABBAGE

SERVES 6

This side dish is cabbage at its best. If you haven't tried cabbage in a while, or you've never roasted it, I encourage you to try this, even if you think you don't like cabbage. I have a feeling this recipe will change your mind.

2 tablespoons coconut oil, melted
1 large head green cabbage
3 tablespoons freshly squeezed lemon juice

1 teaspoon sea salt (Celtic Grey, Himalayan pink, or Redmond Real Salt)
Fresh ground black pepper

Preheat the oven to 450°F. Coat a roasting pan with 1 tablespoon of the coconut oil. Cut the head of cabbage into eight same-size wedges, cutting off the core. Arrange the wedges in a single layer on the roasting pan. Rub the remaining coconut oil on each cabbage wedge, sprinkle the lemon juice evenly over them, and season with the sea salt and pepper to taste.

Roast the cabbage for 15 minutes, remove the pan from the oven, and turn over each wedge carefully. Put back into oven and roast for 10 to 15 more minutes, or until the cabbage is nicely browned and cooked through.

NUTRIENT TOTALS

Calories: 93
Protein: 3 g
Carbohydrate: 13 g

Dietary Fiber: 5 g
Total Sugars: 7 g
Total Fat: 5 g

Saturated Fat: 4 g
Net Carbs: 7 g

BUFFALO CAULIFLOWER BITES
WITH HOT SAUCE

SERVES 4

...sic buffalo wings are one of the most acidic foods you can eat. First, chicken ...s high levels of arachidonic acid, a pro-inflammatory omega-6 fat. Second, they're typically fried in soybean oil, another omega-6 fat. And finally, the classic hot sauce is loaded with chemicals and sugar. This is a healthy swap that tastes great, with an alkaline hot sauce that you'll want to use on everything.

CAULIFLOWER BITES

- 3 tablespoons avocado oil
- 2 teaspoons garlic powder
- 1 teaspoon sea salt (Celtic Grey, Himalayan pink, or Redmond Real Salt), or to taste
- 1 head cauliflower, broken into small florets

HOT SAUCE

- ¼ cup extra-virgin olive oil
- 2 tablespoons paprika
- 1 teaspoon smoked paprika
- ¼ cup chopped white onion
- 1 small garlic clove
- Pinch of cayenne pepper, or to taste
- Pinch of sea salt (Celtic Grey, Himalayan pink, or Redmond Real Salt)
- Freshly ground black pepper

Prepare the cauliflower: Preheat the oven to 450°F. In a large bowl, combine the avocado oil, garlic powder, and sea salt. Toss the cauliflower florets in the mixture, thoroughly coating all the pieces. Next, place the cauliflower florets on a baking sheet and bake for 15 minutes.

While the cauliflower bakes, stir together all the sauce ingredients in a separate bowl, adding black pepper to taste. You can either toss the cauliflower florets in the hot sauce mixture and bake for another 5 to 10 minutes until slightly browned, or place the hot sauce on already baked cauliflower bites, and serve.

NUTRIENT TOTALS

Calories: 268
Protein: 4 g
Carbohydrate: 11.5 g

Dietary Fiber: 4.5 g
Total Sugars: 4 g
Total Fat: 25 g

Saturated Fat: 3 g
Net Carbs: 7 g

AVOCADO KETO WRAP-UPS

SERVES 2

This is a supersimple side dish that can accompany just about any lunch or dinner in minutes. It's a delicious way to get more vitamins, minerals, fiber, and good-for-you fats too.

2 romaine lettuce leaves

1 Hass avocado, peeled, pitted, and diced, or 2 to 3 heaping tablespoons hummus (for homemade, see page 255)

Smashed adzuki beans (optional; Eden Organics is great), for more protein and added delicious flavor

4 large fresh cilantro leaves, chopped

1 tablespoon red onion, diced

Handful of sprouts or microgreens

1 tablespoon freshly squeezed lime juice

Sea salt (Celtic Grey, Himalayan pink, or Redmond Real Salt)

Freshly ground black pepper

Set out each romaine leaf as you would a rice paper roll or a piece of sandwich bread. Smear half of the avocado or hummus into the romaine leaves and add a spoonful of smashed adzuki beans (if using), top with the rest of the diced avocado or hummus, then the cilantro, onion, and sprouts or microgreens. Drizzle the lime juice on top, and season to taste with sea salt and pepper. Roll the leaves to form a wrap or burrito shape and enjoy right away.

NUTRIENT TOTALS

Calories: 120	Dietary Fiber: 5 g	Saturated Fat: 1.5 g
Protein: 2 g	Total Sugars: 1 g	Net Carbs: 2 g
Carbohydrate: 7 g	Total Fat: 11 g	

SHAYNA'S SWEET POTATO FRIES WITH CHIMICHURRI SAUCE

SERVES 6

This recipe was created by my good friend Shayna Taylor, founder of Shayna's Kitchen. It was a hard to pick just one of her recipes—they are all so tasty—but this one stood out. The basil chimichurri sauce is addictive, and you can never go wrong with crispy sweet potato fries that aren't deep-fried (deep frying turns any potato

continues

continued

into a delivery system of unhealthy fats, transforming the spud into a dud). This craveable dish is loaded with minerals and fiber, which will help you detox, reduce cravings, and improve your digestive system function.

SWEET POTATO FRIES

2 pounds sweet potatoes, peeled
Juice of ½ lemon, for soaking
2 tablespoons extra-virgin olive oil
1 teaspoon garlic powder

1 teaspoon paprika
1 teaspoon sea salt (Celtic Grey, Himalayan pink, or Redmond Real Salt)

½ teaspoon freshly ground black pepper

CHIMICHURRI SAUCE

1 cup chopped fresh basil
½ cup fresh parsley leaves
1 small garlic clove

Zest and juice of 1 lemon
6 tablespoons extra-virgin olive oil

1 (1-inch) piece jalapeño pepper, seeds removed (optional)

Prepare the sweet potato fries: Preheat the oven to 400°F. Cut the potatoes into sticks (ideally between ¼ to ½ inch wide and about 3 inches long). Next, fill a bowl with filtered water and add the juice of ½ lemon (releases some of the starches to make the fries extra crispy), then add the potato slices and let them soak for 10 minutes. After soaking, remove the potatoes and lay them out on a clean kitchen towel or paper towel to dry. Once dry, toss them with the olive oil.

Mix together the garlic powder, paprika, salt, and pepper in a small bowl, and then toss with the sweet potato fries. Spread out the potatoes in a single layer on two rimmed baking sheets and bake until browned and crisp on the bottom, about 15 minutes. Then, flip the potato fries over and bake on the other side until crisp, about 10 more minutes.

Prepare the chimichurri sauce: Place all the sauce ingredients in a food processor or blender and blend until smooth. Drizzle over the hot sweet potato fries and serve.

NUTRIENT TOTALS FOR SWEET POTATO FRIES

Calories: 173
Protein: 2.5 g
Carbohydrate: 29 g

Dietary Fiber: 6 g
Total Sugars: 6 g
Total Fat: 4.5 g

Saturated Fat: 0.5 g
Net Carbs: 23 g

NUTRIENTS TOTALS FOR CHIMICHURRI SAUCE

Calories: 126
Protein: 0.5 g
Carbohydrate: 1.5 g

Dietary Fiber: 0.5 g
Total Sugars: 0 g
Total Fat: 13 g

Saturated Fat: 2 g
Net Carbs: 1 g

CINNAMON SWEET POTATOES

SERVES 2

Unlike a lot of sweet potato side dishes out there, this one is nothing but good for you. It uses no dairy products, no added sugar, and definitely no marshmallows to create a sweet and delicious side dish.

2 sweet potatoes, chopped
2 tablespoons coconut oil

1 heaping teaspoon ground cinnamon

Sea salt (Celtic Grey, Himalayan pink, or Redmond Real Salt)

Preheat the oven to 400°F. Toss the sweet potatoes in the coconut oil, cinnamon, and sea salt to taste and transfer to a baking sheet. Roast for 25 to 30 minutes, or until tender.

NUTRIENT TOTALS

Calories: 232	Dietary Fiber: 7 g	Saturated Fat: 12 g
Protein: 2 g	Total Sugars: 5 g	Net Carbs: 19 g
Carbohydrate: 26 g	Total Fat: 14 g	

ROASTED BROCCOLI WITH HUMMUS

SERVES 2 TO 4

Creamy hummus becomes like a vegan sauce when combined with hot, roasted broccoli.

2 cups chopped broccoli
1 tablespoon extra-virgin olive oil
Sea salt (Celtic Grey, Himalayan pink, or Redmond Real Salt)

Freshly ground black pepper
¼ cup plain or flavored hummus (for homemade, see 5-Minute Hummus, page 255)

Preheat the oven to 400°F. Place the broccoli on a baking sheet, toss in the olive oil, and season with sea salt and pepper to taste. Roast for 25 minutes, or until tender and starting to brown. Transfer the roasted broccoli to a bowl and stir in the hummus until the broccoli is coated.

NUTRIENT TOTALS (BASED ON 4 SERVING)

Calories: 69	Dietary Fiber: 2 g	Saturated Fat: 0 g
Protein: 2 g	Total Sugars: 1 g	Net Carbs: 3 g
Carbohydrate: 5 g	Total Fat: 5 g	

GARLIC LEMON ROASTED BRUSSELS SPROUTS

SERVES 4

Brussels sprouts were my number one most-hated vegetable when I was a kid, hands down. But now it's moved to the top of the list and is my very favorite. I like them shredded and raw in salads, and added to stir-fries. But roasting them makes them a crunchy, savory treat—especially when you pair them with garlic, lemon, and olive oil.

1 pound Brussels sprouts, washed, ends removed, and halved

2 to 3 garlic cloves, peeled and minced

2 tablespoons extra-virgin olive oil

2 teaspoons freshly squeezed lemon juice

Pinch of sea salt (Celtic Grey, Himalayan pink, or Redmond Real Salt)

Pinch of freshly ground black pepper

Preheat the oven to 400°F. In a bowl, toss the sprouts with the garlic, olive oil, and lemon juice. Spread onto a baking sheet and season with the sea salt and black pepper.

Bake for about 15 minutes, then toss. Bake for another 10 minutes, remove from the oven, and serve.

NUTRIENT TOTALS

Calories: 124
Protein: 5 g
Carbohydrate: 13 g

Dietary Fiber: 5 g
Total Sugars: 3 g
Total Fat: 7 g

Saturated Fat: 1 g
Net Carbs: 10 g

SNACKS/FOOD TO GO

CLEAN KETO GARLIC DIP

MAKES EIGHT TO TEN ¼-CUP SERVINGS

The base of this dip is sunflower seeds and avocado, which are good sources of plant-based fats, combined with tahini, lemon, olive oil, and fresh herbs—plus garlic, of course! This will be your new favorite dip for fresh cut veggies.

5 to 6 garlic cloves, peeled
1 Hass avocado
½ cup raw sunflower seeds, soaked in water overnight and drained

Juice of 1 lemon
Sea salt (Celtic Grey, Himalayan pink, or Redmond Real Salt)
¼ cup tahini

¼ to ½ cup extra-virgin olive oil
Fresh parsley, for garnish (optional)

Combine the garlic, avocado, sunflower seeds, lemon juice, and sea salt (start with ½ teaspoon) in a food processor and blend. Add the tahini and thoroughly blend again. With the food processor running, pour in the olive oil until the mixture is the texture of hummus: creamy and not too thick. Taste for salt and adjust as needed, then transfer to a bowl and sprinkle with the parsley (if using). Serve with carrot sticks, celery sticks, jicama, cherry tomatoes, cucumber slices, snap peas, or your favorite veggies.

NUTRIENT TOTALS (BASED ON 10 SERVINGS)

Calories: 150
Protein: 3 g
Carbohydrate: 5 g

Dietary Fiber: 2 g
Total Sugars: 0 g
Total Fat: 14 g

Saturated Fat: 2 g
Net Carbs: 3 g

CRISPY CHICKPEAS

SERVES 2 TO 4

If you've tried dehydrated or oven-roasted chickpeas and been disappointed in the texture, you've got to give this recipe a try. By panfrying them in healthy fats, you get a clean keto snack that's seriously crunchy and delicious.

- 1 (15-ounce) can chickpeas, drained and rinsed (Eden Organics is great)
- ¼ cup coconut oil
- Sea salt (Celtic Grey, Himalayan pink, or Redmond Real Salt)
- Red pepper flakes
- Zest of ½ lemon

Roll the chickpeas around on a paper towel or clean cloth to dry them. Heat the coconut oil in a large skillet over medium-high heat. Once hot, add the chickpeas and stand back as they sizzle (some will pop). Cook for 10 minutes, stirring to get an even crisp.

Remove with a slotted spoon and transfer to a dry cloth or paper towel to remove any excess oil. While still hot, season with sea salt and red pepper flakes to taste and the lemon zest. Enjoy right away, or let cool completely before storing in an airtight container for 2 to 3 days.

NUTRIENT TOTALS (BASED ON 4 SERVINGS)

Calories: 223	Dietary Fiber: 6 g	Saturated Fat: 12 g
Protein: 5 g	Total Sugars: 0 g	Net Carbs: 14g
Carbohydrate: 20 g	Total Fat: 14.5 g	

SUPERPOWER ALKALINE TREATS

MAKES 24 SERVINGS

These good-for-you granola balls are grain-free and will keep your energy going all day. They've got it all without the mega-dose of sugar that store-bought granola bars serve up (even the so-called healthy brands). Good fats, plant-based proteins, plenty of fiber, and a touch of sweetness—yum!

- 1 cup raw almond butter
- 6 dates, pitted
- ¼ cup flaxseeds
- ¼ cup cacao nibs
- 1 tablespoon ground cinnamon
- 2 teaspoons pure vanilla extract
- ¼ cup plus 1 tablespoon chia seeds
- 1 cup hemp seeds
- Unsweetened coconut flakes

In a food processor, pulse together the almond butter and dates. Add the flaxseeds, cacao nibs, cinnamon, vanilla, and ¼ cup of the chia seeds and continue to pulse until a ball forms. Roll into 1-inch balls. Combine the hemp seeds, coconut flakes, and remaining tablespoon of chia seeds on a plate and roll the balls in the mixture to coat. Store for up to a week in an airtight container.

NUTRIENT TOTALS

Calories: 158	Dietary Fiber: 4 g	Saturated Fat: 1.5 g
Protein: 7 g	Total Sugars: 1.5 g	Net Carbs: 1 g
Carbohydrate: 5 g	Total Fat: 12.5 g	

MACADAMIA NUT DIP

SERVES 4 TO 6

This dip is a bit like hummus with the added sweet nuttiness of macadamia nuts and goes great with raw veggies. It lasts for about a week in a sealed container in the fridge.

1 cup raw macadamia nuts, soaked in water overnight and drained

3 tablespoons freshly squeezed lemon juice

2 garlic cloves, peeled

2 to 4 tablespoons extra-virgin olive oil

Sea salt (Celtic Grey, Himalayan pink, or Redmond Real Salt)

Freshly ground black pepper

Place all the ingredients, starting with 2 tablespoons of the olive oil, and including sea salt and pepper to taste, in a food processor and puree until smooth. Add more olive oil as needed to reach your desired consistency.

NUTRIENT TOTALS (BASED ON 6 SERVINGS)

Calories: 223	Dietary Fiber: 2 g	Saturated Fat: 3.5 g
Protein: 2 g	Total Sugars: 1 g	Net Carbs: 2 g
Carbohydrate: 4 g	Total Fat: 24 g	

BAKED ZUCCHINI CHIPS WITH COOL DILL DIP

SERVES 2

When I was a kid, a special outing for my family was to go to Little Italy in New York City. Our favorite recipe had fried zucchini on the menu and we always got it. Unfortunately, the restaurant version is loaded with inflammatory fats, barely classifying as a vegetable. These crispy zucchini chips are a perfect swap—with their crunch and the creamy dip, your kids will love them too.

ZUCCHINI CHIPS

- 2 zucchini, thinly sliced (you can use a mandolin)
- 2 tablespoons extra-virgin olive oil
- Sea salt (Celtic Grey, Himalayan pink, or Redmond Real Salt)

DILL DIP

- ½ cup canned full-fat coconut milk (I recommend Native Forest, using the thick cream from top)
- 2 teaspoons freshly squeezed lemon juice
- 1 tablespoon chopped fresh parsley
- 2 tablespoons chopped fresh dill
- 1 garlic clove, minced
- Sea salt (Celtic Grey, Himalayan pink, or Redmond Real Salt)
- Freshly ground black pepper

Prepare the zucchini chips: Thinly slice the zucchini, using a knife or preferably, a mandoline. Blot the zucchini slices with a paper towel to absorb any excess water. Place the zucchini slices on a parchment paper–lined baking sheet. Brush each slice with olive oil and sprinkle with sea salt.

Bake at 225°F for 2 hours (ideal), or at 300°F for 1 hour, or dehydrate in a dehydrator at 115°F for 12 hours (overnight).

Prepare the dill dip: Blend together all the ingredients in a food processor, adding a little water if too thick. Serve with the baked chips.

NUTRIENT TOTALS FOR BAKED ZUCCHINI CHIPS

Calories: 151	Dietary Fiber: 2 g	Saturated Fat: 2 g
Protein: 2 g	Total Sugars: 31 g	Net Carbs: 4 g
Carbohydrate: 6 g	Total Fat: 14 g	

NUTRIENT TOTALS FOR DILL DIP

Calories: 221	Dietary Fiber: 0 g	Saturated Fat: 20 g
Protein: 2 g	Total Sugars: 0 g	Net Carbs: 4 g
Carbohydrate: 4 g	Total Fat: 23 g	

5-MINUTE HUMMUS

MAKES 2 CUPS HUMMUS

You'll never settle for store-bought hummus again once you realize how easy it is to make your own—and how it tastes so much better than anything you can find in the store! Use it on the Roasted Broccoli with Hummus recipe (page 249), or serve with your favorite crudités.

1 (15-ounce) can chickpeas, drained and rinsed (Eden Organics is great)

⅓ cup tahini

1 garlic clove, peeled

2 tablespoons sesame oil

2 tablespoons freshly squeezed lemon juice

Pinch of sea salt (Celtic Grey, Himalayan pink, or Redmond Real Salt)

Pinch of freshly ground black pepper

Put all the ingredients in a food processor and blend until smooth. Depending on your desired consistency, you may need to add a little water; add it 1 to 2 tablespoons at a time so that the hummus doesn't get too runny.

NUTRIENT TOTALS (PER 2-TABLESPOON SERVING)

Calories: 71

Protein: 2 g

Carbohydrate: 6 g

Dietary Fiber: 2 g

Total Sugars: 0.1 g

Total Fat: 4.5 g

Saturated Fat: 0.5 g

Net Carbs: 4 g

EASY CHOOSE-YOUR-OWN-FLAVOR KALE CHIPS

SERVES 1

These crunchy roasted kale chips are a great way to get your greens. The main flavor is garlic; for curry, swap in curry powder for the garlic and melted coconut oil for the olive oil.

1 bunch kale, stemmed, washed, and dried

1 tablespoon extra-virgin olive oil

1 teaspoon garlic powder

2 pinches of sea salt (Celtic Grey, Himalayan pink, or Redmond Real Salt)

Preheat the oven to 300°F. Line a baking sheet with parchment paper.

Take the washed and dried kale, rip the leaves into "chip"-size pieces, and place in a large bowl.

continues

continued

Drizzle the kale with the oil, garlic powder, and sea salt and massage in until evenly covered. Arrange the kale in an even layer on the prepared baking sheet and bake for 10 minutes. Flip the kale pieces over and bake the other side for 10 minutes, or until the edges start to turn a slight brown color. Be careful not to burn.

NUTRIENT TOTALS

Calories: 253	Dietary Fiber: 6 g	Saturated Fat: 2 g
Protein: 12 g	Total Sugars: 0 g	Net Carbs: 15 g
Carbohydrate: 21 g	Total Fat: 16 g	

FAT BOMBS (AND OTHER HEALTHY KETO SNACKS)

CACAO ALMOND FAT BOMBS

MAKES 15 FAT BOMBS

These rich, chocolaty clean-keto fat bombs are made in ice cube trays or mini muffin tins, and you can store them that way in the fridge between cravings. They're full of antioxidants as well as healthy fats.

½ cup coconut oil, melted
¼ cup raw almond butter
¼ cup raw cacao powder

¼ teaspoon ground cinnamon
½ teaspoon pure vanilla extract
5 drops organic liquid stevia

Pinch of sea salt (Celtic Grey, Himalayan pink, or Redmond Real Salt)

Combine all the ingredients, except the sea salt, in a food processor and pulse. Pour into mini muffin tins or ice cube trays to make fifteen equal portions and sprinkle each with sea salt. Refrigerate for at least 10 minutes to solidify, and store in the fridge as well.

NUTRIENT TOTALS

Calories: 97	Dietary Fiber: 1 g	Saturated Fat: 6.7 g
Protein: 1 g	Total Sugars: 0 g	Net Carbs: 1 g
Carbohydrate: 2 g	Total Fat: 10 g	

CHOCOLATE PEPPERMINT MACADAMIA MELTS

MAKES 24 MELTS

If you love a certain Girl Scout cookie, these fat bombs will be your new favorite treat. They sandwich mint in between layers of dark chocolate and macadamia nuts for a taste you're sure to love.

½ cup coconut oil
½ cup raw cacao powder
¼ cup macadamia nuts,
  finely chopped

5 drops peppermint extract or
  food-grade essential oil
5 drops liquid organic stevia,
  or more to taste

Pinch of sea salt (Celtic Grey,
  Himalayan pink, or Redmond
  Rea Salt)

Melt all the ingredients together in a pan over low heat, stirring to prevent burning. Once completely melted, remove from the heat and spoon 2 teaspoons of the mixture each into twenty-four wells of a mini muffin tin or silicone mold, then place in freezer until hardened. Once hardened, remove from the molds and store in a sealed container in the freezer.

NUTRIENT TOTALS

Calories: 124	Dietary Fiber: 2 g	Saturated Fat: 11 g
Protein: 0 g	Total Sugars: 0 g	Net Carbs: 1 g
Carbohydrate: 3 g	Total Fat: 13 g	

CARDAMOM ORANGE CHOCOLATE TRUFFLES

MAKES 10 TO 15 TRUFFLES

Fat bombs are the ultimate guilt-free keto snack. With a great melding of the flavors of chocolate, coconut, cardamom, and orange, this easy-to-make snack will energize you for hours and delight your taste buds. They may be small, but they are delicious.

1 cup raw almond butter
¼ cup coconut oil
2 teaspoons orange zest
⅓ cup raw walnuts
Pinch of ground cardamom
1 tablespoon cacao powder

2 to 4 drops stevia, to taste
½ cup unsweetened shredded coconut
¼ cup unsweetened coconut flakes or shredded coconut, for topping (optional; recommended)
Cacao powder, for topping (optional, instead of coconut topping)

Place all the ingredients, except the optional toppings, in a blender and blend well. Place in the fridge or freezer to solidify (so mixture will be moldable). Form the mixture into ten to fifteen small balls, then roll each ball in the ¼ cup of unsweetened coconut flakes or additional cacao powder (if using). Place in the fridge to set for several hours.

NUTRIENT TOTALS

Calories: 168	Dietary Fiber: 2 g	Saturated Fat: 5.5 g
Protein: 4 g	Total Sugars: 1 g	Net Carbs: 2 g
Carbohydrate: 4 g	Total Fat: 16 g	

RASPBERRY VANILLA KETO BOMBS

MAKES 10 KETO BOMBS

These fat bombs utilize cacao butter, a healthy, edible fat from the cocoa bean. You can buy it at any health food store or online. Store these in the freezer to keep the top raspberry layer frozen until you're ready to enjoy them.

1½ cups coconut oil
¼ cup cacao butter
1¼ cups canned full-fat coconut milk (I recommend Native Forest brand)

1 teaspoon pure vanilla extract
3 drops organic liquid stevia, or to taste
¼ cup frozen or fresh raspberries

Line ten wells of a muffin tin with muffin cups. Set aside.

Melt the coconut oil and cacao butter together in a saucepan over medium heat. Once melted, add 1 cup of the coconut milk and bring to a simmer, about 2 to 3 minutes. Turn off the heat and whisk in the vanilla extract and stevia. Pour the mixture into the prepared muffin pan. Pop into the fridge and allow to set for at least 2 hours, or until solid.

In a blender, combine the remaining ¼ cup of coconut milk and the frozen raspberries and blend until smooth. Add a 2-teaspoon layer of the raspberry mixture to the chilled contents of each muffin well and freeze for 1 hour, or until ready to eat.

NUTRIENT TOTALS

Calories: 339	Dietary Fiber: 0.5 g	Saturated Fat: 32 g
Protein: 0 g	Total Sugars: 0 g	Net Carbs: 0.5 g
Carbohydrate: 1 g	Total Fat: 38 g	

DESSERTS

RAW VEGAN BROWNIES

MAKES 12 BROWNIES

Brownies might sound like a sinful dessert, but without acidic, sugar-heavy ingredients, this version is heavenly. It's so rich and indulgent, and yet it takes only a few minutes to make with six simple ingredients you probably have in your kitchen right now.

½ cup pitted dates
¼ cup warm filtered water

⅔ cup raw cashew butter
½ cup raw cacao powder

½ teaspoon pure vanilla extract
3 tablespoons melted coconut oil

continues

continued

Place the dates in a food processor and pulse until chopped into small pieces. Add up to ¼ cup of the warm water and process until the dates become pastelike, scraping down sides of the food processor as needed. Add the cashew butter, cacao powder, and vanilla and mix until incorporated. With the processor running, add the coconut oil and process until the mixture has a consistent texture (about 1 minute).

Spread in a small, flat, airtight container and refrigerate for at least 2 hours, then cut into small pieces or brownie squares.

NUTRIENT TOTALS

Calories: 151	Dietary Fiber: 3 g	Saturated Fat: 5 g
Protein: 3 g	Total Sugars: 4 g	Net Carbs: 8 g
Carbohydrate: 11 g	Total Fat: 12 g	

CHOCOLATE CHIA PUDDING

SERVES 2 TO 4

Indulging in occasional treats is one of the best things in life, especially if you're indulging the alkaline way with nutrient-rich, low-sugar delights. This pudding is as good as any high-acid dessert, with none of the guilt or weight gain. I made it on *Live with Kelly and Ryan*, where we chatted about how most of us are having dessert for breakfast (when we have muffins, scones, cereals, or pastries). Turns out, this is real dessert you can have for breakfast without wrecking your low-sugar lifestyle.

2 cups coconut water or filtered water

½ cup raw cashews

¼ cup raw cacao powder

2 tablespoons coconut oil

1 tablespoon unsweetened coconut flakes

1 teaspoon ground cinnamon

3 medium-size dates, pitted

⅛ teaspoon sea salt

2 teaspoons pure vanilla extract

6 tablespoons chia seeds

Ground cinnamon, cacao nibs, and/or unsweetened coconut flakes, for garnish (optional)

Place all the ingredients, except the chia seeds and your preferred garnish, in a blender and blend until thoroughly mixed, about 1 minute. Then, on lowest variable speed, add the chia seeds and blend for 1 minute to mix in the chia. If you don't have a variable-speed blender, mix in the chia with a spoon. Transfer to a small, airtight container and refrigerate for at least 5 hours before serving. (To speed up the process, place in freezer for 15 minutes, and it will be ready to eat.) Garnish with cinnamon, cacao nibs, or coconut flakes before serving.

NUTRIENT TOTALS (BASED ON 2 SERVINGS, USING COCONUT WATER)

Calories: 353
Protein: 8 g
Carbohydrate: 26 g

Dietary Fiber: 14 g
Total Sugars: 13.5 g
Total Fat: 24 g

Saturated Fat: 9.5 g
Net Carbs: 12 g

NUTRIENT TOTALS (BASED ON 2 SERVINGS, USING WATER)

Calories: 308
Protein: 7 g
Carbohydrate: 20 g

Dietary Fiber: 10 g
Total Sugars: 4.5 g
Total Fat: 24 g

Saturated Fat: 9 g
Net Carbs: 10 g

PUMPKIN PIE PUDDING

SERVES 2

You can have your pumpkin pie and stay off your acid and sugar! This yummy pudding has plenty of pumpkin flavor, using the chia seeds to create a pudding texture. You'll want to eat this all fall long.

1½ cups unsweetened almond or coconut milk (from a carton, not canned)
¼ cup chia seeds

½ cup pure pumpkin puree (unsweetened)
1 teaspoon ground cinnamon
½ teaspoon ground ginger

½ teaspoon freshly grated nutmeg
Pinch of ground allspice

Mix together all the ingredients in a medium-size bowl and refrigerate for 3 to 4 hours or overnight.

NUTRIENT TOTALS (USING ALMOND MILK)

Calories: 179
Protein: 7 g
Carbohydrate: 15 g

Dietary Fiber: 11 g
Total Sugars: 2 g
Total Fat: 11 g

Saturated Fat: 2.5 g
Net Carbs: 4 g

LOW-CARB CINNAMON APPLES

SERVES 2

Applesauce isn't just for kids! These stewed apples deliver all the comfort of that childhood treat without the added sugar—and they bring healthy fat along with it so that you stay in the fat-burning zone.

2 Granny Smith apples, cored and chopped
2 tablespoons filtered water
1 tablespoon coconut oil
½ teaspoon ground cinnamon

Pinch of sea salt (Celtic Grey, Himalayan pink, or Redmond Real Salt)
¼ teaspoon pure vanilla extract

Placed the chopped apples in a small saucepan along with the water. Cover and cook over medium heat, stirring occasionally. After 5 minutes or so, the apples will become slightly soft and the water will be fully absorbed.

Add the coconut oil and stir it into the chopped apples. Cook for another 5 minutes, stirring every minute or so. Add the cinnamon, sea salt, and vanilla and stir well.

Cook for another few minutes, stirring until the apples reach your desired firmness and consistency.

NUTRIENT TOTALS

Calories: 110
Protein: 0 g
Carbohydrate: 11 g

Dietary Fiber: 3 g
Total Sugars: 8 g
Total Fat: 7 g

Saturated Fat: 6 g
Net Carbs: 8 g

CHOCOLATE FROSTY

SERVES 1

I remember as a kid getting so excited to go through Wendy's drive-through and getting a chocolate frosty. Unfortunately, that beloved treat of my youth is a sugar bomb (and loaded with artificial ingredients), but this is a great replacement that tastes so good, you'll think you're cheating.

¾ cup unsweetened almond or coconut milk from a carton

½ teaspoon pure vanilla extract
1 tablespoon raw cacao powder

½ banana, frozen
Handful of ice cubes

Combine all the ingredients, except the ice, in a blender and blend well. Then, add the ice cubes and pulse until ice is blended, giving you a nice, thick texture.

NUTRIENT TOTALS (USING ALMOND MILK)

Calories: 111
Protein: 1.5 g
Carbohydrate: 16 g

Dietary Fiber: 4 g
Total Sugars: 7.5 g
Total Fat: 4 g

Saturated Fat: 1 g
Net Carbs: 12 g

AVOCADO CHOCOLATE MOUSSE

SERVES 2

This creamy treat is so tasty, it's one of only two recipes I'm including from my first book, *Get Off Your Acid*. (The other is Dr. Daryl's Favorite Salad Dressing, page 234.) I still stand by the claim that this is so rich, creamy, and chocolaty that it's even better than the real thing!

1½ Hass avocados, peeled and pitted
⅔ cup coconut water, ideally raw
1 tablespoon pure vanilla extract

2 tablespoons raw cacao
3 dates, pitted (you can use 5 to make it a little sweeter)

1½ teaspoons sea salt (Celtic Grey, Himalayan pink, or Redmond Real Salt)

Combine all the ingredients in a blender, and blend on high speed, then serve. You can also refrigerate before serving to make a firm mousse. To make a healthy version of Fudgsicles, pour the mousse into ice pop molds and freeze for 30 minutes (if you can wait that long!).

NUTRIENT TOTALS

Calories: 130
Protein: 3 g
Carbohydrate: 11 g

Dietary Fiber: 7 g
Total Sugars: 0.5 g
Total Fat: 13 g

Saturated Fat: 3 g
Net Carbs: 4 g

MACA HOT CHOCOLATE

SERVES 2

Here's another use for the maca you may have bought for the Maca Power Breakfast Shake (page 216). This nourishing treat will warm you up, satisfy your sweet tooth, and boost your energy—all without using sugar.

2 cups unsweetened almond or coconut milk from a carton

1 tablespoon coconut oil

1 tablespoon raw cacao powder

1 teaspoon maca powder

4 pinches of ground cinnamon

Pinch of sea salt (Celtic Grey, Himalayan pink, or Redmond Real Salt)

½ teaspoon ground turmeric (optional)

Pinch of cayenne pepper (optional)

Heat the almond milk and coconut oil together in a medium-size saucepan over low heat. Once heated, transfer to a blender, add the remaining ingredients, blend well until frothy, and serve.

NUTRIENT TOTALS (USING ALMOND MILK)

Calories: 115
Protein: 1.5 g
Carbohydrate: 4 g

Dietary Fiber: 2 g
Total Sugars: 1 g
Total Fat: 10 g

Saturated Fat: 6 g
Net Carbs: 2 g

30-MINUTE APPLE CINNAMON CHIA PUDDING

SERVES 2

As delicious as it is, my Chocolate Chia Pudding needs to be refrigerated for five hours before it's ready to eat—and sometimes you don't have five hours to wait! So, I created this version that sets up in only thirty minutes, so that by the time you've eaten dinner, you can dive in and enjoy a delicious dessert.

2 cups canned full-fat coconut milk (I recommend Native Forest brand)

1 teaspoon pure vanilla extract

2 to 4 pinches of ground cinnamon, plus more for serving

1 green apple, peeled: ½ to blend, ½ diced for topping

2 dates, pitted

5 drops stevia, or more to taste (optional)

½ cup chia seeds

Combine all the ingredients, except the ½ diced apple and chia seeds, in a blender. Blend until smooth. Transfer the mixture to a jar or container with a lid and stir in the chia seeds thoroughly with a spoon, then refrigerate.

After 30 minutes, the chia seeds will have soaked up most of the milk and your pudding will be ready to eat. Top with the diced apple, a pinch of cinnamon, and serve.

NUTRIENT TOTALS

Calories: 331
Protein: 12 g
Carbohydrate: 28 g

Dietary Fiber: 18 g
Total Sugars: 8.5 g
Total Fat: 20 g

Saturated Fat: 3 g
Net Carbs: 10 g

HOMEMADE COCONUT CHOCOLATE SPREAD

SERVES 16 (2 TABLESPOONS PER SERVING)

Nutella is easy to love, until you think about the fact that the store-bought version is loaded with sugar (it's the first ingredient) as well as artificial flavors, dairy, and hydrogenated oils—the perfect storm for weight gain and cravings. Try this healthy swap that tastes so good, you'll think you're cheating!

2 tablespoons coconut oil
2 cups whole raw hazelnuts
6 tablespoons raw cacao powder

½ cup full-fat canned coconut milk (I recommend Native Forest brand)
1 teaspoon pure vanilla extract
2 drops of liquid stevia, or to taste

Pinch of sea salt (Celtic Grey, Himalayan pink, or Redmond Real Salt)

Preheat the oven to 325°F. In a bowl, using 1 tablespoon of the coconut oil, and roll and cover the hazelnuts thoroughly with the oil. Transfer the hazelnuts to a baking sheet and roast in the oven for 10 to 12 minutes. You want the nuts to be dark brown, but be careful not to burn.

Remove from the oven, and when cool enough to handle, dampen some paper towels and rub off the somewhat bitter skins. An alternative way to remove the skins is to put the hazelnuts in a mason jar, add the lid, and shake—the papery skins will fall right off.

Place the skinless nuts in a food processor or a high-powered blender with the remaining tablespoon of coconut oil. Grind until a smooth nut butter consistency is reached, usually 4 to 5 minutes. Add the cacao, coconut milk, vanilla extract, stevia, and sea salt to the mixture and blend for another minute, or until all the ingredients are combined and smooth. Transfer to a mason jar, and store in the fridge for several weeks.

NUTRIENT TOTALS

Calories: 145
Protein: 2.5 g
Carbohydrate: 4 g

Dietary Fiber: 3 g
Total Sugars: 1 g
Total Fat: 14 g

Saturated Fat: 4 g
Net Carbs: 1 g

Resources

<u>Alkamind Daily Omega-3.</u> I'm very proud of the fish oil I've developed; it has an exact 2:1 ratio of EPA to DHA and we organically purify it three times—most companies do this only once (or not at all). It's also molecular distilled, an expensive purification process that removes all metals and contaminants as it concentrates the fish oil, meaning, you take *less* to get *more*. Whereas some supplement companies require you to take eight to twelve softgels a day to get the recommended 3,000 mg, with ours, you have to take only three.

<u>Alkamind Acid-Kicking Greens.</u> This highly alkalizing blend of twenty-one raw and organic vegetables, grasses, herbs, low-sugar fruits, and nutrient-rich superfoods helps you gain energy, lose weight, fight inflammation, and optimize your health on a daily basis. One scoop (dissolved in water or unsweetened coconut water) delivers five servings of organic greens in thirty seconds.

<u>Alkamind Acid-Kicking Minerals.</u> Our Acid-Kicking Minerals powder contains the top four acid-fighting minerals, in a medical grade and in their most bioavailable form. Because they're in powdered form, the

minerals bypass the digestive tract, quickly absorbing into the bloodstream. It has the ideal 1:1 ratio of magnesium to calcium, plus potassium and sodium bicarbonate to crush sugar cravings, alleviate stress, promote better sleep and faster recovery, and eliminate reflux.

Alkamind Acid-Kicking Protein Power. This premium vegan protein powder contains the top three core alkaline proteins— hemp, pea, and sacha inchi—plus healthy plant-based keto fats to promote lean muscle and turn your body into a fat-burning machine. Most protein powders use acidic ingredients, such as whey, sugar, artificial sweeteners, and fillers. Our protein powder is doctor-formulated and uses nothing but the most premium plant-based organic alkaline ingredients to help you **burn fat and build lean muscle.** Available in both vanilla coconut and creamy chocolate flavors.

Alkamind Black Seed Oil. My favorite antioxidant is black seed oil, which is three times more anti-inflammatory than turmeric and up to one thousand times more active an antioxidant than vitamin E, elderberry, and echinacea. This formulation has the highest concentration of thymoquinone of any other black seed oils, making it the most powerful natural anti-inflammatory and antioxidant you can put in your body.

Alkamind Acid-Kicking Coffee Alkalizer. Neutralizes the acid in your morning cup of coffee with the four most powerful alkalizing minerals; premium keto fats to suppress hunger, promote weight loss, and improve energy and performance; Himalayan pink salt with eighty-four trace minerals to crush cravings; and fat-burning enzymes to boost metabolism and burn off your stored body fat. The Coffee Alkalizer comes in three acid-kicking flavors—salted caramel, vanilla, and mocha.

Alkamind Omega-3 Acid Inflammation At-Home Test Kit. Just like an at-home glucose test, this test takes less than sixty seconds and requires only one drop of blood from your finger that you send in a prestamped envelope back to the lab. In two weeks, you'll be emailed a detailed report, telling you the following information:

- **Omega-3 Index:** How deficient you are in omega-3 fatty acids
- **Cell Inflammation Balance:** Your omega-6/omega-3 ratio
- **Cell Toxicity Index:** How toxic your cells are from carbohydrate metabolism
- **Four Cognitive Function Brain Assessments:** Memory capacity, sustained attention, cognitive flexibility, and processing speed
- **Plus . . .** a summary of results, list of recommendations, and a longevity trajectory index.

RESOURCES FROM OTHER SOURCES
Magnesium Red Blood Cell Test

requestatest.com

A normal range is 4.2–6.8 ng/dL; ideally, it's at least 6.

Revitin Probiotic Toothpaste

revitin.com

Dr. Curatola (who talks about the importance of nourishing your oral microbiome on page 153) created a prebiotic-rich toothpaste filled with essential oils, vitamins, enzymes, and minerals that feeds the good bacteria in your mouth. It also whitens teeth as it reduces plaque, gum bleeding, and inflammation of the gums more than standard other brands do.

BrainTap

braintap.com

Dr. Patrick Porter created BrainTap technology to help people tap into their mind's full potential through light, sound, and frequency. It's a quick and easy way to relax, reboot, and revitalize by simply optimizing your brain's peak potential—anytime, anywhere. Backed by neuroscience and research, BrainTap is proven to help people who experience high stress, difficulty sleeping, low energy, addiction, and other lifestyle challenges.

You can get a free fifteen-day trial by going to **getoffyourstress.com**—it takes ten seconds to get a username and password, then download the free BrainTap Pro app, and listen to it in bed before sleep or any other time.

Shayna's Kitchen Matcha Powder

shaynaskitchen.com

I was introduced to the power and deliciousness of matcha by my good friend, model, blogger, and chef Shayna Taylor. Her company, Shayna's Kitchen, sells ceremonial-grade Japanese matcha that has 120 times more antioxidants than ordinary green tea and helps you get into a fat-burning state. Stirring the powder into tea is also a meditative, stress-reducing ritual.

Anna Kaiser Studios

annakaiserstudios.com

If you love the 8-Minute Acid-Kicking Workout Anna Kaiser created for *Get Off Your Sugar* (see page 173) and want more, here's your source! This subscription service brings Anna Kaiser's always changing workouts right to your home.

Redmond Real Salt

realsalt.com

This is my go-to, favorite sea salt. It comes from the Great Salt Lake in Utah. I love it because it has eighty-four trace minerals, which help crush cravings for sugar. This unrefined, ancient salt has been mined since 1958 from an ancient seabed protected from pollution. It's the only pink salt mined in America.

Gopal's Sprouted Almond Butter

gopalshealthfoods.com

This is our go-to, everyday almond butter. It's made from sprouted almonds to remove antinutrients, such as lectins, which makes its nutrients more bioavailable to your body; this also makes it creamier and more delicious (with no need to stir in oil that's settled on the top).

Jem Almond Butter

jemorganics.com

When we're looking for a little extra oomph, we love these flavored almond butters. They are so decadent. Our favorite flavors are organic cinnamon red maca, organic salted caramel, and organic cashew cardamom. We spread it on green apples with cinnamon for the kids; you don't need a lot of it and it has great flavor.

Synergy Science Molecular Hydrogen Echo Water System

synergyscience.com

This is an amazing filtration system that, in addition to removing chemicals and fluoride, also adds molecular hydrogen into your water. (I have one at home and at my office—that's how much I love it.) If you don't want to invest in the filter, Synergy Science also sells molecular hydrogen drops that you can add to your water. Molecular hydrogen, which reduces oxidative stress and inflammation, has over 750 studies that demonstrate benefits for over 170 diseases. Water that has molecular hydrogen added to it has -450 mV of electrical potential to stimulate anaerobic microflora in the gut, and can outpace the damaging effects of an antibiotic. The founder of this company is Dr. Paul Barattiero, who cowrote the chapter on hydration in my first book, *Get Off Your Acid*. He's a very good friend of mine as well as a speaker in *The Truth About Cancer* documentary.

Sovereign Silver

sovereignsilver.com

This is the silver hydrosol that Dr. Robert Scott Bell uses in his leaky gut protocol (which he was gracious enough to let me share on page 25). In addition to helping your GI tract heal, it's an immunomodulator, with antibacterial, antifungal, and antiviral properties. When you spray it in your mouth and your nose, it helps stop viral replication. I use the spray on my kids' hands as a form of hand sanitizer; it doesn't contain the antibacterial chemicals that most standard hand sanitizers have, which decimate the friendly bacterial population on your skin.

Acknowledgments

CHELSEA—MY ALKALINE GODDESS! WORDS CANNOT EXPRESS THE GRATITUDE I have for you and all you do—for me, for our children, and for what we are building together. You've been there every step of the way, not only holding my hand, but leading by example. You give all of yourself and more, and you keep smiling through it all. Thank you for keeping me grounded, strong, focused, and rooted in love.

Brayden and Alea—I'm so grateful to watch you grow. My heart has never been more full with love. You inspire me every day. The work I do is truly for you, so that you can inherit a better life and a better world. I am so proud to be your father, and I cannot wait to see the bright futures ahead of you. Thank you for your hugs, snuggles, and love. You are my "why."

Mom—As I get older, I realize more and more what a real-life superhero you were as I grew up, and are now to me and our family. It's impossible to thank you for everything you've done for all of us. I couldn't have asked for a better mom, and my words can never express my gratitude and love. Thank you for your constant support and always being there for me.

Dad—I miss you more than ever, and I can't believe it's been three years since you've passed. I know you're with me in spirit every single day, guiding me, loving me, and helping me make the right decisions as you always have. Thank you Kahuna, for inspiring me and instilling the courage in me to go after my dreams.

Tony, Brandon, and family—We've been through so much together and you will each always have a huge space in my heart. Blood truly is thicker than anything else.

My entire Pittsburgh family—I'm endlessly grateful to you, and not just for the love of my life. I couldn't ask for a better family to become a part of.

Kelly Ripa—You define the word *balance*. I am continually impressed and inspired by you. You Kick Acid in every area of your life, from supermom, to your work, to working out, to the way you strength eat. You are a role model to me and so many others, and I am forever grateful to you for helping me get this message out to the world.

Ryan Seacrest—One of the hardest working people I know. It's so inspiring how you take care of so much, including your physical health. Thank you for being so supportive of me and my message. I appreciate you deeply.

Anna Kaiser—You're a warrior and a trailblazer. Thank you for creating the most efficient and effective total body workout that gets the best results in the shortest period of time. Every time I take your exercise class, I drown in my sweat, and I never feel better! You've changed my life in so many ways, and inspired me to become a better version of myself. I'll always treasure our friendship and will always stand strong by your side.

Kate Hanley—To my writing partner; you are so truly gifted at what you do!

Thank you for your patience, the countless hours and phone calls, keeping me focused and on track, and for bringing out the best in the finished product. I couldn't have done it without you.

I am so grateful to the insightful, talented group at **Hachette Books, especially Michael Clark and Iris Bass, with special thanks to Renée Sedliar**, my amazing editor. Thank you for believing in me, first with *Get Off Your Acid*, and now with *Get Off Your Sugar*. It is an incredible honor to work with someone who gets it in the way that you do.

Thank you to my agent, **Ellen Scordato from Stonesong**, for believing in me from day one, and for always standing up for me and my vision. Thank you for helping me find the perfect publisher. None of this would have been possible without your steadfast advocacy.

Thank you to my press team from **Pace Publications, especially Annie Scranton and Lindsay Ferraro Bennett**, for your incredible support and commitment. You're on a mission with me to bring this information to the world, and I am so grateful to partner with such strong voices.

Fran Drescher—Thank for being a warrior, for your trust and confidence in having me on the Cancer Schmancer Medical Advisory Board, and for all you do to help people become informed on better ways to fight cancer, and to prevent it through healthy living.

Dorinda Medley—From the moment we first met, I've watched your powerful and inspiring health transformation. You are constantly seeking ways to better yourself physically and emotionally, tapping into your powerful purpose to make it happen. You glow with health from the inside out, and I truly value the close friendship we've developed along the way.

Kelly Dodd and Luann de Lesseps— My acid-kicking Real Housewives crew! Thanks for ardently believing in the value of my work, and beautifully sharing your trust in me with the world. You are both strong and incredibly good-hearted women, and I am so honored to have gotten to know you on a deeper level. I'm proud to call you my friends.

Dr. Bob Hoffman—Thank you for all of the coaching, guidance, and wisdom. When times get filled with stress, you have always helped bring me right back to focus on my outcome and what's most important.

Dr. Dan Pompa, Trevor King, JJ Virgin, Jorge Cruise, Dr. Gerry Curatola, Dr. Patrick Porter, Dr. Robert Scott Bell, Dr. Paul Barattiero, Stu Gelbard, Dr. Dan Murphy, Liana Werner-Gray, Ty Bollinger, Dr. David Jockers, Michael Collins, Darin Olien, Dr. Jane Goldberg, Peggy Higgins, Ellen Lovelace, Ross Bridgeford, and Marcus and Wesley Eave—My cutting-edge experts who have become like family, thank you for leading the way as you stand up for what you know to be true. Each of you inspire my work and make it better. Thank you for sharing your wisdom and your friendship.

Petra Nemcova, Shayna Taylor, Garrett and Nicole McNamara, Bobbi Brown, Shannon Elizabeth, Sara Bliss, Tamsen Fadal, Aviva Drescher, Jeffrey Casciano, and Kimberlyn Parris—You are all wellness gurus in your own beautiful, unique ways. Thank you for your impassioned support, and thank you for teaching me so much.

Josh Shaw—You are my most trusted business advisor. It's impossible to count all the ways that you've helped me in my career. I am forever grateful for your guidance. Thanks for always having my back.

Mark Birnbaum, John Decker, Ron Tumpowsky, Jason Strauss, and Anthony Whitehurst—We go back a long way, but you have become more than friends over the years. You are my business mentors and teachers. Thank you for always being there.

Ernest Lupinacci—You are a creative genius, and I don't know where I'd be without your vision. I am so thankful to have you by my side as my chief brand officer. From *Get Off Your Acid* to Acid-Kicking Coffee, you are a true Acid-Kicker!

Chris Cook and Marissa Heitshusen— Thank you for making my vision a reality in graphic design and on social media. You know what I want before I do, and I'm grateful.

Luana Natalicio—My right hand; thank you for always going above and beyond, handling urgent tasks, even on your days off, and always making sure I appear to have it all together. I cannot thank you enough.

Traci Bermingham—You are the most resourceful person I know. You've been there by my side since the first day we met, and have always had my back. You define the ultimate team player, and Chelsea and I are honored to have you as our dear friend. Thank you for the amazing work you do while always keeping everyone on the team calm. We would be lost without you!

Katherine Copeland—You are such a gifted copywriter. Thank you for articulating my vision, the mission we are on, and this lifestyle. Our audience is healthier because of you.

Judi and Chip Hale—You started out as clients and have grown to be close friends. Your transformative journey to amazing health inspires Chelsea and me every day, and we are so grateful to have you both in our lives.

Too many to name but nonetheless near and dear to my heart are my patients and followers of @getoffyouracid and @drdarylgioffre. You are my tribe. Thank you for your constant and never-ending support, your curiosity for the sake of improving yourselves, and for showing the world what health looks like when you kick acid and get off your sugar!

Notes

CHAPTER 1: WHY SUGAR IS SO EASY TO LOVE AND SO HARD TO GIVE UP

1. "New CDC Report: More Than 100 Million Americans Have Diabetes or Prediabetes," CDC, July 18, 2017, https://www.cdc.gov/media/releases/2017/p0718-diabetes-report.html.

2. Emelia J. Benjamin et al., "Heart Disease and Stroke Statistics—2019 Update: A Report from the American Heart Association," *Circulation* 139, no. 10 (2019): e56–e528, https://doi .org/10.1161/CIR.0000000000000659.

3. "How Many People Are Affected by/at Risk for Obesity & Overweight?" National Institute of Child Health and Human Development, accessed May 2, 2019, https://www.nichd.nih.gov /health/topics/obesity/conditioninfo/risk.

4. Alice Walton, "How Much Sugar Are Americans Eating? [Infographic]" *Forbes*, August 30, 2012, https://www.forbes.com/sites/alicegwalton/2012/08/30/how-much-sugar-are-americans -eating-infographic.

5. B. M. Popkin and C. Hawkes, "The Sweetening of the Global Diet, Particularly Beverages: Patterns, Trends, and Policy Responses for Diabetes Prevention," *Lancet Diabetes & Endocrinology* 4, no. 2 (2015): 174–186, https://doi.org/10.1016/S2213-8587(15)00419-2.

6. Joseph Mercola, "Why Cutting Down on Sugar Might Be the Best Health Insurance Available," April 23, 2016, https://articles.mercola.com/sites/articles/archive/2016/04/23/cut-down -sugar-consumption.aspx.

7. "Dietary Guidelines 2015–2020: Executive Summary," US Department of Health and Human Services and the US Department of Agriculture, May 21, 2019, https://health.gov /dietaryguidelines/2015/guidelines/executive-summary.

8. "Guideline: Sugars Intake for Adults and Children," World Health Organization, March 4, 2015, https://www.who.int/publications-detail/9789241549028.

9. "Added Sugars," American Heart Association, accessed May 21, 2019, https://www.heart.org/en/healthy-living/healthy-eating/eat-smart/sugar/added-sugars.

10. *Here & Now* staff, NPR, "How the Food Industry Helps Engineer Our Cravings," December 16, 2015, https://www.npr.org/sections/thesalt/2015/12/16/459981099/how-the-food-industry-helps-engineer-our-cravings.

11. Erin Fothergill et al., "Persistent Metabolic Adaptation 6 Years After 'The Biggest Loser' Competition," *Obesity* 24, no. 8 (2016): 1612–1619, https://doi.org/10.1002/oby.21538.

12. S. W. Ng, M. M. Slining, and B. M. Popkin, "Use of Caloric and Noncaloric Sweeteners in US Consumer Packaged Foods, 2005–2009," *Journal of the Academy of Nutrition and Dietetics* 112, no. 11 (2012): 1828–1834, https://doi.org/10.1016/j.jand.2012.07.009.

13. J. J. DiNicolantonio, J. H. O'Keefe, and S. C. Lucan, "Added Fructose," *Mayo Clinic Proceedings* 90, no. 3 (2015): 372–381, https://doi.org/10.1016/j.mayocp.2014.12.019.

14. Sayed Hossein Davoodi et al., "Calorie Shifting Diet Versus Calorie Restriction Diet: A Comparative Clinical Trial Study," *International Journal of Preventive Medicine* 5, no. 4 (2014): 447–456.

15. Patrice D. Cani et al., "Metabolic Endotoxemia Initiates Obesity and Insulin Resistance," *Diabetes* 56, no. 7 (2007): 1761–1772, https://doi.org/10.2337/db06-1491.

16. P. Cani et al., "Changes in Gut Microbiota Control Metabolic Endotoxemia-Induced Inflammation in High-Fat Diet-Induced Obesity and Diabetes in Mice," *Diabetes* 57, no. 6 (2008): 1470–1481, https://doi.org/10.2337/db07-1403.

CHAPTER 2: HOW SUGAR DRAINS YOUR WHOLE-BODY HEALTH

1. K. R. Magnusson et al., "Relationships Between Diet-Related Changes in the Gut Microbiome and Cognitive Flexibility," *Neuroscience* 300 (2015): 128–140, https://doi.org/10.1016/j.neuroscience.2015.05.016.

2. H. P. Weingarten and D. Elston, "Food Cravings in a College Population," *Appetite* 17, no. 3 (1991): 167–175, https://doi.org/10.1016/0195-6663(91)90019-o.

3. Ting-Li Han, Richard D. Cannon, and Silas G. Villas-Bôas, "The Metabolic Basis of Candida Albicans Morphogenesis and Quorum Sensing," *Fungal Genetics and Biology* 48, no. 8 (2011): 747–763, https://doi.org/10.1016/j.fgb.2011.04.002.

4. Lisa Richards, CNC, "Why Does Candida Really Need Sugar?" September 17, 2017, https://www.thecandidadiet.com.

5. E. J. Rentz, "Viral Pathogens and Severe Acute Respiratory Syndrome: Oligodynamic Ag+ for Direct Immune Intervention," *Journal of Nutritional and Environmental Medicine* 13, no. 2 (2003): 109–118, https://doi.org/10.1080/13590840310001594061.

6. Atsushi Goto et al., "High Hemoglobin A1c Levels Within the Non-Diabetic Range Are Associated with the Risk of All Cancers," *International Journal of Cancer* 138, no. 7 (2016): 1741–1753, https://doi.org/10.1002/ijc.29917.

7. Atsushi Goto et al., "Hemoglobin A1c Levels and the Risk of Cardiovascular Disease in People Without Known Diabetes: A Population-Based Cohort Study in Japan," *Medicine* 94, no. 7 (2015): e785, https://doi.org/10.1097/MD.0000000000000785.

8. R. Brookmeyer et al., "Forecasting the Prevalence of Preclinical and Clinical Alzheimer's Disease in the United States," *Alzheimer's & Dementia* 14, no. 2 (2018): 121–129, https://doi.org/10.1016/j.jalz.2017.10.009.

9. K. Gudala et al., "Diabetes Mellitus and Risk of Dementia: A Meta-Analysis of Prospective Observational Studies," *Journal of Diabetes Investigation* 4, no. 6 (2013): 640–650, https://doi.org/10.1111/jdi.12087.

10. R. O. Roberts et al., "Relative Intake of Macronutrients Impacts Risk of Mild Cognitive Impairment or Dementia," *Journal of Alzheimer's Disease* 32, no. 2 (2012): 329–339, https://doi.org/10.3233/JAD-2012-120862.

11. J. V. Pottala et al., "Higher RBC EPA + DHA Corresponds with Larger Total Brain and Hippocampal Volumes," *Neurology* 82, no. 5 (2014): 435–442. https://doi.org/10.1212/WNL.0000000000000080.

12. Kuan-Pin Su, Ping-Tao Tseng, and Pao-Yen Lin, "Association of Use of Omega-3 Polyunsaturated Fatty Acids with Changes in Severity of Anxiety Symptoms," *JAMA Network Open* 1, no. 5 (2018): e182327, https://doi.org/10.1001/jamanetworkopen.2018.2327.

13. H. N. Yassine et al., "Association of Serum Docosahexaenoic Acid with Cerebral Amyloidosis," *JAMA Neurology* 73, no. 10 (2016): 1208–1216, https://doi.org/10.1001/jamaneurol.2016.1924.

14. Ingrid B. Helland et al., "Maternal Supplementation with Very-Long-Chain n-3 Fatty Acids During Pregnancy and Lactation Augments Children's IQ at 4 Years of Age," *Pediatrics* 111, no. 1 (2003): e39–e44, https://doi.org/10.1542/peds.111.1.e39.

15. A. B. Camara, I. D. de Souza, and R. J. S. Dalmolin, "Sunlight Incidence, Vitamin D Deficiency, and Alzheimer's Disease," *Journal of Medicinal Food* 21, no. 9 (2018): 841–848, https://doi.org/10.1089/jmf.2017.0130; Catherine Feart et al., "Associations of Lower Vitamin D Concentrations with Cognitive Decline and Long-Term Risk of Dementia and Alzheimer's Disease in Older Adults," *Alzheimer's & Dementia* 13, no. 11 (2017): 1207–1216, https://doi.org/10.1016/j.jalz.2017.03.003.

16. Guosong Liu et al., "Efficacy and Safety of MMFS-01, A Synapse Density Enhancer, for Treating Cognitive Impairment in Older Adults: A Randomized, Double-Blind, Placebo-Controlled Trial," *Journal of Alzheimer's Disease* 49, no. 4 (2015): 971–990, https://doi.org/10.3233/JAD-150538.

17. Mark A. Reger et al., "Effects of β-Hydroxybutyrate on Cognition in Memory-Impaired Adults," *Neurobiology of Aging* 25, no. 3 (2004): 311–314, https://doi.org/10.1016/S0197-4580(03)00087-3.

18. H. Van Praag, "Neurogenesis and Exercise: Past and Future Directions," *Neuromolecular Medicine* 10, no. 2 (2008): 128–140, https://doi.org/10.1007/s12017-008-8028-z.

19. G. Livingston et al., "Dementia Prevention, Intervention, and Care," *Lancet* 390, no. 10113 (2017): 2673–2734.

20. S. Müller et al., "Relationship Between Physical Activity, Cognition, and Alzheimer Pathology in Autosomal Dominant Alzheimer's Disease," *Alzheimer's & Dementia* 14, no. 11 (2018): 1427–1437, https://doi.org/10.1016/j.jalz.2018.06.3059.

21. E. B. Ansell et al., "Cumulative Adversity and Smaller Gray Matter Volume in Medial Prefrontal, Anterior Cingulate, and Insula Regions," *Biological Psychiatry* 72, no. 1 (2012): 57–64, https://doi.org/10.1016/j.biopsych.2011.11.022.

22. L. Schwabe, O. T. Wolf, and M. S. Oitzl, "Memory Formation Under Stress: Quantity and Quality," *Neuroscience & Biobehavioral Reviews* 34, no. 4 (2010): 584–591, https://doi.org/10.1016/j.neubiorev.2009.11.015.

23. E. E. Powell et al., "The Natural History of Nonalcoholic Steatohepatitis: A Follow-up Study of Forty-Two Patients for Up to 21 Years," *Hepatology* 11, no. 1 (1990): 74-80, https://doi.org/10.1002/hep.1840110114; G. C. Farrell and C. Z. Larter, "Nonalcoholic Fatty Liver Disease: From Steatosis to Cirrhosis," *Hepatology* 43, no. 2, supplement 1 (2006): S99–S112, https://doi.org/10.1002/hep.20973.

24. Jorge Rezzonico et al., "Introducing the Thyroid Gland as Another Victim of the Insulin Resistance Syndrome," *Thyroid* 18, no. 4 (2008): 461–464, https://doi.org/10.1089/thy.2007.0223.

25. M. Inoue-Choi et al., "Sugar-Sweetened Beverage Intake and the Risk of Type I and Type II Endometrial Cancer Among Postmenopausal Women," *Cancer Epidemiology, Biomarkers & Prevention* 22, no. 12 (2013): 2384–2394, https://doi.org/10.1158/1055-9965.EPI-13-0636.

26. J. E. Chavarro et al., "A Prospective Study of Dietary Carbohydrate Quantity and Quality in Relation to Risk of Ovulatory Infertility," *European Journal of Clinical Nutrition* 63, no. 1 (2009): 78–86, https://doi.org/10.1038/sj.ejcn.1602904.

27. "Facts About Heart Disease in Women," American Heart Association, accessed May 23, 2019, https://www.goredforwomen.org/fight-heart-disease-women-go-red-women-official-site/about-heart-disease-in-women/facts-about-heart-disease.

28. Q. Yang et al., "Added Sugar Intake and Cardiovascular Diseases Mortality Among US Adults," *JAMA Internal Medicine* 174, no. 4 (2014): 516–524, https://doi.org/10.1001/jamainternmed.2013.13563.

CHAPTER 4: OUTSMART CRAVINGS

1. M. P. Pase et al., "Cocoa Polyphenols Enhance Positive Mood States but Not Cognitive Performance: A Randomized, Placebo-Controlled Trial," *Journal of Psychopharmacology* 27, no. 5 (2013): 451–458, https://doi.org/10.1177/0269881112473791.

2. E. T. Rolls and C. McCabe, "Enhanced Affective Brain Representations of Chocolate in Cravers vs. Non-Cravers," *European Journal of Neuroscience* 26 (2007): 1067–1076, https://doi.org/10.1111/j.1460-9568.2007.05724.x.

3. H. M. Savignac et al., "Prebiotic Feeding Elevates Central Brain Derived Neurotrophic Factor, N-methyl-D-aspartate Receptor Subunits and D-serine," *Neurochemistry International* 63, no. 8 (2013): 756–764, https://doi.org/10.1016/j.neuint.2013.10.006.

4. K. Schmidt et al., "Prebiotic Intake Reduces the Waking Cortisol Response and Alters Emotional Bias in Healthy Volunteers," *Psychopharmacology* 232, no. 10 (2015): 1793–1801, https://doi.org/10.1007/s00213-014-3810-0.

5. J. A. Parnell and R. A. Reimer, "Prebiotic Fibres Dose-Dependently Increase Satiety Hormones and Alter Bacteroidetes and Firmicutes in Lean and Obese JCR: LA-cp Rats," *British Journal of Nutrition* 107, no. 4 (2012): 601–613, https://doi.org/10.1017/S0007114511003163.

6. Robert H. Lustig, MD, *Fat Chance: Beating the Odds Against Sugar, Processed Food, Obesity, and Disease* (New York: Avery, 2013), 41.

7. Q. Yang, "Gain Weight by 'Going Diet?' Artificial Sweeteners and the Neurobiology of Sugar Cravings: Neuroscience 2010," *Yale Journal of Biology and Medicine* 83, no. 2 (2010): 101–108.

8. S. P. Fowler et al., "Fueling the Obesity Epidemic? Artificially Sweetened Beverage Use and Long-Term Weight Gain," *Obesity* 16 (2008): 1894–1900, https://doi.org/10.1038/oby.2008.284.

9. Yang, "Gain Weight by 'Going Diet?'"

10. Susan S. Schiffman and Kristina I. Rother, "Sucralose, A Synthetic Organochlorine Sweetener: Overview of Biological Issues," *Journal of Toxicology and Environmental Health, Part B* 16, no. 7 (2013): 399–451, https://doi.org/10.1080/10937404.2013.842523.

11. M. B. Abou-Donia et al., "Splenda Alters Gut Microflora and Increases Intestinal p-glycoprotein and Cytochrome p-450 in Male Rats," *Journal of Toxicology and Environmental Health, Part A* 71, no. 21 (2008): 1415–1429, https://doi.org/10.1080/15287390802328630.

12. D. Dhurandhar, V. Bharihoke, and S. Kalra, "A Histological Assessment of Effects of Sucralose on Liver of Albino Rats," *Morphologie* 102, no. 338 (2018): 197–204, https://doi.org/10.1016/j.morpho.2018.07.003.

13. M. Y. Pepino et al., "Sucralose Affects Glycemic and Hormonal Responses to an Oral Glucose Load," *Diabetes Care* 36, no. 9 (2013): 2530–2535, https://doi.org/10.2337/dc12-2221.

14. Nora Gedgaudas, *Primal Body, Primal Mind: Beyond the Paleo Diet for Total Health and a Longer Life* (Vermont: Healing Arts Press, 2011), 139.

15. D. Harpaz et al., "Measuring Artificial Sweeteners Toxicity Using a Bioluminescent Bacterial Panel," *Molecules* 23, no. 10 (2018): 2454, https://doi.org/10.3390/molecules23102454.

CHAPTER 5: THE FIRST 7 DAYS: DETOX YOUR MIND, YOUR PANTRY, AND YOUR BODY

1. Y. Gu et al., "Sugary Beverage Consumption and Risk of Alzheimer's Disease in a Community-Based Multiethnic Population," presentation, 2018 Alzheimer's Association International Conference, Chicago, July 22–26, 2018.

2. C. W. Leung et al., "Soda and Cell Aging: Associations Between Sugar-Sweetened Beverage Consumption and Leukocyte Telomere Length in Healthy Adults from the National Health and Nutrition Examination Surveys," *American Journal of Public Health* 104, no. 12 (2014): 2425–2431, https://doi.org/10.2105/AJPH.2014.302151.

CHAPTER 6: STEP 1 (DAYS 1–3): RE-MINERALIZE

1. W. Li et al., "Elevation of Brain Magnesium Prevents Synaptic Loss and Reverses Cognitive Deficits in Alzheimer's Disease Mouse Model," *Molecular Brain* 7 (2014): 65, https://doi.org/10.1186/s13041-014-0065-y.

2. Inna Slutsky et al., "Enhancement of Learning and Memory by Elevating Brain Magnesium," *Neuron* 65, no. 2 (2010): 165–177, https://doi.org/10.1016/j.neuron.2009.12.026.

3. A. Trauinger et al., "Oral Magnesium Load Test in Patients with Migraine," *Headache* 42 (2002): 114–119, https://doi.org/10.1046/j.1526-4610.2002.02026.x; A. Mauskop and B. M. Altura, "Role of Magnesium in the Pathogenesis and Treatment of Migraine," *Clinical Neuroscience* 5, no. 1 (1998): 24–27.

4. A. Peikert, C. Wilimzig, and R. Köhne-Volland, "Prophylaxis of Migraine with Oral Magnesium: Results from a Prospective, Multi-Center, Placebo-Controlled and Double-Blind Randomized Study," *Cephalalgia* 16, no. 4 (1996): 257–263, https://doi.org/10.1046/j.1468-2982.1996.1604257.x.

5. D. Feskanich et al., "Milk, Dietary Calcium, and Bone Fractures in Women: A 12-Year Prospective Study," *American Journal of Public Health* 87, no. 6 (1997): 992–997, https://doi.org/10.2105/ajph.87.6.992.

6. "Sodium/Potassium Ratio Important for Health," *Harvard Health Letter*, September 2011, https://www.health.harvard.edu/heart-health/sodiumpotassium-ratio-important-for-health.

7. Inna Slutsky et al., "Enhancement of Synaptic Plasticity through Chronically Reduced Ca2+ Flux during Uncorrelated Activity," *Neuron* 44, no. 5 (2004): 835–849, https://doi.org/10.1016/j.neuron.2004.11.013.

8. Felice N. Jacka et al., "Association Between Magnesium Intake and Depression and Anxiety in Community-Dwelling Adults: The Hordaland Health Study," *Australian and New Zealand Journal of Psychiatry* 43, no. 1 (2009): 45–52, https://doi.org/10.1080/00048670802534408.

CHAPTER 7: STEP 2 (DAYS 4–6): ADD MORE HEALTHY FATS

1. "Iowa State University Researcher Finds Further Evidence That Fats and Oils Help to Unlock Full Nutritional Benefits of Veggies," Iowa State University News Service, October 9, 2017, https://www.news.iastate.edu/news/2017/10/09/saladvegetablesandoil.

2. "Fructose Alters Hundreds of Brain Genes, Which Can Lead to a Wide Range of Diseases," EurekAlert!, April, 22, 2016, https://www.eurekalert.org/pub_releases/2016-04/uoc—fah042116.php.

3. R. Agrawal and F. Gomez-Pinilla, "'Metabolic Syndrome' in the Brain: Deficiency in Omega-3 Fatty Acid Exacerbates Dysfunctions in Insulin Receptor Signalling and Cognition," *Journal of Physiology* 590, no. 10 (2012): 2485, https://doi.org/10.1113/jphysiol.2012.230078.

4. Gary Taubes, "Guest Post: Vegetable Oils, (Francis) Bacon, Bing Crosby, and the American Heart Association," Cardio Brief, http://www.cardiobrief.org/2017/06/16/guest-post-vegetable-oils-francis-bacon-bing-crosby-and-the-american-heart-associatio; Melissa Clark,

"Once a Villain, Coconut Oil Charms the Health Food World," *New York Times*, March 1, 2011, https://www.nytimes.com/2011/03/02/dining/02Appe.html?pagewanted=all.

CHAPTER 8: STEP 3 (DAYS 7–9): GET PROTEIN SMART

1. Pablo Hernández-Alonso et al., "High Dietary Protein Intake Is Associated with an Increased Body Weight and Total Death Risk," *Clinical Nutrition* 35, no. 2 (2016): 496–506, https://doi.org/10.1016/j.clnu.2015.03.016.

2. D. S. Goldfarb and R. L. Coe, "Prevention of Recurrent Nephrolithiasis," *American Family Physician* 60, no. 8 (1999): 2269–2276.

3. Uriel S. Barzel and Linda K. Massey, "Excess Dietary Protein Can Adversely Affect Bone," *Journal of Nutrition* 128, no. 6 (1998): 1051–1053, https://doi.org/10.1093/jn/128.6.1051; Chander Rekha Anand and Hellen M. Linkswiler, "Effect of Protein Intake on Calcium Balance of Young Men Given 500 mg Calcium Daily," *Journal of Nutrition* 104, no. 6 (1974): 695–700, https://doi.org/10.1093/jn/104.6.695.

4. Jacy Reese, "US Factory Farming Estimates," Sentience Institute, updated April 11, 2019, https://www.sentienceinstitute.org/us-factory-farming-estimates.

5. D. W. Lamming et al., "Restriction of Dietary Protein Decreases mTORC1 in Tumors and Somatic Tissues of a Tumor-Bearing Mouse Xenograft Model," *Oncotarget* 6, no. 31 (2015): 31233–31240, https://doi.org/10.18632/oncotarget.5180.

6. Ronni Chernoff, "Protein and Older Adults," *Journal of the American College of Nutrition* 23, no. 6, supplement (2004): 627S–630S, https://doi.org/10.1080/07315724.2004.10719434.

7. N. S. Rizzo et al., "Nutrient Profiles of Vegetarian and Nonvegetarian Dietary Patterns," *Journal of the Academy of Nutrition and Dietetics* 113, no. 12 (2013): 1610–1619, https://doi.org/10.1016/j.jand.2013.06.349.

8. M. Tharrey et al., "Patterns of Plant and Animal Protein Intake Are Strongly Associated with Cardiovascular Mortality: The Adventist Health Study-2 Cohort," *International Journal of Epidemiology* 47, no. 5 (2018): 1603–1612, https://doi.org/10.1093/ije/dyy030.

9. Teresia Goldberg et al., "Advanced Glycoxidation End Products in Commonly Consumed Foods," *Journal of the Academy of Nutrition and Dietetics* 104, no. 8 (2004): 1287–1291, https://doi.org/10.1016/j.jada.2004.05.214.

10. Alison Goldin et al., "Advanced Glycation End Products," *Circulation* 114, no. 6 (2006): 597–605, https://doi.org/10.1161/CIRCULATIONAHA.106.621854.

11. Teresa Norat and Elio Riboli, "Meat Consumption and Colorectal Cancer: A Review of Epidemiologic Evidence," *Nutrition Reviews* 59, no. 2 (2001): 37–47, https://doi.org/10.1111/j.1753-4887.2001.tb06974.x; Walter C. Willett et al., "Relation of Meat, Fat, and Fiber Intake to the Risk of Colon Cancer in a Prospective Study among Women," *New England Journal of Medicine* 323 (1990): 1664–1672, https://doi.org/10.1056/NEJM199012133232404.

12. G. J. Brewer, "Iron and Copper Toxicity in Diseases of Aging, Particularly Atherosclerosis and Alzheimer's Disease," *Experimental Biology and Medicine* 232, no. 2 (2007): 323–335.

13. D. Bujnowski et al., "Longitudinal Association Between Animal and Vegetable Protein Intake and Obesity Among Men in the United States: The Chicago Western Electric Study," *Journal of the American Dietetic Association* 111, no. 8 (2011): 1150–1155.e1, https://doi.org /doi:10.1016/j.jada.2011.05.002.

14. GRAIN, IATP, and Heinrich Boll Foundation, "Big Meat and Dairy's Supersized Climate Footprint," GRAIN, November 7, 2017, https://www.grain.org/article/entries/5825-big-meat -and-dairy-s-supersized-climate-footprint.

15. J. Poore and T. Nemecek. "Reducing Food's Environmental Impacts Through Producers and Consumers," *Science* 360, no. 6392 (2018): 987–992, https://doi.org/10.1126/science.aaq 0216.

16. D. Akramiene et al., "Effects of Beta-Glucans on the Immune System," *Medicina* 43, no. 8 (2007): 597–606.

17. Jane G. Goldberg. "Almonds: Raw or Rocket Fuel?" December 2, 2015. http://drjane goldberg.com/almonds-raw-or-rocket-fuel.

CHAPTER 9: STEP 4 (DAYS 10–12): SPICE THINGS UP

1. Farzaneh Saberi et al., "Effect of Ginger on Relieving Nausea \and Vomiting in Pregnancy: A Randomized, Placebo-Controlled Trial," *Nursing and Midwifery Studies* 3, no. 1 (2014): e11841, https://doi.org/10.17795/nmsjournal11841.

2. J. L. Ryan et al., "Ginger (Zingiber officinale) Reduces Acute Chemotherapy-Induced Nausea: A URCC CCOP Study of 576 patients," *Support Care Cancer* 20, no. 7 (2012): 1479–1489, https://doi.org/10.1007/s00520-011-1236-3.

3. R. W. Allen et al., "Cinnamon Use in Type 2 Diabetes: An Updated Systematic Review and Meta-analysis," *Annals of Family Medicine* 11, no. 5 (2013): 452–459, https://doi.org/10.1370 /afm.1517.

4. A. Pengelly et al., "Short-Term Study on the Effects of Rosemary on Cognitive Function in an Elderly Population," *Journal of Medicinal Food* 15, no. 1 (2012): 10–17, https://doi .org/10.1089/jmf.2011.0005.

5. Kosmetische MEDIZIN et al., "Fenugreek + Micronutrients: Efficacy of a Food Supplement Against Hair Loss," *Kosmetische Medizin* 27, no. 4 (2006).

CHAPTER 10: STEP 5 (DAYS 13–15): TIME YOUR MEALS

1. Adrienne R. Barnosky et al., "Intermittent Fasting vs Daily Calorie Restriction for Type 2 Diabetes Prevention: A Review of Human Findings," *Translational Research* 164, no. 4 (2014): 302–311, https://doi.org/10.1016/j.trsl.2014.05.013.

2. S. Klein et al., "Effect of Short- and Long-Term Beta-Adrenergic Blockade on Lipolysis During Fasting in Humans," *American Journal of Physiology* 257, no. 1, part 1 (1989): E65–73.

3. J. J. DiNicolantonio and M. McCarty, "Autophagy-Induced Degradation of Notch1, Achieved Through Intermittent Fasting, May Promote Beta Cell Neogenesis: Implications for

Reversal of Type 2 Diabetes," *Open Heart* 6 (2019): e001028, https://doi.org/10.1136/openhrt-2019-001028.

4. A. T. Hutchison et al., "Time-Restricted Feeding Improves Glucose Tolerance in Men at Risk for Type 2 Diabetes: A Randomized Crossover Trial," *Obesity* 27 (2019): 724–732, https://doi.org/10.1002/oby.22449.

5. Dan Pompa, *Beyond Fasting* (Revelation Health, LLC, 2017), 68.

6. Sarah J. Mitchell et al., "Daily Fasting Improves Health and Survival in Male Mice Independent of Diet Composition and Calories," *Cell Metabolism* 29, no. 1 (2019): 221–228.e3, https://doi/org/10.1016/j.cmet.2018.08.011.

7. T. Shimazu et al., "Suppression of Oxidative Stress by β-hydroxybutyrate, an Endogenous Histone Deacetylase Inhibitor," *Science* 339, no. 6116 (2013): 211–214, https://doi.org/10.1126/science.1227166.

8. M. Kogevinas et al., "Effect of Mistimed Eating Patterns on Breast and Prostate Cancer Risk (MCC-Spain Study)," *International Journal of Cancer*, 143 (2018): 2380–2389, https://doi:10.1002/ijc.31649.

9. University of Washington Study, reported in *Integrated and Alternative Medicine Clinical Highlights* 4, no. 1 (2002): 16.

CHAPTER 11: STEP 6 (DAYS 16–18): SUPPLEMENT YOUR EFFORTS

1. Donald Davis, Melvin Epp, and Hugh Riordan, "Changes in USDA Food Composition Data for 43 Garden Crops, 1950 to 1999," *Journal of the American College of Nutrition* 23, no. 6 (2004): 669–682, https://doi.org/10.1080/07315724.2004.10719409.

2. S. L. McDonnell et al., "Serum 25-Hydroxyvitamin D Concentrations ≥40 ng/ml Are Associated with >65% Lower Cancer Risk: Pooled Analysis of Randomized Trial and Prospective Cohort Study," [published correction: *PLoS One* 13, no. 7 (2018): e0201078] *PLoS One* 11, no. 4 (2016): e0152441, https://doi.org/10.1371/journal.pone.0152441.

3. Alexander Nazaryan, "Is Cancer Lurking in Your Toothpaste? (And Your Soap? And Your Lipstick?)," *Newsweek*, September 4, 2014, https://www.newsweek.com/2014/09/26/cancer-lurking-your-toothpaste-and-your-soap-and-your-lipstick-268322.html.

CHAPTER 12: STEP 7 (DAYS 19–21): AMP UP YOUR WORKOUT

1. Stoyan Dimitrov, Elaine Hulteng, and Suzi Hong, "Inflammation and Exercise: Inhibition of Monocytic Intracellular TNF Production by Acute Exercise via β2-Adrenergic Activation," *Brain, Behavior, and Immunity* 61 (2017): 60–68, https://doi.org/10.1016/j.bbi.2016.12.017.

2. Christian Werner et al., "Physical Exercise Prevents Cellular Senescence in Circulating Leukocytes and in the Vessel Wall," *Circulation* 120, no. 24 (2009): 2438–2447, https://doi.org/10.1161/CIRCULATIONAHA.109.861005.

3. David W. Hill, "Morning–Evening Differences in Response to Exhaustive Severe-Intensity Exercise," *Applied Physiology, Nutrition, and Metabolism* 39 (2014): 248–254, https://doi.org/10.1139/apnm-2013-0140.

4. Jeff S. Volek et al., "Metabolic Characteristics of Keto-Adapted Ultra-endurance Runners," *Metabolism—Clinical and Experimental* 65, no. 3 (2015): 100–110. https://doi.org /10.1016/j.metabol.2015.10.028.

5. Nina Mohorko et al., "Weight Loss, Improved Physical Performance, Cognitive Function, Eating Behavior, and Metabolic Profile in a 12-Week Ketogenic Diet in Obese Adults," *Nutrition Research* 62 (2019): 64–77, https://doi.org/10.1016/j.nutres.2018.11.007.

6. Paul Lee et al., "Irisin and FGF21 Are Cold-Induced Endocrine Activators of Brown Fat Function in Humans" *Cell Metabolism* 19, no. 2 (2014): 302–309, https://doi.org/10.1016/j.cmet .2013.12.017.

7. Emma E. A. Cohen et al., "Rowers' High: Behavioural Synchrony Is Correlated with Elevated Pain Thresholds," *Biology Letters* 6, no. 1 (2009), https://doi.org/10.1098/rsbl.2009.0670.

8. A. Bhattacharya et al., "Body Acceleration Distribution and O2 Uptake in Humans During Running and Jumping," *Journal of Applied Physiology* 49, no. 5 (1980): 881–887, https://doi .org/10.1152/jappl.1980.49.5.881.

9. F. F. Reichert et al., "The Role of Perceived Personal Barriers to Engagement in Leisure-Time Physical Activity," *American Journal of Public Health* 97, no. 3 (2007): 515–519, https://doi.org/10.2105/AJPH.2005.070144.https://doi.org/10.2105/AJPH.2005.070144.

10. Paul H. Falcone et al., "Caloric Expenditure of Aerobic, Resistance, or Combined High-Intensity Interval Training Using a Hydraulic Resistance System in Healthy Men," *The Journal of Strength & Conditioning Research* 29, no. 3 (2015): 779–785, https://doi.org/10.1519 /JSC.0000000000000661.

11. Hailee L. Wingfield et al., "The Acute Effect of Exercise Modality and Nutrition Manipulations on Post-Exercise Resting Energy Expenditure and Respiratory Exchange Ratio in Women: A Randomized Trial," *Sports Medicine—Open* 1 (2015): 11, https://doi.org/10.1186 /s40798-015-0010-3.

12. T. J., Hazell et al., "Two Minutes of Sprint-Interval Exercise Elicits 24-hr Oxygen Consumption Similar to That of 30 Min of Continuous Endurance Exercise," *International Journal of Sport Nutrition and Exercise Metabolism* 22, no. 4 (2012): 276–283, https://doi.org/10.1123 /ijsnem.22.4.276.

13. M. Wewege et al., "The Effects of High-Intensity Interval Training vs. Moderate-Intensity Continuous Training on Body Composition in Overweight and Obese Adults: A Systematic Review and Meta-analysis," *Obesity Reviews* 18, no. 6 (2017): 635–646, https://doi.org/10.1111 /obr.12532.

14. M. Heydari, J. Freund, and S. H. Boutcher, "The Effect of High-Intensity Intermittent Exercise on Body Composition of Overweight Young Males," *Journal of Obesity* 2012 (2012): 480467, https://doi.org/10.1155/2012/480467.

15. Romeo B. Batacan Jr. et al., "Effects of High-Intensity Interval Training on Cardiometabolic Health: A Systematic Review and Meta-analysis of Intervention Studies," *British Journal of Sports Medicine* 51, no. 6 (2017): 494–503, https://doi.org/10.1136/bjsports-2015-095841.

16. N. Shaban, K. A. Kenno, and K. J. Milne, "The Effects of a 2 Week Modified High Intensity Interval Training Program on the Homeostatic Model of Insulin Resistance (HOMA-IR) in

Adults with Type 2 Diabetes," *Journal of Sports Medicine and Physical Fitness* 54, no. 2 (2014): 203–209.

17. C. Jelleyman et al., "The Effects of High Intensity Interval Training on Glucose Regulation and Insulin Resistance: A Meta-analysis," *Obesity Reviews* 16, no. 11 (2015): 942–961, https://doi.org/10.1111/obr.12317; Chueh-Lung Hwang et al., "Novel All-Extremity High-Intensity Interval Training Improves Aerobic Fitness, Cardiac Function and Insulin Resistance in Healthy Older Adults," *Experimental Gerontology* 82 (2016): 112–119, https://doi.org/10.1016/j.exger.2016.06.009.

18. Matthew M. Robinson et al., "Enhanced Protein Translation Underlies Improved Metabolic and Physical Adaptations to Different Exercise Training Modes in Young and Old," *Cell Metabolism* 25, no. 3 (2017): 581–592, https://doi.org/10.1016/j.cmet.2017.02.009.

CHAPTER 13: YOUR LIFE AFTER SUGAR

1. Josiane L. Broussard et al., "Impaired Insulin Signaling in Human Adipocytes After Experimental Sleep Restriction: A Randomized, Crossover Study," *Annals of Internal Medicine* 157, no. 8 (2012): 549–557, https://doi.org/10.7326/0003-4819-157-8-201210160-00005.

2. Karine Spiegel et al., "Brief Communication: Sleep Curtailment in Healthy Young Men Is Associated with Decreased Leptin Levels, Elevated Ghrelin Levels, and Increased Hunger and Appetite," *Annals of Internal Medicine* 141, no. 11 (2004): 846–850, https://doi.org/10.7326/0003-4819-141-11-200412070-00008.

3. Heather M. Ochs-Balcom et al., "Short Sleep Is Associated with Low Bone Mineral Density and Osteoporosis in the Women's Health Initiative," *Journal of Bone Mineral Research* 35, no. 2 (2019), https://doi.org/10.1002/jbmr.3879.

4. Honglong Cao et al., "Circadian Rhythmicity of Antioxidant Markers in Rats Exposed to 1.8 GHz Radiofrequency Fields," *International Journal of Environmental Research and Public Health* 12, no. 2 (2015): 2071–2087, https://doi.org/10.3390/ijerph120202071.

5. Ingrid Nesdal Fossum et al., "The Association Between Use of Electronic Media in Bed Before Going to Sleep and Insomnia Symptoms, Daytime Sleepiness, Morningness, and Chronotype," *Behavioral Sleep Medicine* 12, no. 5 (2014): 343–357, https://doi.org/10.1080/15402002.2013.819468.

Index

ginger
  Detox Tea, 220
  Dr. Green Detox Smoothie,
    215–216
  Grain-Free Granola, 222
  Green Detox Juice, 219
  health benefits, 130
  how to eat it, 130–131
  Morning Fat Burner Tonic,
    219–220
  Pumpkin Pie Pudding, 261
  Skinny Mint Green
    Smoothie, 217
  -Tomato Soup, Spicy
    Moroccan, 225–226
gluconeogenesis, 7, 48
glucose (monosaccharide),
  55
glucose, blood. *See* blood
  glucose
glutathione, 157
glycation, 25–29
glyphosate, 148
Granola, Grain-Free, 222
grazing on food, 41
Green Curry with Summer
  Veggies, 238–239
green foods, mineral-rich, 99
greenhouse gasses, 120
green juice, effect on taste
  buds, 63
greens. *See also specific greens*
  Chilled Green Detox Soup,
    225
  Perfect Salad in a Jar, 234
  Salad with Spicy Salsa
    Verde, 230
gum disease, 153–154
gut bacteria
  altering, to reduce cravings,
    53–54
  effect of antibiotics on,
    114
  effect of sugar on, 21–25
  resetting, by fasting, 139
gymnema, 57

H

habits, forming, 38, 185
Hashimoto's disease, 32, 156
hazelnuts
  Homemade Coconut
    Chocolate Spread, 265
HDL cholesterol, 45, 103
headaches, 87, 91
healthy fats. *See also specific
    types of fats*
  adding to diet, tips for,
    111–112
  benefits of, 102–103
  good/better/best sources of,
    110–111
  as percentage of daily
    calories, 41
  in step 2 of program,
    101–112
  stocking pantry with, 77
  turning off hunger with, 144
  types of, 104–105
  types to start eating,
    108–109
heart disease, 1, 34–35
heart rate variability (HRV),
  161
hedonic hunger, 49
hemoglobin A1C test, 26–27,
  45
hemp seeds
  health benefits, 122
  Superpower Alkaline
    Treats, 252–253
herbicides, 148
herbs. *See also specific herbs*
  adding to drinks, 135
  fresh, storing, 135
  health benefits, 129–136
  stocking pantry with, 77
  top ten, for optimizing
    health, 130–134
Hibbeln, Joseph, 106
high blood pressure, 26, 34
high-fructose corn syrup, 7,
  56

high-intensity, low-impact
  interval training
  (HILIIT), 172
high-intensity interval
  training (HIIT), 170–172
high-sensitivity C-reactive
  protein test, 45
Himalayan pink salt, 92
homeostasis, 40
homocysteine blood test, 45
hormones. *See also specific
    hormones*
  causing sugar cravings,
    48–49
  effect of sugar on, 31–33
hummus
  5-Minute, 255
  Roasted Broccoli with, 249
hunger. *See also* cravings;
    sugar cravings
  biohacks for, 146
  caused by constant eating,
    138
  caused by high leptin levels,
    66
  hedonic, 49
  mistaken for dehydration,
    55, 141
  suppressing, 49, 144, 146
hyperthyroidism, 32
hypothyroidism, 32, 156

I

identify your why, 71–72
incantations, 72–73
infertility, 33
inflammation
  from acidic environment, 10
  effects of sugar on, 26
  excess calcium and, 88
  linked to chronic diseases,
    11
  markers of, 45
  reducing, with fasting, 140
  reducing, with fat burning,
    40

Maca Hot Chocolate, 264
Maca Power Breakfast Shake, 216
magnesium
    citrate, 150
    deficiencies, 51, 52, 149
    dosage recommendations, 149–150
    glycinate, 150
    health benefits, 149, 158
    importance of, 29, 87–88
    low levels of, 91
    in red blood cells, 45, 149
    sources of, 149
    testing levels of, 149
    threonate, 150
Magnesium Miracle, The (Dean), 86
maltose, 56
mammalian target of rapamycin (mTOR) pathway, 115
Manning, Drew, 164
MCT oil, 105
meals. *See also* intermittent fasting
    before bedtime, 140–142, 198
    daily number of, 42
    serving sizes at, 188
    supereasy, ideas for, 194
    timing of, 137–146
meat, 7, 10, 52
Mediterranean diet, 19
medium-chain triglycerides (MCTs), 30, 105
melatonin, 197
menstrual periods, 33, 145
mental stress, 73–74
Mercola, Joseph, 53
metabolic mitochondrial fitness, 140
metabolic syndrome, 32, 34
metabolism, 166, 171
methanol, 62

Michels, Karin, 111
microbiome
    altering, to reduce cravings, 53–54
    antibiotics and, 114
    effect of sugar on, 21–25
    resetting, with fasting, 139
microcirculation, 160
migraines, 87
mind detox, 68–73
mineral deficiencies
    cravings caused by, 51–53
    high rates of, 86–87
    signs of, 90–91
minerals. *See also* mineral deficiencies; *specific minerals*
    for digestion process, 141–142
    importance of, 86
    mineral-rich green foods, 99
    other mineral superstars, 98
    in step 1 of program, 85–100
    top four minerals, 87
    top ten mineral-rich foods, 93–98
    trace, 51, 52, 90
mineral salts deficiency, 51, 52
Mint Green Smoothie, Skinny, 217
mitochondria, 140, 166
mitophagy, 40
molecular hydrogen (H2), 157
monk fruit, about, 60
monosaccharides, 55–56
monounsaturated fats, 104–105
Moskowitz, Howard, 4
motivation, for exercise, 168
Mousse, Avocado Chocolate, 263
"muffin top," 138–139
muscles
    cramping in, 89, 91, 164

loss of, from insufficient protein, 165
magnesium for, 87–88
preserving, with HIIT, 172
spasms in, 91
mushrooms, 53–54, 121–122

N

N-acetyl cysteine (NAC), 157
natural sweeteners, 60–61
net carbs, 13–14, 75
neurogenesis, 30
neuroinflammation, 28
neuroplasticity, 168
neurotransmitters, 160
neurotrophins, 30
nighttime snacks, resisting, 142
nonalcoholic fatty liver disease (NAFLD), 31
nonalcoholic liver cirrhosis, 31
nonalcoholic steatohepatitis (NASH), 31
nonshivering thermogenesis, 166
nut butters. *See also* almond butter
    stocking pantry with, 77
    types of, 108–109
nut milks, types of, 109
nutrient density, meaning of, 95
nutrients. *See also specific types*
    fat-soluble, 103
    nutrient-dense foods, 53
    nutrition deficiencies, 51–53
nutritional yeast, note about, 53–54, 121
nutrition labels, 11–15
nuts. *See also specific nuts*
    baru, about, 110
    Grain-Free Granola, 222

spinach
    Basil Soup, Creamy, 226
    Chickpea Veggie Frittata,
        223
    Chocolate Almond
        Smoothie, 215
    Coco-Berry Smoothie,
        217–218
    The Crimson Kicker, 218
    Dr. Green Detox Smoothie,
        215–216
    Green Detox Juice, 219
    health benefits, 93–94
    Pomegranate and White
        Bean Salad with Tarragon
        Dressing, 231–232
    Skinny Mint Green
        Smoothie, 217
    Spread, Homemade Coconut
        Chocolate, 265
sprouts, 93
squash. *See also* zucchini
    Pumpkin Pie Pudding, 261
    spaghetti, health benefits,
        97
squats, 180
statin drugs, 88, 152
stevia, about, 60
strength training, 162
stress
    chronic, 31
    effect on body, 67–68
    effect on sugar cravings, 3
    mental, 73–74
    physical, 78–81
    relieving, 31, 194–196
    three types of, 67
stress eating, 5, 199
subcutaneous fat, 138–139
sucralose, 62
sucrose, 7, 55–56
sugar
    added, harmful effects of, 7
    "added," on labels, 11
    in beverages, 14
    in breakfast foods, 14

in condiments, 15
consumption of, 2–3, 16
dietary sources of, 7–10
different names for, 11,
    12–13
disaccharides, 55–56
effect on endocrine system,
    31–33
effect on liver, 31
estimating amount per
    serving, 11–12
identifying, on nutrition
    labels, 11–15
impact on health, xiv, 7,
    10–11, 21–35
link with cancer, 33–34
link with heart disease,
    34–35
link with inflammation, 26
monosaccharides, 55–56
in our food culture, xv
six truths about, 5–10
in snacks, 14
two main categories of,
    55–56
types of, 7
sugar addiction
    breaking, health benefits
        from, xviii
    power of, xiv–xv, 3–5
    quiz on, 8–10
    science behind, 6
sugar-burning system
    effect on fat burning, 6
    effect on sugar cravings,
        6–7
    self-assessment quiz, 43–44
sugar cravings, 47–64. *See
    also* sugar cravings,
    crushing
caused by artificial
    sweeteners, 61–63
caused by stress and poor
    diet, 6
hormones responsible for,
    48–49

mineral deficiencies
    behind, 51, 91
role of gut bacteria in, 23
sugar cravings, crushing
    by avoiding fructose, 55–56
    biohacks for, 53–54, 57
    with craving-smashing
        snacks, 50–51
    with fiber-rich foods, 60
    with low-sugar swaps,
        54–55
    with natural sweeteners,
        60–61
    by restoring sensitivity to
        sweetness, 49–50
    simple ideas for, 196–197
    with three-step snack rule,
        55
    with whole fruit, 57–59
sulfonamide antibiotics, 25
sun exposure, 151–152
superbusy schedules,
    193–194
Superpower Alkaline Treats,
    252–253
supplements, 147–158
    brain-supporting, 29–30
    consulting doctor about,
        148
    supporting players,
        154–157
    top five, for overall health,
        149–153
    top three, for brain health,
        158
    why they are needed, 148
sweeteners, 60–63
sweet potato(es)
    Cinnamon, 249
    Fries, Shayna's, with
        Chimichurri Sauce,
        247–248
    roasted, preparing, 194
switching lunges, 178
sympathetic nervous system,
    161, 162, 195

T

tacos, adzuki bean, preparing, 194

tahini
Clean Keto Garlic Dip, 251
5-Minute Hummus, 255
Spicy Moroccan Tomato-Ginger Soup, 225–226

Tao of Natural Breathing, The (Lewis), 195

taste buds, retraining, 49–50

tea
Detox, 220
Jorge's Flat-Belly, 144
Morning Fat Burner Tonic, 219–220

technology detox, 73–74

television, 142, 197

telomeres, 77, 104, 140, 161

Thai Spring Roll Veggie Bowl, 241–242

3:6:5 Power Breath, 74

thyroid cancer, 32

thyroid hormone, 32–33

thyroid issues, 156

tomato(es)
Creamy Spinach Basil Soup, 226
Ginger Soup, Spicy Moroccan, 225–226
Mediterranean Chopped Salad, 233
Mexican Spice Immune-Boosting Green Bowl, 243–244
Perfect Salad in a Jar, 234
Salad with Spicy Salsa Verde, 230

tooth decay, 153

toothpaste, 153–154

toxic soil, 148

trampolines, 169–170

trans fats, 103

travel, and eating out, 193

triceps dip, 181

triclosan, 154

triglycerides, 7, 45, 55

Truffles, Cardamom Orange Chocolate, 258

turmeric
Detox Tea, 220
health benefits, 131
how to eat it, 131
making more bioavailable, 131
Quinoa Power Bowl, 244
Vegan Protein Boneless Broth, 227–228

20/4 eating pattern, 143

type 2 diabetes
causes of, 7
dementia and, 28–29
precursor to, 32
preventing or reversing, with fasting, 139
red meat and, 120

type 3 diabetes (aka Alzheimer's), 28

U

uric acid, 35

urine ketone strips, 42

V

vaginal yeast infections, 23–25

vegan and vegetarian diets
compatibility with Get Off Your Sugar program, 18
foods excluded in, 18
omega-3 supplements for, 150–151
protein amounts for, 117

Vegan Protein Boneless Broth, 227–228

vegetables. *See also specific vegetables*
Farmer's Lentil Soup, 228–229
Green Curry with Summer Veggies, 238–239
as percentage of daily calories, 41

stocking pantry with,

Thai Spring Roll Veggie Bowl, 241–242

Vegan Protein Boneless Broth, 227–228

vinegar
apple cider, health benefits, 57
Morning Fat Burner Tonic, 219–220

Virgin, JJ, 3

visceral fat, 102, 138, 171

vitamin A deficiency, 53

vitamin B_{12}, 52, 121

vitamin C, 157

vitamin D
for brain health, 29
for calcium absorption, 88
deficiencies in, 53
general health benefits, 151–152
for immunity and bone health, 45
recommended dosage, 152
testing levels of, 152

vitamin D_2, 152

vitamin D_3, 152

vitamin D_{12}, 155

vitamin K_2, 88, 152

vitamins, B complex. *See* B vitamins

W

walking, 55, 74, 161

walnuts
Cardamom Orange Chocolate Truffles, 258
Raw Zucchini Pesto Pasta, 237–238

Warburg, Otto, 103

water
at bedtime, 141
for hard workouts, 172
Jorge's Flat-Belly, 145
to ride out cravings, 55

watercress, 95